Food Supplements and Functional Foods Assessment for Health and Nutrition—Volume II

Food Supplements and Functional Foods Assessment for Health and Nutrition—Volume II

Collection Editors

Laura Domínguez Díaz
Montaña Cámara
Virginia Fernández-Ruiz

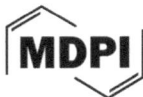

Basel • Beijing • Wuhan • Barcelona • Belgrade • Novi Sad • Cluj • Manchester

Collection Editors

Laura Domínguez Díaz
Complutense University of Madrid (UCM)
Madrid
Spain

Montaña Cámara
Complutense University of Madrid (UCM)
Madrid
Spain

Virginia Fernández-Ruiz
Complutense University of Madrid (UCM)
Madrid
Spain

Editorial Office
MDPI AG
Grosspeteranlage 5
4052 Basel, Switzerland

This is a reprint of the Topical Collection, published open access by the journal *Nutrients* (ISSN 2072-6643), freely accessible at: https://www.mdpi.com/journal/nutrients/topical_collections/Food_Supplements_Assessment_Nutrition.

For citation purposes, cite each article independently as indicated on the article page online and as indicated below:

Lastname, A.A.; Lastname, B.B. Article Title. *Journal Name* **Year**, *Volume Number*, Page Range.

ISBN 978-3-7258-1881-5 (Hbk)
ISBN 978-3-7258-1882-2 (PDF)
https://doi.org/10.3390/books978-3-7258-1882-2

© 2024 by the authors. Articles in this book are Open Access and distributed under the Creative Commons Attribution (CC BY) license. The book as a whole is distributed by MDPI under the terms and conditions of the Creative Commons Attribution-NonCommercial-NoDerivs (CC BY-NC-ND) license (https://creativecommons.org/licenses/by-nc-nd/4.0/).

Contents

About the Editors vii

Preface ix

Brigitta Plasek, Zoltán Lakner and Ágoston Temesi
I Believe It Is Healthy—Impact of Extrinsic Product Attributes in Demonstrating Healthiness of Functional Food Products
Reprinted from: Nutrients 2021, 13, 3518, https://doi.org/10.3390/nu13103518 1

Marie-Josèphe Amiot, Christian Latgé, Laurence Plumey and Sylvie Raynal
Intake Estimation of Phytochemicals in a French Well-Balanced Diet
Reprinted from: Nutrients 2021, 13, 3628, https://doi.org/10.3390/nu13103628 17

Elżbieta Studzińska-Sroka, Agnieszka Galanty, Anna Gościniak, Mateusz Wieczorek, Magdalena Kłaput, Marlena Dudek-Makuch, et al.
Herbal Infusions as a Valuable Functional Food
Reprinted from: Nutrients 2021, 13, 4051, https://doi.org/10.3390/nu13114051 29

Jieping Yang, Venu Lagishetty, Patrick Kurnia, Susanne M. Henning, Aaron I. Ahdoot and Jonathan P. Jacobs
Microbial and Chemical Profiles of Commercial Kombucha Products
Reprinted from: Nutrients 2022, 14, 670, https://doi.org/10.3390/nu14030670 45

Monika Turska, Piotr Paluszkiewicz, Waldemar A. Turski and Jolanta Parada-Turska
A Review of the Health Benefits of Food Enriched with Kynurenic Acid
Reprinted from: Nutrients 2022, 14, 4182, https://doi.org/10.3390/nu14194182 61

Ricardo López-Rodríguez, Laura Domínguez, Virginia Fernández-Ruiz and Montaña Cámara
Extracts Rich in Nutrients as Novel Food Ingredients to Be Used in Food Supplements: A Proposal Classification
Reprinted from: Nutrients 2022, 14, 3194, https://doi.org/10.3390/nu14153194 84

Maja Bensa, Irena Vovk and Vesna Glavnik
Resveratrol Food Supplement Products and the Challenges of Accurate Label Information to Ensure Food Safety for Consumers
Reprinted from: Nutrients 2023, 15, 474, https://doi.org/10.3390/nu15020474 103

Anna Puścion-Jakubik, Natalia Bartosiewicz and Katarzyna Socha
Is the Magnesium Content in Food Supplements Consistent with the Manufacturers' Declarations?
Reprinted from: Nutrients 2021, 13, 3416, https://doi.org/10.3390/nu13103416 125

Laura Domínguez, Virginia Fernández-Ruiz and Montaña Cámara
Micronutrients in Food Supplements for Pregnant Women: European Health Claims Assessment
Reprinted from: Nutrients 2023, 15, 4592, https://doi.org/10.3390/nu15214592 135

Marta Czarnowska-Kujawska, Joanna Klepacka, Olga Zielińska and María de Lourdes Samaniego-Vaesken
Characteristics of Dietary Supplements with Folic Acid Available on the Polish Market
Reprinted from: Nutrients 2022, 14, 3500, https://doi.org/10.3390/nu14173500 148

Laura Domínguez, Virginia Fernández-Ruiz, Patricia Morales, María-Cortes Sánchez-Mata and Montaña Cámara
Assessment of Health Claims Related to Folic Acid in Food Supplements for Pregnant Women According to the European Regulation
Reprinted from: *Nutrients* **2021**, *13*, 937, https://doi.org/10.3390/nu13030937 . . . . **159**

About the Editors

Laura Domínguez Díaz

Dr. Laura Domínguez Díaz is an Assistant Professor in the Food Science and Nutrition Department of the Faculty of Pharmacy at the Complutense University of Madrid. She is a member of the UCM Research Group ALIMNOVA - Novel Foods. Scientific, Technological and Social aspects (Ref.: 951505). In 2016, she received her bachelor's degree in pharmaceutical studies and was awarded the "Fundación Rafael Folch" Award. Then, she completed her master's degree in food safety with Honorable Mention (2017) and her PhD in pharmacy (2022), being granted the First Extraordinary Doctorate Award by Complutense University of Madrid. Her research is focused on the analysis of foods of plant origin, functional foods, and food supplements (nutrients, bioactive compounds), as well as their legal implications in terms of labeling, nutritional and health claims, and food safety.

Montaña Cámara

Dr. Montaña Cámara is Head Professor in the Food Science and Nutrition Department of the Faculty of Pharmacy at the Complutense University of Madrid. She is the research lead of the UCM Research Group ALIMNOVA - Novel Foods. Scientific, Technological and Social aspects (Ref.: 951505), and the Corresponding Academic of the Royal National Academy of Pharmacy. She is the Co-director of the UCM master's in food safety and Co-chair of the study group on Functional Foods, Bioactives and Human Health at the Royal Complutense College of Harvard. She is also a member of the EFSA Experts NDA Panel (Nutrition, Novel Foods ¬ Allergens). She has received awards such as the Royal Academy of Pharmacy Research (1989), Antama Foundation Scientific Communication (2014), Bernard Bierch Award – Melcoptor Award (2018), UCM Technology and Knowledge Transfer, Area of Biomedical and Health Sciences (2020) and FIAB Award, Health Sciences (2021).

Virginia Fernández-Ruiz

Dr. Virginia Fernández-Ruiz is Full Professor in the Food Science and Nutrition Department of the Faculty of Pharmacy at Complutense University of Madrid. Her research focuses on the chemical and sensory food analysis of foods with plant origin, as well as consumer studies, novel foods and health. She is a member of the UCM Research Group ALIMNOVA - Novel Foods. Scientific, Technological and Social aspects (Ref.: 951505) and a Scientific Technical Advisor in food sensory analysis for ENAC (National Accreditation Entity), as well as a signatory of all international agreements of EA, ILAC and IAF (International Accreditation Forum). She is a member of the Association for Sensory Analysis (AEPAS) and the European Society for Sensory Science (E3S). She has received the Young Researcher Award (2012), UCM Technology and Knowledge Transfer Award, Area of Biomedical and Health Sciences (2020), and Innovation Award from the Wine Technology Platform in the II Edition of the PTV award from Innovation (2020).

Preface

Developed societies are shifting their perception of food, with consumers increasingly seeking food products that offer more than basic nutrients and the satisfaction of appetite. They desire foods that enhance their nutritional well-being, health, and quality of life by reducing the risk of disease and promoting the adequate functioning of bodily systems. Preventing non-communicable diseases associated with unhealthy diets is currently one of the most critical global public health challenges. In this sense, food supplements and functional foods are gaining importance, as they contain functional ingredients that positively impact human health.

In this reprint of the Topical Collection "*Food Supplements and Functional Foods Assessment for Health and Nutrition*", up-to-date reviews and original research articles concerning the characterization of the nutritional composition and phytochemicals of functional foods and food supplements, as well as its legal implications in terms of labeling, nutrition and health claims, are presented. In addition, the evaluation of the functional effects and potential health benefits of different ingredients (nutrients and bioactive compounds) present in these functional products; consumers' perception, behavior, and/or attitudes towards functional products; and food policies (regulatory frameworks, laws, rules, official guidelines) are also topics covered in this reprint.

We would like to extend our heartfelt thanks and appreciation to the MDPI Reprint staff; the editorial team of *Nutrients*, with a special reference to Ms. Lilian Gao for her great support and assistance; the reviewers for their invaluable work during the peer-review process; and the talented scientists for their insightful contributions.

Laura Domínguez Díaz, Montaña Cámara, and Virginia Fernández-Ruiz
Collection Editors

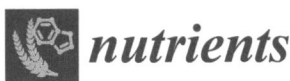

Article

I Believe It Is Healthy—Impact of Extrinsic Product Attributes in Demonstrating Healthiness of Functional Food Products

Brigitta Plasek *, Zoltán Lakner and Ágoston Temesi

Institute of Economics Science, Department of Food Chain Management, Hungarian University of Agriculture and Life Sciences, Villányi Road 29-43, 1118 Budapest, Hungary; Lakner.Zoltan.Karoly@uni-mate.hu (Z.L.); Temesi.Agoston@uni-mate.hu (Á.T.)
* Correspondence: Plasek.Brigitta@uni-mate.hu

Abstract: Due to the high proportion of impulse purchases and the short time devoted to purchase decisions, packaging and other extrinsic attributes are becoming increasingly important in demonstrating the health benefits of a functional food item to consumers as plausibly as possible. Our research aims at identifying the role of extrinsic features (claims related to ingredients and health claims, organic or domestic origin, as well as the shape and color of packaging), gathered in the course of in-depth literature analysis, in the case of a functional smoothie. Our online consumer questionnaire was completed by 633 respondents, and the answers were assessed by choice based conjoint analysis. Our results show that each examined attribute plays a role in the assessment of health effects. The color blue has the biggest impact on making the consumer believe in the health benefits of the product. This is followed by the indication of organic origin, then the statement emphasizing the natural quality of the ingredients. The assessment of the specific extrinsic attributes is affected by consumers' general health interest level, their involvement with food items, and their various demographic features.

Keywords: functional foods; healthy eating; credibility; extrinsic attributes; conjoint analysis

1. Introduction

A significant proportion of purchases are impulse purchases, and packaging plays a key role in this type of purchase [1–3]. Various factors can serve as bases for impulse purchases [4], such as a promotion, personal characteristics, the shop environment, demographic, situational, and social factors [5] and also the perceived health effect of the product. The assessment of the healthiness of food products is a critical factor influencing the success of food-related businesses [6], and for functional foods this effect is of vital importance. A key issue for companies developing functional foods is to be able to use the short purchasing decision situation to show the customer the benefits of the product [7], including its health benefits, as a competitive advantage of these products lies in their additional health benefits on top of the basic nutritional effects [8]. Pramudya and Seo [9] maintain that packaging is one of the most important extrinsic features that influence consumer perception and decision-making.

Assessing the impact on health is a particularly difficult task for the consumer as healthiness is a kind of credence attribute [10–12]. According to Verbeke [13], credence attributes are "product characteristics that can neither be directly perceived nor verified by consumers". A unique feature of them is that they are difficult to assess even after consumption [14,15]. Nevertheless, the product is assessed as a complex whole, based on intrinsic and extrinsic attributes [16,17]. Research has shown that consumer assessment of the health impact of a product is influenced by several extrinsic [18] and intrinsic attributes [19], as well as non-product-specific factors: e.g., prior knowledge of the consumer [20–22]. Such an intrinsic factor is the various ingredients found in a product [23–29] as well as the taste and other sensory features of the product [30–34]. At the same time, consumers tend to

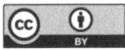

use extrinsic characteristics instead of other factors as an indicator of product quality [35] and they have to rely on them in a shopping environment. The first purchase made by a consumer also heavily depends on these extrinsic attributes [36,37]. Extrinsic features are important in that they allow the product to adapt to changing consumer needs without the manufacturer making any changes to the product itself [19,38].

In addition to playing an important role in the assessment of product quality, extrinsic cues are also features that significantly influence consumer decision-making, and help the assessment of the expected performance, safety, and social acceptance of the product [39], and their role is also important when examining perceived healthiness as well [40,41].

2. Aim of Research

Our research aim is to examine which extrinsic features, when combined, result in a product that most plausibly shows the consumer that it has a beneficial impact on health. We included attributes based on our literature reviews [42,43]: we examine various claims related to ingredients, health claims, the effect of organic and domestic (Hungarian) origin, as well as the effect of the shape and color of packaging. While our aim was to identify a packaging combination that would convincingly show a health effect, we also aimed to determine the weight of the different factors and characteristics identified by previous research and to rank them in order of importance. Although previous research has already looked at the factors that we are now ranking, we thought it was important that we also investigated which factors are most important in determining the health impact of the functional test product.

The aim of our research was also to clarify the contradictory findings on the shape and color of packaging in the literature. Based on the results of previous research, the shape of the packaging is also a factor influencing the assessment of healthiness [44–46]. The shape of the packaging may indicate the physique desired by the consumer [46], and may influence calorie consumption, and thus the perceived effect on health [47]. In addition to the humanoid form, square and rounder packaging were foregrounded in several studies [48–50]; however, their results hardly provide a basis to identify a shape which shows consumers the most that the product is beneficial to health.

In addition to the shape of the packaging, its color is also a factor influencing perceived healthiness [50–54]. According to several studies, the colors blue and green make a positive contribution to the assessment of the healthiness of a product [51,54]. Some results suggest that the color red conveys a kind of prohibition to consumers [52], it does not make them feel that the product is healthier, rather, it makes them think that the product is unhealthy. According to the research results of Huang and Lu [51], respondents perceived a blue-packaged product to be healthier than a red-packaged one. At the same time, for certain products the color red still contributes to the assessment of perceived healthiness [50,54].

Our research also aimed to assess the differences between consumer groups in terms of their perception of health impacts. Research has highlighted the relationship between consumer characteristics (gender, age, level of education) and the assessment of functional foods [55–57]. Several studies have concluded that women are more open to functional foods than men, and those with a higher education level and the older age group have a completely different attitude towards the perception of functional foods than those with a lower education level or those who are younger in age [56–61]. Several previous studies examining purchase intention for functional foods foreground consumers' health awareness, attention to health and health motivations among the influencing factors [62–66]. This research repeatedly highlights the important impact of consumer health motivations, thus for example Bornkessel, et al. [67] pinpoint health motivations as the factor which most influences awareness of functional food ingredients. In addition to the importance of health motivations; Steinhauser, Janssen and Hamm [66] also found that consumers with higher health motivation spent more time studying health claims and nutrition claims, but it did not affect their purchase intention. Our research aim is related to consumers' health interest, as measured by the items of the General Health Interest Scale constructed by Roinien and colleagues [68].

In addition to influencing the purchase intention of functional foods [69], food involvement also plays a role in the assessment of the healthiness of different products [70]. Although indirectly, the different levels of food involvement contribute to consumers' food choices, including how healthy the chosen products are [71]. Involvement, however, contributes not only to the different assessment of perceived healthiness, but also to the processing of nutritional information [72] and to the different utilization of extrinsic features, for example. For consumers with lower involvement, extrinsic features facilitate a simplified assessment process [73]. To measure food involvement, we used the items of the Food involvement scale developed by Brunsø, et al. [74], which is an element of the modified food-related lifestyle model.

2.1. Hypothesis Building

2.1.1. The Role of Claims Related to Ingredients, Health Claims and Nutrition Claims

In our research, we examine whether the highlighting of ingredients with separate claims has an impact on the assessment of health effects; we also examine the influence of the natural quality of an ingredient, the added protein content, or the high vitamin content on consumers.

Research shows that consumers consider natural foods healthier than processed products [75,76]; also, the naturalness of a product is an indicator of perceived healthiness for consumers [21]. Wąsowicz, Styśko-Kunkowska and Grunert [54] maintain that consumers consider healthy products to be natural, among other things. Related to the natural character of a product, we examine the effect of the claim "with natural ingredients."

The two other claims we examine in our research relate to vitamin content and protein content. The research results of Rizk and Treat [29] show that in addition to other ingredients, some consumers are influenced by the protein content of a product in the perception of its healthiness, while others ignore protein and other ingredients when making a decision [24]. To assess the significance of this ingredient, we examine the claim "26 g protein per portion".

Vitamins and minerals also influence consumers in their assessment of health effects; some consumer segments specifically prefer foods rich in vitamins and minerals [23]. We examine the effect of emphasizing vitamin content through the claim "rich in vitamin C", which is a claim widely used by manufacturers in the soft drinks market.

Health claims and nutrition claims are important influencing factors in helping consumers to assess health effect [51,77], though Orquin and Scholderer [78] showed that health claims have only a small impact on the assessment of health effect. Using such claims can greatly influence consumers in their perception of a product [79], although certain consumer groups are skeptical about them and ignore them [80]. Research related to health claims has examined the effect of various health claims on the assessment of the healthiness of a product [81], how credible they are and in what form they are credible to consumers [82–84].

Research on ingredients has shown that consumers mostly pay attention to the product ingredients that nutritionists emphasize in relation to a healthy diet, such as the content of sugar, salt, fat and omega-3 fatty acids [26–29,85]. Health claims also play an important role in the perception of healthiness [86]; at the same time, too much information can make consumers skeptical [87,88], making the role of health claims questionable. Based on the results of several studies, we can state that using nutrition claims and health claims will make the consumer perceive the product as more beneficial to health [89–92], although skepticism arising in consumers [93] may offset this effect. Thus, we assume that health claims will have a positive effect on the perceived healthiness of a product, although to a lesser extent than the other examined characteristics. Based on all this, our first hypothesis is the following:

Hypothesis 1 (H1). A claim related to an ingredient has a stronger influence on the assessment of the health benefits of a food product than displaying a health claim.

2.1.2. Organic Origin

According to the results of several studies, the organic origin of products has a positive effect on the assessment of the healthiness of a product [25,94–97]. Health-conscious consumers also tend to be more open to organic food while typically ignoring the health-related messages of functional food products [80].

Hypothesis 2 (H2). Of all the factors examined, the organic origin will have the strongest impact on perceived healthiness.

2.1.3. Domestic Origin

Information on the place of origin of a food item may play an important role in consumer decisions and the assessment of the product [98,99]. Puduri, et al. [100] maintain that consumers prefer information on country of origin because they are concerned about the health effects of foreign products. If the consumer's perception of a given country is positive, it also affects the perception of the product from there [101]. Previous research has also shown a relationship between country of origin and the assessment of health effect. It is both a significant influencing factor for foods in general [25], and specifically for functional foods [102]. In our fifth hypothesis we assume that although domestic origin has a positive effect on the assessment of healthiness, it is not the most significant factor.

Hypothesis 3 (H3). Information on domestic origin has a positive effect on the assessment of the health benefits of a product.

3. Materials and Methods

3.1. Data Collection

Our data collection methodology was an online consumer survey, which yielded 633 respondents between November and December 2020. Data collection took place on the university's social media interface through paid advertisement. Respondents provided written consent for their answers to be analyzed. The distribution of the sample by demographic and other characteristics is shown in Table 1.

Table 1. Respondents' demographic and other characteristics (n = 633).

Variables		Sample Composition
		%
Gender	male	26.2
	female	73.8
Age group	18–25 years	25.4
	26–35 years	19.6
	36–45 years	15.2
	46–55 years	15.2
	56 years and older	24.6
Education	max 8 years of elementary school/trade school/vocational school	9.1
	secondary school diploma	47.6
	higher education degree	43.6

Table 1. Cont.

Variables		Sample Composition %
Place of living	Capital	28.4
	Greater capital area	11.2
	Countryside town (not in the greater area)	44.2
	Village/settlement outside of the greater area	16.1
Perceived income status	very tight/tight	21
	average	53.2
	good/very good	25.8
Person responsible for grocery shopping in the household	Respondent	47.4
	Other	6.3
	Shared	46.3
Size of household	1 person	14.1
	2 persons	38.2
	3 persons	21.8
	4 persons	14.5
	5 or more persons	11.4

A big advantage of online sampling is time- and cost-effectiveness [103]; yet, it also involves drawbacks, such as lower response rate or non-representative samples [104]. Our research did not aim at a representative sample, and as a result of online sampling, the distribution of the respondents is biased in several respects, such as the respondents' education or gender.

The questionnaire used in the consumer survey can be divided into three main parts. In the first part, we asked respondents to choose between the products with different designs. Then, we asked respondents to evaluate attitude statements which later provided a basis for differentiating between the individual consumer groups. The claims related to healthy lifestyle were measured using elements of the General Health Interest scale [68], whereas food-related consumer involvement was measured using the corresponding scale of the Food related lifestyle model [74]. The third part of the questionnaire included demographic questions.

3.2. Choice-Based Conjoint Analysis

Conjoint analysis is a widely used method in behavioral research [105], used, among others, to assess consumer preferences. To achieve our research aim, we performed choice-based conjoint analysis, during which we showed respondents choice-sets with two product combinations each, from which they could choose one, simulating a scenario close to a real choice situation [106].

To examine the individual levels, we used a smoothie product for several reasons. The market for functional drinks has been increasing in recent years [107], and smoothies have become an alternative to healthy eating for consumers [108]. In our analysis, we examined the effects of 6 attributes: claims related to ingredients (4 levels), organic origin (2 levels), health claims (3 levels), shape of packaging (3 levels), color of packaging (3 levels) and domestic origin (2 levels). These factors are based on two in-depth literature reviews, which revealed several product-specific and non-product-specific characteristics that influence functional food-related credibility and the assessment of the health effects of a product [42,43]. When completing the questionnaire, respondents always had to choose the picture which they thought presented a product more beneficial to health. The questionnaire did not have a no choice option. Figure 1 summarizes the attributes and their levels.

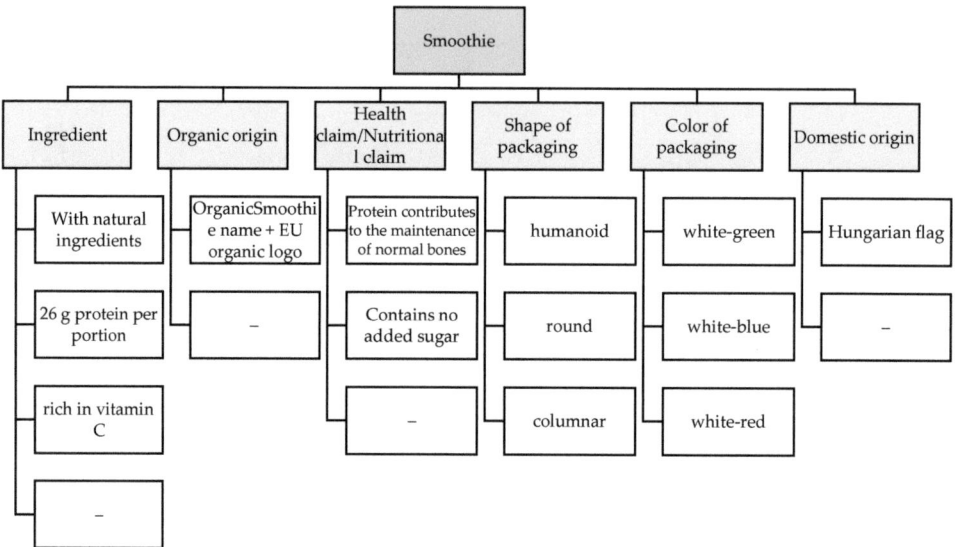

Figure 1. Summary of attributes and levels.

To create the choice sets, we used Aizaki and Nishimura's [109] 5-step description, and based on this, the R statistics software [110]. Accordingly, we first created full factorial design with the help of the AlgDesign package. However, given the extremely large number of combinations thus obtained (4 × 2 × 3 × 3 × 3 × 2 = 432), we used orthogonal design, which allows for the examination of the main effects without having to examine all the combinations that exist [111]. Accordingly, 16 combinations were used in the next steps, in 16 choice sets, comparing two product combinations in each case.

Random utility theory states that consumers make rational decisions, maximizing the utility of their decisions. According to the theory, perceived utility (U_j) can be divided into two parts, systematic utility (V_j), and a random component (ε_j) [112], and can be described with the following equation:

$$U_j = V_j + \varepsilon_j$$

Based on the attributes and levels used in our research, the representative component of utility can be described using the following equation:

$$V_j = \beta_I Ing_j + \beta_O Org_j + \beta_H Hcl_j + \beta_S Sha_j + \beta_C Col_j + \beta_{Ori} Ori_j$$

where, V_j is the representative component of utility in the case of j smoothie (j = A,B, A—option 1, B—option 2), the value of Org_j is 1 if an organic product features in the given j combination; if not, then it is 0. The value of Ori_j is also 1 if an indication of Hungarian origin appears in the given j combination; if not, then it is 0. Ing_j, HCl_j, Sha_j, Col_j indicate a claim related to an ingredient, a health claim, shape of packaging and color used with j smoothie. $\beta_I, \beta_O, \beta_H, \beta_S, \beta_C, \beta_{Ori}$ are unknown parameters associated with Ing_j, Org_{j-}, HCl_{j-}, Sha_j, Col_j and Ori_j.

Figure 2 provides an example of the choice sets as they appeared in the online questionnaire.

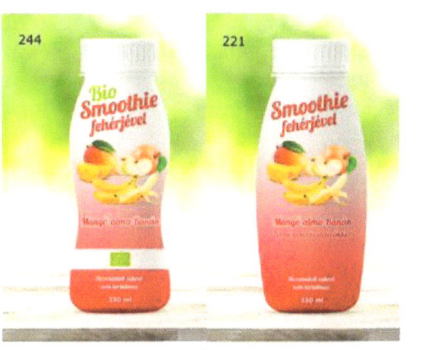
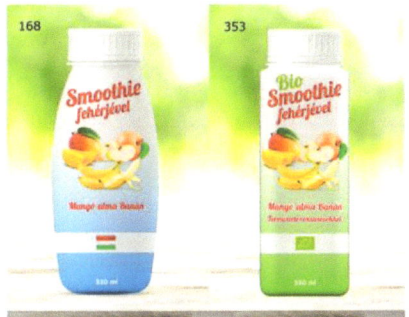

Figure 2. Examples of choice sets.

4. Results

Our main research aim was to identify the extrinsic attribute combination which results in a product that most convincingly shows the consumer that it contains a beneficial impact on health. We summarize the results of the conditional logit model analysis for the whole sample in Table 2. In the model, the last category of each attribute is a reference category with a coefficient value of 0, so they do not appear in the table.

Table 2. Results of the conditional logit model.

Level of attribute	Coefficients	Exp (coef)	se (coef)	z-value
Attribute—Claim Related to an Ingredient				
With natural ingredients [a]	0.698 **	2.010	0.046	15.168
Rich in vitamin C [a]	0.469 **	1.599	0.065	7.211
26 g protein per portion [a]	0.280 **	1.324	0.066	4.254
Attribute—Organic				
OrganicSmoothie name + EU organic logo [b]	1.016 **	2.761	0.033	30.596
Attribute—health claim				
With no added sugar [c]	0.529 **	1.698	0.05	10.476
Protein contributes to the maintenance of normal bones [c]	−0.087 n.s.	0.917	0.059	−1.458
Attribute—shape				
columnar [d]	0.315 **	1.37	0.053	5.959
round [d]	0.046 n.s.	1.047	0.048	0.959
Attribute—color				
white-blue [e]	1.385 **	3.992	0.153	9.037
white-green [e]	0.627 **	1.873	0.089	7.004
Attribute—origin				
Hungarian flag [f]	0.606 **	1.833	0.0572	10.602

[a]—reference category: packaging with no claim on an ingredient; [b]—reference category—nonorganic product; [c]—reference category—packaging with no health claim; [d]—reference category—humanoid shape; [e]—reference category—white—red; [f]—reference category—packaging without a Hungarian flag; ** $p < 0.01$, n.s.—non-significant.

As the results in Table 2 show, each attribute contributes to the assessment of the health effect of the product to some extent and there was a significant feature for each. Considering the obtained coefficients on the whole, the assessment of health effect is most supported by the color white-blue, as well as organic origin of the product. Based on this, we were able to partially verify our second hypothesis, as the second most influential factor is organic origin.

In our research, we examined different types of claims, such as claims related to ingredients and health claims. The use of all ingredient claims helps to assess the health effects of a product. However, whereas the use of the claim "26 g protein per portion" increases the degree of credibility by 1.3 times (Exp coef = 1.32), and the claim "rich in vitamin C" by 1.6 times (Exp coef = 1.6), the claim "with natural ingredients" doubles it (Exp coef = 2.01) compared to not displaying such a claim. Our results confirm our first hypothesis, in which we assumed that the use of ingredient claims makes the health effect more credible than health claims.

Scrutinizing health claims and nutritional claims, not all examined factors showed a significant effect. Whereas the applied nutritional claim ("Contains no added sugar") contributes to a more authentic demonstrations of the health benefits of the product, the effect of the examined health claim is not significant. When displaying this nutritional claim on the packaging, consumers are 1.7 times more likely (Exp coef = 1.69) to consider a product beneficial to health than without such a claim on the packaging.

Examining shape, we concluded that using the columnar shape is the most advantageous, while there is no significant difference between the assessment of the health effect of the round and humanoid shape. If instead of the humanoid shape, the manufacturer uses the columnar shape to package a functional smoothie, consumers are 1.4 times more likely (Exp coef = 1.37) to assess the product as beneficial to their health. If the manufacturer uses the color white-blue instead of white-red as the emphasized color of the packaging, it is four times (Exp coef = 3.99) as likely that the consumer will consider the product to be beneficial to their health as if the manufacturer had used the color white-red. This ratio is also significant in the case of the color white-green, where the consumer is nearly twice as likely (Exp coef = 1.87) to assess a white-green-packaged functional smoothie to be beneficial to health than a white-red one.

An indication of domestic origin also makes the health benefits of a product more credible, which confirms our third hypothesis. A functional smoothie with an indication of domestic origin on the packaging is nearly twice as likely (Exp coef. = 1.83) to be perceived by the consumer as beneficial to health than a product without such an indication.

Based on the results in Table 2, the product combination considered to be the healthiest is the one that is organic, white-blue in color, includes the statement "with natural ingredients", an indication of domestic origin, a nutritional claim, and is square shaped.

The Effects of Individual Characteristics on Valuation

In addition to surveying the whole sample, we assumed that the different characteristics of consumers would result in differences in the assessment of the individual levels. We examined the influence of consumers' general health interest level, involvement with food, and the different demographic features on the assessment of healthiness. We assessed the differences between women and men, those with higher and lower level of education, and those aged under 36 and those 36 years old or older. When examining General Health Interest, we split the sample into two: respondents with a below average and those with an above average GHI level, based on averaging the values given to the scales. Based on the mean values, we divided the sample into two parts with roughly equal number of elements, then coded it into the table used for the conditional logit model with codes 0 and 1. The code 0 indicated a below average GHI level, and 1 indicated an above average 1. We also proceeded similarly with involvement.

Based on the description of Aizaki and Nishimura [109], we supplemented the command line run on the whole sample in R with the various criteria and examined the significant discrepancies. The results thus obtained are summarized in Table 3, in which the rows where we found a significant difference are highlighted.

Table 3. Results of the conditional logit model: Interaction effects.

Level of attribute	Interaction effect	Coefficients	Exp (coef)	se (coef)	z-value
Attribute—Claim Related to Ingredient					
With natural ingredients [a]	:gender	0.216 *	1.240	0.106	2.021
	:education	0.262 *	1.299	0.135	1.931
Rich in vitamin C [a]	:gender	0.407 **	1.502	0.149	2.726
26 g protein per portion [a]	:education	0.262 *	1.299	0.135	1.931
Attribute—Organic					
OrgSmoothie name + EU organic logo [b]	:General health interest	−0.128 *	0.88	0.068	−1.872
	:involvement	0.214 **	1.239	0.069	3.090
Attribute—Health claim					
Contains no added sugar [c]	:age	0.502 **	1.652	0.106	4.719
Protein contributes to the maintenance of normal bones [c]	:age	0.281 **	1.324	0.125	2.251
Attribute—Shape					
round [d]	:General health interest	−0.131 *	0.877	0.078	−1.669
	:education	−0.229 **	0.795	0.078	−2.937
columnar [d]	:gender	0.239 **	1.27	0.12	1.996

[a]—reference category: packaging with no claim on an ingredient; [b]—reference category—nonorganic product; [c]—reference category—packaging with no health claim; [d]—reference category—humanoid shape; * $p < 0.1$, ** $p < 0.05$;

According to the gender, age, and education of respondents, we found significant differences at several points.

The gender of the respondent influences the assessment of the different levels for two of the six attributes. Women assess the health impact even more credible than men if the manufacturer uses columnar packaging instead of humanoid (Exp coef = 1.27), and women also ascribe greater importance to the statements "Rich in vitamin C" (Exp coef = 1.5) and "With natural ingredients" (Exp coef = 1.29).

The age of the respondent gains importance in relation to health claims. Respondents under the age of 36 are more likely to believe the health benefits of a smoothie containing either a nutritional claim or a health claim than the older age group (Exp. coef = 1.65; 1.32). Education plays an important role in the case of two ingredient claims and a shape. As opposed to the manufacturer not using such a claim, respondents with a higher education judged the claims "With natural ingredients" and "26 g protein per portion" equally (Exp coef = 1.29 in both cases) more useful when assessing the impact on health than those with a lower education. On the other hand, compared to humanoid packaging, respondents with a higher education are less likely to believe that a product with a round shape packaging is beneficial to health (Exp coef = 0.79) than those with a lower education.

We obtained interesting results related to organic origin. Consumers with a higher general health interest are less likely to believe that an organic product is beneficial to health than those with less such interest (Exp coef = 0.88). Furthermore, those with a higher food involvement level are more likely to consider an organic functional smoothie beneficial to their health than the less involved (Exp coef = 1.239). Those with a higher general health interest also assessed the round shape differently: compared to a humanoid shape, they consider it less credible (Exp coef = 0.87) that a product with a round shape is beneficial to health than respondents with a lower GHI level.

5. Discussion

Extrinsic cues play a prominent role in the assessment of a product. Although the effect on health is a kind of credence attribute, its assessment is strongly influenced by extrinsic product features. In our research, we aimed to determine the extent to which different characteristics used on the packaging influence the consumer assessment of the health impact of a product. Another aim of ours was to clarify the conflicting results found in the literature regarding the shape and color of the packaging. We examined six extrinsic attributes: claims related to ingredients, organic origin, health claims, the shape and color of packaging, and domestic origin. Our results show that of the extrinsic characteristics examined, it is the color white-blue followed by organic origin that have the greatest effect on the consumer's belief in the health benefits of a product.

By showing that the color white-blue has the strongest influencing effect, we confirm the results of previous research [54] that also highlight this color, with the addition that white-blue contributes four times more effectively to the assessment of healthiness than white-red. This is supported by the results of research by Reutner and his colleagues [52], which demonstrates that the use of red tends to influence consumer perceptions of products that are perceived as unhealthy. Thus, we can rather support the prohibitive nature of the color red. Organic origin should be highlighted in the sense that, although previous research has consistently shown it to be a strong factor influencing perceptions of health impact [25,94–97], it has not been the most important factor in our case. The fact that organic origin is the second most influential factor is presumably due to the health halo effect associated with it, which makes consumers perceive such products as healthier [113,114]. These two factors are followed by a claim related to ingredients (With natural ingredients) and the indication of domestic origin. That the perception of products is influenced by the inclusion of information on domestic origin has been confirmed by several studies [98–102], and the results of our research contribute to this by ranking the importance of this information. In the order of importance, health claims/nutritional claims are only the fifth of the six elements, and only the nutritional claim showed significant effect, the tested health claim did not. We confirm the results of previous research that consumers may be skeptical about these claims [54,80,93] and also supports the findings of Orquin and Scholderer [78] that health claims have only a small influence on perceptions of healthiness. The form of packaging is also a factor that has been studied in several previous studies [46–50], but its importance in assessing the credibility of the health impact is, based on our results, small compared to the factors studied. Shape has the least influence on the assessment of healthiness, and although previous research has suggested the use of a rounder shape [50], our result suggest that the square shape is more effective.

The non-significant effect is probably due to consumer skepticism, confirming previous research results which showed that consumers may become skeptical about health claims [80,93]. Regarding color, in line with some previous results [51,54], the significant effect of the color white-blue can be highlighted, which, of the examined colors, can contribute the most to consumer belief that the product has a beneficial effect on health.

In addition to the fact that the manufacturer should pay attention to these differences between target groups, we also conclude that the most prominent factor, the color white-blue, positively influences the assessment of the effect on health regardless of the examined consumer criteria and attitudes, and we can draw a similar conclusion in relation to the indication of domestic origin.

At the same time, it is important that manufacturers know their target groups, as the assessment of further attributes varies depending on involvement with food, the level of general health interest, and the different demographic criteria. We found significant differences between consumers with below average and above average general health interest, and between consumers with different involvement levels. When assessing healthiness, organic origin is more important for consumers who are involved above average than for those below average. Claims related to ingredients were assessed differently by women and men, and by respondents with lower and higher education: women are more likely to believe that a smoothie containing the claim "With natural ingredients" or "Rich in vitamin C" is beneficial to health than men. Furthermore, the same is true for those with a higher education rather than a lower education for the former claim or the claim "26 g protein per portion".

Our results are useful to companies producing functional foods, because in addition to collecting the main extrinsic characteristics that affect perceived healthiness, we also determined their weight. It all helps manufacturers to most effectively imply the healthiness of a product, which is of great relevance in the case of functional foods, to consumers during the purchasing process. A functional food producing company's marketing strategy must consider the health benefits of its products, among many other aspects. If a company knows the strength of each of the factors that significantly influence health impact, it can make better decisions about which aspects to change even though they may require changes to other elements of the marketing strategy, and which aspects to leave unchanged because of other factors influencing the marketing strategy.

Our results show that it is not the nutritionally valuable sources of information that most influence consumers' perceptions of product healthiness, which raises the importance of the work of nutritionists and dieticians. As credible communicators [115], they have an important role to play in ensuring that health-conscious consumers are more conscious when making a purchase, and seek and evaluate the right information.

6. Limitations

In accordance with the Total Food Quality model of Grunert, et al. [116], which treats price as a separate category outside of extrinsic features, we did not explicitly include price among the examined factors in our research. However, price can be a significant influencing factor, so it would be worth exploring this in a future study.

Our research is based on two in-depth literature analyses, but it is important to note that the factors under investigation, such as color, can also have other meanings. The two reviews focused specifically on perceived healthiness and this research was not designed to explore other present-tense aspects.

7. Conclusions

In our research, following an analysis of the literature, five characteristics that influence the perception of a product's health impact have been identified, namely the shape and color of the packaging, health claims, claims related to the ingredients of the product and the impact of domestic origin. Our aim was to rank the characteristics in order of which most influence whether a consumer believes a functional food to be beneficial to health. We also aimed to determine the weight of different characteristics in the assessment of health impact. According to our results, among all the six examined attributes there are characteristics which significantly influences the credibility of the health effect. Our results show that consumers are most likely to believe that product is beneficial to their health if it is primarily white and blue, organic and contains an ingredient claim. These are followed to a lesser extent by the indication of domestic origin and the nutritional claim, and least influenced by the form of the packaging. However, we found that in the perception of health effect even the shape that resembled the humanoid shape differed significantly from the columnar shape. In addition, we consider it an important part of our results to point out that while health claims do not significantly affect the credibility of the health effect, nutritional claims do. The smoothie with the simplest packaging was the least likely to be perceived by respondents as having health benefits. This means that consumers were least likely to believe that the packaging was beneficial to health if it was red-white, not organic, did not contain any ingredient claims or health claims, did not have a domestic origin label and was angular in shape.

In the functional food market, a significant proportion of products are withdrawn by companies shortly after launch. The results of our research may help manufacturers to create and present packaging in a combination that consumers are more likely to believe has positive health benefits.

Although our research results have shown which features contribute the most to making the consumer believe that a product has a beneficial effect on health, the question arises whether the combined use of so much information would be good corporate practice. It is possible that packaging with much less information more effectively presents the healthiness of the product to the consumer. Further research may aim to gauge how much information a manufacturer should use on the packaging to convey a sufficiently credible effect on health to the consumer.

Author Contributions: Conceptualization, B.P. and Á.T.; formal analysis, B.P.; investigation, B.P.; resources, B.P. and Á.T.; data curation, B.P.; methodology, B.P., Á.T. and Z.L.; writing—original draft preparation, B.P.; writing—review and editing, Á.T.; visualization, B.P.; supervision, Á.T. and Z.L.; funding acquisition, Á.T. All authors have read and agreed to the published version of the manuscript.

Funding: This research received no external funding.

Institutional Review Board Statement: Not applicable.

Informed Consent Statement: Informed consent was obtained from all subjects involved in the study.

Data Availability Statement: The data presented in this study are available on request from the corresponding author.

Conflicts of Interest: The authors declare no conflict of interest.

References

1. Mehta, K.; Phillips, C.; Ward, P.; Coveney, J.; Handsley, E.; Carter, P. Marketing foods to children through product packaging: Prolific, unhealthy and misleading. *Public Health Nutr.* **2012**, *15*, 1763–1770. [CrossRef]
2. Page, R.; Montgomery, K.; Ponder, A.; Richard, A. Targeting children in the cereal aisle: Promotional techniques and content features on ready-to-eat cereal product packaging. *Am. J. Health Educ.* **2008**, *39*, 272–282. [CrossRef]
3. Pulker, C.E.; Chew Ching Li, D.; Scott, J.A.; Pollard, C.M. The impact of voluntary policies on parents' ability to select healthy foods in supermarkets: A qualitative study of australian parental views. *Int. J. Environ. Res. Public Health* **2019**, *16*, 3377. [CrossRef] [PubMed]
4. Waani, R.C.; Tumbuan, W.J.A. The influence of price discount, bonus pack, and in-store display on impulse buying decision in hypermart kairagi manado. *J. EMBA J. Ris. Ekon. Manaj. Bisnis Dan Akunt.* **2015**, *3*, 420–428. [CrossRef]
5. Zulfiqar, J.; Ambreen, G.; Bushra, M.F. A comprehensive literature review of impulse buying behavior. *J. Adv. Res. Soc. Behav. Sci.* **2018**, *11*, 94–104.
6. Hur, J.; Jang, S.S. Anticipated guilt and pleasure in a healthy food consumption context. *Int. J. Hosp. Manag.* **2015**, *48*, 113–123. [CrossRef]
7. Gonzalez, M.-P.; Thornsbury, S.; Twede, D. Packaging as a tool for product development: Communicating value to consumers. *J. Food Distrib. Res.* **2007**, *38*, 61–66. [CrossRef]
8. Diplock, A.; Charuleux, J.-L.; Crozier-Willi, G.; Kok, F.; Rice-Evans, C.; Roberfroid, M.; Stahl, W.; Vina-Ribes, J. Functional food science and defence against reactive oxidative species. *Br. J. Nutr.* **1998**, *80*, S77–S112. [CrossRef]
9. Pramudya, R.C.; Seo, H.-S. Hand-feel touch cues and their influences on consumer perception and behavior with respect to food products: A review. *Foods* **2019**, *8*, 259. [CrossRef]
10. Barreiro Hurlé, J.; Gracia Royo, A.; de Magistris, T. Market implications of new regulations: Impact of health and nutrition information on consumer choice. *Span. J. Agric. Res.* **2009**, *7*, 257–268. [CrossRef]
11. Barreiro-Hurlé, J.; Gracia, A.; De-Magistris, T. Using latent classes to determine consumer heterogeneity in nutritional label valuation. *Food Econ. Acta Agric. Scand. Sect. C* **2008**, *5*, 178–193. [CrossRef]
12. Roosen, J.; Marette, S.; Blanchemanche, S.; Verger, P. The effect of product health information on liking and choice. *Food Qual. Prefer.* **2007**, *18*, 759–770. [CrossRef]
13. Verbeke, W.; Demey, V.; Bosmans, W.; Viaene, J. Consumer versus producer expectations and motivations related to "superior" quality meat: Qualitative research findings. *J. Food Prod. Mark.* **2005**, *11*, 27–41. [CrossRef]
14. Darby, M.R.; Karni, E. Free competition and the optimal amount of fraud. *J. Law Econ.* **1973**, *16*, 67–88. [CrossRef]
15. Grunert, K.G.; Bredahl, L.; Brunsø, K. Consumer perception of meat quality and implications for product development in the meat sector—A review. *Meat Sci.* **2004**, *66*, 259–272. [CrossRef]
16. Ophuis, P.A.O.; Van Trijp, H.C. Perceived quality: A market driven and consumer oriented approach. *Food Qual. Prefer.* **1995**, *6*, 177–183. [CrossRef]
17. Veale, R.; Quester, P.; Karunaratna, A. The role of intrinsic (sensory) cues and the extrinsic cues of country of origin and price on food product evaluation. Proceedings of 3rd International Wine Business and Marketing Research Conference, Refereed Paper. Montpellier, France, 6–8 July 2006; pp. 6–8.

18. Rao, A.R.; Monroe, K.B. The effect of price, brand name, and store name on buyers' perceptions of product quality: An integrative review. *J. Mark. Res.* **1989**, *26*, 351–357. [CrossRef]
19. Olson, J.C.; Jacoby, J. Cue Utilization in The Quality Perception Process. In Proceedings of the Third Annual Conference of the Association for Consumer Research, Chicago, IL, USA, 3–5 November 1972; pp. 167–179.
20. Grubor, A.; Djokic, N.; Djokic, I.; Kovac-Znidersic, R. Application of health and taste attitude scales in Serbia. *Br. Food J.* **2015**, *117*, 840–860. [CrossRef]
21. Hartmann, C.; Hieke, S.; Taper, C.; Siegrist, M. European consumer healthiness evaluation of 'Free-from'labelled food products. *Food Qual. Prefer.* **2018**, *68*, 377–388. [CrossRef]
22. Wijayaratne, S.P.; Reid, M.; Westberg, K.; Worsley, A.; Mavondo, F. Food literacy, healthy eating barriers and household diet. *Eur. J. Mark.* **2018**, *52*, 2449–2477. [CrossRef]
23. Brečić, R.; Mesić, Ž.; Cerjak, M. Importance of intrinsic and extrinsic quality food characteristics by different consumer segments. *Br. Food J.* **2017**, *119*, 845–862. [CrossRef]
24. Bucher, T.; Müller, B.; Siegrist, M. What is healthy food? Objective nutrient profile scores and subjective lay evaluations in comparison. *Appetite* **2015**, *95*, 408–414. [CrossRef] [PubMed]
25. Cavallo, C.; Piqueras-Fiszman, B. Visual elements of packaging shaping healthiness evaluations of consumers: The case of olive oil. *J. Sens. Stud.* **2017**, *32*, e12246. [CrossRef]
26. Lazzarini, G.A.; Zimmermann, J.; Visschers, V.H.; Siegrist, M. Does environmental friendliness equal healthiness? Swiss consumers' perception of protein products. *Appetite* **2016**, *105*, 663–673. [CrossRef]
27. Pires, M.A.; de Noronha, R.L.F.; Trindade, M.A. Understanding consumer's perception and acceptance of bologna sausages with reduced sodium content and/or omega-3 addition through conjoint analysis and focus group. *J. Sens. Stud.* **2019**, *34*, e12495. [CrossRef]
28. Polizer Rocha, Y.J.; Lapa-Guimarães, J.; de Noronha, R.L.F.; Trindade, M.A. Evaluation of consumers' perception regarding frankfurter sausages with different healthiness attributes. *J. Sens. Stud.* **2018**, *33*, e12468. [CrossRef]
29. Rizk, M.T.; Treat, T.A. Perceptions of food healthiness among free-living women. *Appetite* **2015**, *95*, 390–398. [CrossRef] [PubMed]
30. Anders, S.; Schroeter, C. Estimating the effects of nutrition label use on Canadian consumer diet-health concerns using propensity score matching. *Int. J. Consum. Stud.* **2017**, *41*, 534–544. [CrossRef]
31. Carrete, L.; Arroyo, P. Social marketing to improve healthy dietary decisions. *Qual. Mark. Res.* **2014**, *17*, 239–263. [CrossRef]
32. Labbe, D.; Rytz, A.; Godinot, N.; Ferrage, A.; Martin, N. Is portion size selection associated with expected satiation, perceived healthfulness or expected tastiness? A case study on pizza using a photograph-based computer task. *Appetite* **2017**, *108*, 311–316. [CrossRef]
33. Marino, R.; Della Malva, A.; Seccia, A.; Caroprese, M.; Sevi, A.; Albenzio, M. Consumers' expectations and acceptability for low saturated fat 'salami': Healthiness or taste? *J. Sci. Food Agric.* **2017**, *97*, 3515–3521. [CrossRef]
34. Vasiljevic, M.; Pechey, R.; Marteau, T.M. Making food labels social: The impact of colour of nutritional labels and injunctive norms on perceptions and choice of snack foods. *Appetite* **2015**, *91*, 56–63. [CrossRef]
35. Richardson, P.S.; Dick, A.S.; Jain, A.K. Extrinsic and intrinsic cue effects on perceptions of store brand quality. *J. Mark.* **1994**, *58*, 28–36. [CrossRef]
36. Meillon, S.; Urbano, C.; Guillot, G.; Schlich, P. Acceptability of partially dealcoholized wines–Measuring the impact of sensory and information cues on overall liking in real-life settings. *Food Qual. Prefer.* **2010**, *21*, 763–773. [CrossRef]
37. Speed, R. Choosing between line extensions and second brands: The case of the Australian and New Zealand wine industries. *J. Prod. Brand Manag.* **1998**, *7*, 519–536. [CrossRef]
38. Akdeniz, B.; Calantone, R.J.; Voorhees, C.M. Effectiveness of marketing cues on consumer perceptions of quality: The moderating roles of brand reputation and third-party information. *Psychol. Mark.* **2013**, *30*, 76–89. [CrossRef]
39. Bearden, W.O.; Shimp, T.A. The use of extrinsic cues to facilitate product adoption. *J. Mark. Res.* **1982**, *19*, 229–239. [CrossRef]
40. Bolha, A.; Blaznik, U.; Korošec, M. Influence of Intrinsic and Extrinsic Food Attributes on Consumers' Acceptance of Reformulated Food Products: A Systematic Review. *Slov. J. Public Health* **2020**, *60*, 72. [CrossRef] [PubMed]
41. Rondoni, A.; Millan, E.; Asioli, D. Consumers' preferences for intrinsic and extrinsic product attributes of plant-based eggs: An exploratory study in the United Kingdom and Italy. *Br. Food J.* ahead of print. **2021**. [CrossRef]
42. Plasek, B.; Lakner, Z.; Temesi, Á. Factors that Influence the Perceived Healthiness of Food. *Nutrients* **2020**, *12*, 1881. [CrossRef]
43. Plasek, B.; Temesi, Á. The credibility of the effects of functional food products and consumers' willingness to purchase/willingness to pay—Review. *Appetite* **2019**, *143*, 104398. [CrossRef]
44. Schnurr, B. Too cute to be healthy: How cute packaging designs affect judgments of product tastiness and healthiness. *J. Assoc. Consum. Res.* **2019**, *4*, 363–375. [CrossRef]
45. van Ooijen, I.; Fransen, M.L.; Verlegh, P.W.; Smit, E.G. Signalling product healthiness through symbolic package cues: Effects of package shape and goal congruence on consumer behaviour. *Appetite* **2017**, *109*, 73–82. [CrossRef]
46. Yarar, N.; Machiels, C.J.; Orth, U.R. Shaping up: How package shape and consumer body conspire to affect food healthiness evaluation. *Food Qual. Prefer.* **2019**, *75*, 209–219. [CrossRef]
47. Koo, J.; Suk, K. The effect of package shape on calorie estimation. *Int. J. Res. Mark.* **2016**, *33*, 856–867. [CrossRef]
48. Fenko, A.; Lotterman, H.; Galetzka, M. What's in a name? The effects of sound symbolism and package shape on consumer responses to food products. *Food Qual. Prefer.* **2016**, *51*, 100–108. [CrossRef]

49. Festila, A.; Chrysochou, P. Implicit communication of food product healthfulness through package design: A content analysis. *J. Consum. Behav.* **2018**, *17*, 461–476. [CrossRef]
50. Marques da Rosa, V.; Spence, C.; Miletto Tonetto, L. Influences of visual attributes of food packaging on consumer preference and associations with taste and healthiness. *Int. J. Consum. Stud.* **2019**, *43*, 210–217. [CrossRef]
51. Huang, L.; Lu, J. The impact of package color and the nutrition content labels on the perception of food healthiness and purchase intention. *J. Food Prod. Mark.* **2016**, *22*, 191–218. [CrossRef]
52. Reutner, L.; Genschow, O.; Wänke, M. The adaptive eater: Perceived healthiness moderates the effect of the color red on consumption. *Food Qual. Prefer.* **2015**, *44*, 172–178. [CrossRef]
53. Tijssen, I.; Zandstra, E.H.; de Graaf, C.; Jager, G. Why a 'light'product package should not be light blue: Effects of package colour on perceived healthiness and attractiveness of sugar-and fat-reduced products. *Food Qual. Prefer.* **2017**, *59*, 46–58. [CrossRef]
54. Wąsowicz, G.; Styśko-Kunkowska, M.; Grunert, K.G. The meaning of colours in nutrition labelling in the context of expert and consumer criteria of evaluating food product healthfulness. *J. Health Psychol.* **2015**, *20*, 907–920. [CrossRef]
55. Ares, G.; Gámbaro, A. Influence of gender, age and motives underlying food choice on perceived healthiness and willingness to try functional foods. *Appetite* **2007**, *49*, 148–158. [CrossRef] [PubMed]
56. Kraus, A.; Annunziata, A.; Vecchio, R. Sociodemographic factors differentiating the consumer and the motivations for functional food consumption. *J. Am. Coll. Nutr.* **2017**, *36*, 116–126. [CrossRef]
57. Vorage, L.; Wiseman, N.; Graca, J.; Harris, N. The Association of Demographic Characteristics and Food Choice Motives with the Consumption of Functional Foods in Emerging Adults. *Nutrients* **2020**, *12*, 2582. [CrossRef] [PubMed]
58. De Jong, N.; Ocke, M.C.; Branderhorst, H.A.; Friele, R. Demographic and lifestyle characteristics of functional food consumers and dietary supplement users. *Br. J. Nutr.* **2003**, *89*, 273–281. [CrossRef]
59. Urala, N. Functional Foods in Finland: Consumers' Views, Attitudes and Willingness to Use. *VTT Publications* **2005**.
60. Verbeke, W. Consumer acceptance of functional foods: Socio-demographic, cognitive and attitudinal determinants. *Food Qual. Prefer.* **2005**, *16*, 45–57. [CrossRef]
61. Verneau, F.; La Barbera, F.; Furno, M. The role of health information in consumers' willingness to pay for canned crushed tomatoes enriched with Lycopene. *Nutrients* **2019**, *11*, 2173. [CrossRef]
62. Barauskaite, D.; Gineikiene, J.; Fennis, B.M.; Auruskeviciene, V.; Yamaguchi, M.; Kondo, N. Eating healthy to impress: How conspicuous consumption, perceived self-control motivation, and descriptive normative influence determine functional food choices. *Appetite* **2018**, *131*, 59–67. [CrossRef]
63. Kljusurić, J.G.; Čačić, J. Changes of young consumers' perception regarding functional food-case of Croatia. *J. Hyg. Eng. Des.* **2014**, *7*, 61–65.
64. Krutulyte, R.; Grunert, K.G.; Scholderer, J.; Lähteenmäki, L.; Hagemann, K.S.; Elgaard, P.; Nielsen, B.; Graverholt, J.P. Perceived fit of different combinations of carriers and functional ingredients and its effect on purchase intention. *Food Qual. Prefer.* **2011**, *22*, 11–16. [CrossRef]
65. Siegrist, M.; Shi, J.; Giusto, A.; Hartmann, C. Worlds apart. Consumer acceptance of functional foods and beverages in Germany and China. *Appetite* **2015**, *92*, 87–93. [CrossRef]
66. Steinhauser, J.; Janssen, M.; Hamm, U. Who buys products with nutrition and health claims? A purchase simulation with eye tracking on the influence of consumers' nutrition knowledge and health motivation. *Nutrients* **2019**, *11*, 2199. [CrossRef]
67. Bornkessel, S.; Bröring, S.; Omta, S.O.; van Trijp, H. What determines ingredient awareness of consumers? A study on ten functional food ingredients. *Food Qual. Prefer.* **2014**, *32*, 330–339. [CrossRef]
68. Roininen, K.; Lähteenmäki, L.; Tuorila, H. Quantification of consumer attitudes to health and hedonic characteristics of foods. *Appetite* **1999**, *33*, 71–88. [CrossRef]
69. Ares, G.; Besio, M.; Giménez, A.; Deliza, R. Relationship between involvement and functional milk desserts intention to purchase. Influence on attitude towards packaging characteristics. *Appetite* **2010**, *55*, 298–304. [CrossRef]
70. Gomez, P.; Schneid, N.; Delaere, F. How often should I eat it? Product correlates and accuracy of estimation of appropriate food consumption frequency. *Food Qual. Prefer.* **2015**, *40*, 1–7. [CrossRef]
71. Barker, M.; Lawrence, W.; Woadden, J.; Crozier, S.; Skinner, T. Women of lower educational attainment have lower food involvement and eat less fruit and vegetables. *Appetite* **2008**, *50*, 464–468. [CrossRef] [PubMed]
72. Grunert, K.G.; Wills, J.M.; Fernández-Celemín, L. Nutrition knowledge, and use and understanding of nutrition information on food labels among consumers in the UK. *Appetite* **2010**, *55*, 177–189. [CrossRef]
73. Xie, Y.; Grebitus, C.; Davis, G.C. Can the new label make a difference? Comparing consumer attention towards the current versus proposed Nutrition Facts panel. In Proceedings of the AAEA & WAEA Joint Annual Meeting, San Francisco, CA, USA, 26–28 July 2015.
74. Brunsø, K.; Birch, D.; Memery, J.; Temesi, Á.; Lakner, Z.; Lang, M.; Dean, D.; Grunert, K.G. Core dimensions of food-related lifestyle: A new instrument for measuring food involvement, innovativeness and responsibility. *Food Qual. Prefer.* **2021**, *91*, 104192. [CrossRef]
75. Aschemann-Witzel, J.; Grunert, K.G. Influence of 'soft'versus 'scientific'health information framing and contradictory information on consumers' health inferences and attitudes towards a food supplement. *Food Qual. Prefer.* **2015**, *42*, 90–99. [CrossRef]
76. Rozin, P.; Spranca, M.; Krieger, Z.; Neuhaus, R.; Surillo, D.; Swerdlin, A.; Wood, K. Preference for natural: Instrumental and ideational/moral motivations, and the contrast between foods and medicines. *Appetite* **2004**, *43*, 147–154. [CrossRef]

77. Stancu, V.; Lähteenmäki, L.; Grunert, K.G. The role of time constraints in consumer understanding of health claims. *Food Qual. Prefer.* **2021**, *94*, 104261. [CrossRef]
78. Orquin, J.L.; Scholderer, J. Consumer judgments of explicit and implied health claims on foods: Misguided but not misled. *Food Policy* **2015**, *51*, 144–157. [CrossRef]
79. Hirogaki, M. Estimating consumers' willingness to pay for health food claims: A conjoint analysis. *Int. J. Innov. Manag. Technol.* **2013**, *4*, 541. [CrossRef]
80. Gineikiene, J.; Kiudyte, J.; Degutis, M. Functional, organic or conventional? Food choices of health conscious and skeptical consumers. *Balt. J. Manag.* **2017**, *12*, 139–152. [CrossRef]
81. Chrysochou, P.; Grunert, K.G. Health-related ad information and health motivation effects on product evaluations. *J. Bus. Res.* **2014**, *67*, 1209–1217. [CrossRef]
82. Grunert, K.G.; Lähteenmäki, L.; Boztug, Y.; Martinsdóttir, E.; Ueland, Ø.; Åström, A.; Lampila, P. Perception of health claims among Nordic consumers. *J. Consum. Policy* **2009**, *32*, 269–287. [CrossRef]
83. Hoefkens, C.; Verbeke, W. Consumers' health-related motive orientations and reactions to claims about dietary calcium. *Nutrients* **2013**, *5*, 82–96. [CrossRef] [PubMed]
84. Masson, E.; Debucquet, G.; Fischler, C.; Merdji, M. French consumers' perceptions of nutrition and health claims: A psychosocial-anthropological approach. *Appetite* **2016**, *105*, 618–629. [CrossRef]
85. Shan, L.C.; De Brún, A.; Henchion, M.; Li, C.; Murrin, C.; Wall, P.G.; Monahan, F.J. Consumer evaluations of processed meat products reformulated to be healthier–A conjoint analysis study. *Meat Sci.* **2017**, *131*, 82–89. [CrossRef]
86. Grunert, K.G. *Consumer Trends and New Product Opportunities in The Food Sector*; Wageningen Academic Publishers: Wageningen, The Netherlands, 2017.
87. Singer, L.; Williams, P.; Ridges, L.; Murray, S.; McMahon, A. Consumer reactions to different health claim formats on food labels. *Food Aust.* **2006**, *58*, 92–97.
88. Verbeke, W.; Scholderer, J.; Lähteenmäki, L. Consumer appeal of nutrition and health claims in three existing product concepts. *Appetite* **2009**, *52*, 684–692. [CrossRef] [PubMed]
89. Acton, R.B.; Hammond, D. Do Consumers Think Front-of-Package "High in" Warnings are Harsh or Reduce their Control? A Test of Food Industry Concerns. *Obesity* **2018**, *26*, 1687–1691. [CrossRef] [PubMed]
90. Carabante, K.M.; Ardoin, R.; Scaglia, G.; Malekian, F.; Khachaturyan, M.; Janes, M.E.; Prinyawiwatkul, W. Consumer acceptance, emotional response, and purchase intent of rib-eye steaks from grass-fed steers, and effects of health benefit information on consumer perception. *J. Food Sci.* **2018**, *83*, 2560–2570. [CrossRef] [PubMed]
91. Machín, L.; Aschemann-Witzel, J.; Curutchet, M.R.; Giménez, A.; Ares, G. Does front-of-pack nutrition information improve consumer ability to make healthful choices? Performance of warnings and the traffic light system in a simulated shopping experiment. *Appetite* **2018**, *121*, 55–62. [CrossRef]
92. Miraballes, M.; Gámbaro, A. Influence of Images on the Evaluation of Jams Using Conjoint Analysis Combined with Check-All-That-Apply (CATA) Questions. *J. Food Sci.* **2018**, *83*, 167–174. [CrossRef] [PubMed]
93. Annunziata, A.; Vecchio, R.; Kraus, A. Awareness and preference for functional foods: The perspective of older I talian consumers. *Int. J. Consum. Stud.* **2015**, *39*, 352–361. [CrossRef]
94. Apaolaza, V.; Hartmann, P.; Echebarria, C.; Barrutia, J.M. Organic label's halo effect on sensory and hedonic experience of wine: A pilot study. *J. Sens. Stud.* **2017**, *32*, e12243. [CrossRef]
95. Prada, M.; Garrido, M.V.; Rodrigues, D. Lost in processing? Perceived healthfulness, taste and caloric content of whole and processed organic food. *Appetite* **2017**, *114*, 175–186. [CrossRef] [PubMed]
96. Tleis, M.; Callieris, R.; Roma, R. Segmenting the organic food market in Lebanon: An application of k-means cluster analysis. *Br. Food J.* **2017**, *119*, 1423–1441. [CrossRef]
97. Xie, B.; Wang, L.; Yang, H.; Wang, Y.; Zhang, M. Consumer perceptions and attitudes of organic food products in Eastern China. *Br. Food J.* **2015**, *117*, 1105–1121. [CrossRef]
98. Götze, F.; Brunner, T.A. Sustainability and country-of-origin. *Br. Food J.* **2020**, *122*, 291–308. [CrossRef]
99. Hoffmann, N.C.; Symmank, C.; Mai, R.; Stok, F.M.; Rohm, H.; Hoffmann, S. The influence of extrinsic product attributes on consumers' food decisions: Review and network analysis of the marketing literature. *J. Mark. Manag.* **2020**, *36*, 888–915. [CrossRef]
100. Puduri, V.; Govindasamy, R.; Onyango, B. Country of origin labelling of fresh produce: A consumer preference analysis. *Appl. Econ. Lett.* **2009**, *16*, 1183–1185. [CrossRef]
101. Papadopoulos, N.; Heslop, L. Country equity and country branding: Problems and prospects. *J. Brand Manag.* **2002**, *9*, 294–314. [CrossRef]
102. Dobrenova, F.V.; Grabner-Kräuter, S.; Terlutter, R. Country-of-origin (COO) effects in the promotion of functional ingredients and functional foods. *Eur. Manag. J.* **2015**, *33*, 314–321. [CrossRef]
103. Wright, K.B. Researching Internet-based populations: Advantages and disadvantages of online survey research, online questionnaire authoring software packages, and web survey services. *J. Comput. Mediat. Commun.* **2005**, *10*, JCMC1034. [CrossRef]
104. Rice, S.; Winter, S.R.; Doherty, S.; Milner, M. Advantages and disadvantages of using internet-based survey methods in aviation-related research. *J. Aviat. Technol. Eng.* **2017**, *7*, 5. [CrossRef]
105. Green, P.E.; Srinivasan, V. Conjoint analysis in consumer research: Issues and outlook. *J. Consum. Res.* **1978**, *5*, 103–123. [CrossRef]

106. Hair, J.F.; Black, W.C.; Babin, B.J.; Anderson, R.E. *Multivariate data analysis*; Pearson New International Edition; Pearson Education Limited: London, UK, 2014; Volume 1, p. 2.
107. Statista.com. Market value of functional beverages worldwide from 2010 to 2019. Available online: https://www.statista.com/statistics/979839/market-size-of-functional-drinks-worldwide/ (accessed on 1 March 2021).
108. Serpa-Guerra, A.M.; Velásquez-Cock, J.A.; Barajas-Gamboa, J.A.; Vélez-Acosta, L.M.; Gómez-Hoyos, B.; Zuluaga-Gallego, R. Development of a fortified drink from the mixture of small colombian native fruits. *Dyna* **2018**, *85*, 185–193. [CrossRef]
109. Aizaki, H.; Nishimura, K. Design and analysis of choice experiments using R: A brief introduction. *Agric. Inf. Res.* **2008**, *17*, 86–94. [CrossRef]
110. Team, R.C. *R: A Language and Environment for Statistical Computing*; R Foundation for Statistical Computing: Vienna, Austria, 2013.
111. ibm.com. Generating an Orthogonal Design. Available online: https://www.ibm.com/support/knowledgecenter/SSLVMB_sub/statistics_mainhelp_ddita/spss/conjoint/idh_orth.html (accessed on 27 November 2020).
112. Cascetta, E. Methods for the evaluation and comparison of transportation system projects. In *Transportation Systems Analysis*; Springer: Boston, MA, USA, 2009; pp. 621–681. [CrossRef]
113. Besson, T.; Lalot, F.; Bochard, N.; Flaudias, V.; Zerhouni, O. The calories underestimation of "organic" food: Exploring the impact of implicit evaluations. *Appetite* **2019**, *137*, 134–144. [CrossRef] [PubMed]
114. Her, E.; Seo, S. Health halo effects in sequential food consumption: The moderating roles of health-consciousness and attribute framing. *Int. J. Hosp. Manag.* **2017**, *62*, 1–10. [CrossRef]
115. Patch, C.S.; Tapsell, L.C.; Williams, P.G. Overweight consumers' salient beliefs on omega-3-enriched functional foods in Australia's Illawarra region. *J. Nutr. Educ. Behav.* **2005**, *37*, 83–89. [CrossRef]
116. Grunert, K.G.; Larsen, H.H.; Madsen, T.K.; Baadsgaard, A. *Market Orientation in Food and Agriculture*; Springer Science & Business Media: Boston, MA, USA, 1996.

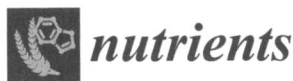

Article

Intake Estimation of Phytochemicals in a French Well-Balanced Diet

Marie-Josèphe Amiot [1,*], Christian Latgé [2], Laurence Plumey [3] and Sylvie Raynal [4]

1. INRAE, MoISA, University of Montpellier, CIHEAM-IAMM, CIRAD, Institut Agro-Montpellier SupAgro, IRD, Campus La Gaillarde, 2 Place Pierre Viala, 34000 Montpellier, France
2. Pierre Fabre Laboratories, Langlade-3 Avenue Hubert Curien-BP 13 562, CEDEX 1, 31035 Toulouse, France; christian.latge@pierre-fabre.com
3. NUTRITION CO&CO, 11 Avenue des Vignes, 92210 St Cloud, France; laurence.plumey@free.fr
4. Naturactive, Pierre Fabre Laboratories, 29 Avenue du Sidobre, 81106 Castres, France; sylvie.raynal@pierre-fabre.com
* Correspondence: marie-josephe.amiot-carlin@inrae.fr; Tel.: +33-(0)4-99-61-22-16

Abstract: Phytochemicals contribute to the health benefits of plant-rich diets, notably through their antioxidant and anti-inflammatory effects. However, recommended daily amounts of the main dietary phytochemicals remain undetermined. We aimed to estimate the amounts of phytochemicals in a well-balanced diet. A modelled diet was created, containing dietary reference intakes for adults in France. Two one-week menus (summer and winter) were devised to reflect typical intakes of plant-based foods. Existing databases were used to estimate daily phytochemical content for seven phytochemical families: phenolic acids, flavonoids (except anthocyanins), anthocyanins, tannins, organosulfur compounds, carotenoids, and caffeine. The summer and winter menus provided 1607 and 1441 mg/day, respectively, of total polyphenols (phenolic acids, flavonoids, anthocyanins, and tannins), the difference being driven by reduced anthocyanin intake in winter. Phenolic acids, flavonoids (including anthocyanins), and tannins accounted for approximately 50%, 25%, and 25% of total polyphenols, respectively. Dietary carotenoid and organosulfur compound content was estimated to be approximately 17 and 70 mg/day, respectively, in both seasons. Finally, both menus provided approximately 110 mg/day of caffeine, exclusively from tea and coffee. Our work supports ongoing efforts to define phytochemical insufficiency states that may occur in individuals with unbalanced diets and related disease risk factors.

Keywords: Mediterranean diet; phytonutrients; dietary recommendations; healthy diet; polyphenols; flavonoids; carotenoids; organosulfur; caffeine

1. Introduction

A healthy diet is considered to be one that provides adequate calories and nutrients to meet an individual's needs for energy, growth, and repair, and to prevent diet-related non-communicable diseases. A diverse range of foods from several different food groups should be included. Plant-derived foods, such as whole grains, fruits, vegetables, nuts, and seeds, form an essential part of healthy diets.

Healthy, plant-rich diets (including Mediterranean-type or DASH (Dietary Approaches to Stop Hypertension) diets) have been reported to cover all of the macro- and micronutrients considered essential to health [1]. They are particularly rich in monounsaturated and polyunsaturated fatty acids and antioxidants, which regulate lipid and glucose metabolism, counteract oxidative stress, reduce inflammation, and support endothelial function [2]. Adherence to a Mediterranean diet has been associated with comparatively low rates of cardiovascular and cerebrovascular disease, diabetes, cancer, and cognitive decline [3–8].

Additionally, numerous studies have described the health benefits of foods rich in phytochemicals, also named bioactive compounds or phytonutrients or phytomicroconstituents, which are bioactive secondary metabolites found in plants, and in foods, drinks, and condiments derived from them [9,10]. Phytochemicals are chemically diverse compounds that can be classified into distinct families: polyphenols (phenolic acids, flavonoids (including anthocyanins), and tannins), carotenoids (for example, beta-carotene, lycopene, lutein, and zeaxanthin), organosulfur compounds (for example, isothiocyanates, indoles, allyl sulfur compounds, and sulforaphane), and phytosterols (for example, sitosterol, campesterol, stigmasterol, sitostanol, campestanol, and stigmastanol) [11]. Table 1 lists examples of foods that are high, medium, or low in each of these phytochemical families, although it must be noted that harvesting, processing, storage, and cooking can reduce the phytochemical content of food.

Table 1. Foods and drinks considered to have high, medium, and low levels of different families of phytochemicals [11]. Reference ranges describing high, medium, and low phytochemical levels differ between phytochemical families, and are therefore shown alongside each family above the list of foods. The units of measurement for these reference ranges are mg per 100 g (for foods) or mg per 100 mL (for drinks).

Phytochemical Class	High	Medium	Low
Phenolic acids	100–650	45–100	5–45
	Flax and sunflower seeds, yams, red chicory, filter coffee, artichokes, prunes, mushrooms, endive, mangos, Jerusalem artichokes, raspberries	Cherries, chia seeds, dark chocolate (70–85% cocoa), pineapple, wholegrain wheat, flageolet beans, white beans, lentils, split peas	Watermelon, red beans, cashew nuts, walnuts, coriander (cilantro), potatoes, peaches, carrots, black tea, broccoli, dates, basil, apples, white rice, blackcurrants, quinces, green tea, nectarines, peaches, red wine, red bell peppers (capsicum), pears, strawberries, apricots, turnips, grapefruit, cauliflower
Flavonoids (except anthocyanins)	50–250	10–50	1–10
	Dark chocolate (70–85% cocoa), parsley, black tea, dill, shallots, fennel, green tea, red chicory, rocket, mint, grapefruit, cress, thyme	Red wine, blackberries, oranges, soy, kale, lemons, chia seeds, cranberries, onions, black grapes, artichokes, chives, asparagus, mandarins, blueberries, pecan nuts, buckwheat, cherries, olives, blackcurrants, turnips, pistachio nuts, broccoli, spinach, apricots, prunes, endive	Peaches, apples, almonds, figs, raspberries, green bell peppers (capsicum), Brussels sprouts, strawberries, bananas, nectarines, pears, coriander (cilantro), blackcurrants, hazelnuts, flat beans, flageolet beans, white beans, lentils, split peas, green beans, celery, garlic, leeks, white grapes, lettuce, kiwifruit, black radishes, chickpeas, quinces, persimmons, mangos, yellow bell peppers (capsicum), squash, potatoes, tomatoes, courgettes, flax seeds, cashew nuts, white cabbage, cauliflower, watermelon
Anthocyanins	45–210	10–45	1–10
	Red cabbage, blueberries, blackcurrants, red chicory, blackberries, aubergines (eggplants), cranberries, red radishes, raspberries	Currant berries, cherries, strawberries, red wine, pecan nuts	Pistachio nuts, hazelnuts, red beans, prunes, walnuts, almonds, apples, nectarines, pears, peaches, dates
Tannins	100–600	10–100	1–10
	Blackcurrants, red beans, hazelnuts, pecan nuts, cranberries, pistachios, red cabbage, plums, blueberries, almonds, peanuts, strawberries, apples	White and black grapes, peach, walnuts, currant berries, pears, apricots, raspberries, nectarines, red wine, blackberries, cherries, dates, mangos	Buckwheat, green tea, quinces, black tea, bananas, kiwifruit, cashew nuts
Carotenoids	5–20	2.5–5	1–2.5
	Spinach, carrots, parsley, kale, red chicory, basil, squash, yams, cress, lettuce, coriander (cilantro)	Arugula, watermelon, pistachio nuts, chives, leeks, thyme, tomatoes, persimmons, olives, peas	Red bell peppers (capsicum), grapefruit, apricots, melon, Brussels sprouts, broccoli, fennel, asparagus, flat beans, red cabbage, avocados
Sulfur compounds	>1000	100–250	10–100
	Onions, leeks	Brussels sprouts, garlic, black radishes, kale	Red radishes, red cabbage, broccoli, green cabbage, white cabbage, cauliflower

Table 1. Cont.

Phytochemical Class	High	Medium	Low
Caffeine	50–100	10–50	<10
	Espresso, filter coffee	Energy drinks, black tea, green tea	Cola drinks
Phytosterols	>200	50–200	3–50
	Vegetable oils (corn, sunflower, soybean)	Almonds, peanuts, corn (maize), oats, wheat	Cauliflower, broccoli, carrots, tomatoes, apples, bananas, grapes, oranges

Dietary polyphenols are present in numerous plant-derived foods and beverages, their quantities differing according to the plant species, varietal, environmental factors (for example, climate and soil), and cultural practices. This family includes phenolic acids (for example, hydroxybenzoic and hydroxycinnamic acids), flavonoids, and tannins. Flavonoids, such as flavones, flavonols, flavanones, and flavanes (also called flavanols or catechins) are present in high amounts in dark chocolate (70–85% cocoa), black and green teas, herbs (for example, parsley, dill, shallots, fennel, mint, and thyme), salad vegetables (for example, red chicory, rocket, and cress), and grapefruit. Anthocyanins, a subtype of flavonoids, are water-soluble pigments that contribute to the red, purple, or blue color of plants and products derived from them. Thus, they are found in high quantities in berries (for example, blueberries, blackcurrants, blackberries, cranberries, and raspberries) and in red varieties of cabbage, chicory, and radish. Tannins are grouped into two main categories, namely hydrolyzable tannins (gallotannins and ellagitannins) and non-hydrolyzable, or condensed tannins (proanthocyanidins). Tannins are found in high quantities in berries (for example, blackcurrants, cranberries, blueberries, and strawberries), nuts (for example, hazelnuts, pecans, pistachios, almonds, and peanuts), stone fruits (for example, plums), red beans, and red cabbage.

Leafy greens and orange vegetables are the richest sources of carotenoids. The most abundant carotenoid is beta-carotene, which is hydrolyzed in vivo to vitamin A (hence its alternative name, provitamin A). However, other carotenoids, such as lycopene (a red pigment present in red tomatoes and grapefruit), lutein (found in green vegetables such as spinach and lettuce), and zeaxanthin (found in corn (maize)) are not metabolized to vitamin A.

Dietary sulfur compounds are divided into two classes: allyl sulfur compounds (for example, alliin), which are abundant in alliaceous vegetables, such as onions (*Allium cepa*) and garlic (*Allium sativum*); and glucosinolates, which are found in cruciferous vegetables, especially broccoli. During culinary processing and after ingestion, allyl sulfur compounds and glucosinolates undergo transformation to highly bioactive compounds (diallyl mono-, di- or tri-sulfides, sulforaphanes, and isothiocyanates) that have antioxidant and detoxifying properties [12].

A phytochemical index (PI), based on 24 h intake recall, has been proposed for use in epidemiological studies of diseases in which diet is a causative factor [13]. The PI is the percentage of dietary calories derived from foods that are rich in phytochemicals. Diets with a higher PI have been associated with a lower prevalence of cardiometabolic disorders, including abdominal obesity, hyperglycemia, hypertension, hypertriglyceridemia, and metabolic syndrome [13]. Although the PI is a useful global indicator, it does not consider the amounts of individual phytochemicals or phytochemical families that are present in a healthy diet; indeed, there is currently no sufficiently sophisticated estimation method that allows dietary phytochemical content to be readily quantified in a clinical setting. We therefore undertook a study to determine levels of different phytochemicals in a well-balanced French diet, in order to inform and support public health objectives and recommendations in France.

2. Materials and Methods

We designed two typical weekly seasonal menus, one for summer and one for winter, included plant-based foods commonly found in current French diets (see Tables S1 and S2 in the Supplementary Materials). The menus were consistent with the current recommendations of the French National Agency for Food, Environmental and Occupational Health and Safety (ANSES; Agence Nationale de Sécurité Sanitaire Alimentation, Environnement, Travail) [14] and with the scientific literature [15]. Additionally, the menus were designed to include all essential macro- and micronutrients, and to account for seasonal variations in the availability of plant foods. We then prepared tables of the phytochemical content of each food, and used these to estimate the expected phytochemical intake per day for each menu.

Portion sizes were determined for each food category in accordance with French dietary habits, guidelines from the Groupe d'Étude des Marchés en Restauration Collective et Nutrition (GEM-RCN; French Collective Study Group on Catering and Nutrition) [16] and Programme National Nutrition Santé (PNNS; the French National Health Nutrition Programme) [17], and the opinion of the authors.

For each of the menus, the amount of each food category (FC) consumed daily (i.e., FCy, measured in grams) was calculated using the following formula:

$$FCy = FF \times z \times PS$$

where FF (frequency factor) is a multiplier reflecting the frequency of intake (FF: Frequency factors = 1 per day, 0.143 per week, and 0.033 per month), z denotes the total number of servings, and PS is the portion size in grams.

A database of the phytochemical content of 116 plant foods (mainly fruits and vegetables) was created. The phytochemicals of interest were phenolic acids, flavonoids (including anthocyanins, which were considered separately); tannins; organosulfur compounds; carotenoids; and caffeine. The phytochemical content of individual foods was obtained from the US Department of Agriculture for carotenoids and flavonoids (including anthocyanidins) [18–20]; Phenol-Explorer for total polyphenols and phenolic acids [21–23]; and published scientific literature for tannins and organosulfur compounds [24]. Data for organosulfur compounds found in garlic and onion, regrouped in the same category, were also added. Other data were derived from consumption studies, such as the study of the average consumption of fruits and vegetables in France [14], as well as research on phytochemicals reported by Tennant et al. in 2014 [25].

Our analysis focused on phytochemicals with proven health benefits at amounts that can be readily obtained by dietary intake. Thus, we did not include phytosterols, because the beneficial effects of these compounds require a level of intake (for example, >3 g/day for phytosterols) that can only be achieved by dietary supplementation. Conversely, caffeine was included as a family in its own right because it accounts for a significant proportion of daily phytochemical intake, has well-documented health benefits, and is routinely included in nutritional recommendations such as those issued by ANSES [14].

Deviations of each phytochemical that result from an aggregation of numerous-level values associated to the variability of plant food products and their consumption frequencies are taken into account in our values. Moreover, some phytochemicals (i.e., carotenoids) supplied by consuming animal-origin foods such as fish, eggs, milk, and meats were not integrated in calculations. Animal food products were included in our menus to balance the caloric intake, but not retained, because their contribution was very low in comparison to that of the plant food products.

3. Results

For each menu, the weekly number of portions, and the estimated daily amounts of each food category, are shown in Table 2. The estimated daily amounts of phytochemicals associated with each menu are shown in Table 3.

Table 2. Menu analysis, according to the number of portions of each food category consumed per week and the amount (expressed in grams) of each food category consumed per day.

Food Category	Examples	Portions per Week		Amounts per Day (g)	
		Summer Menu	Winter Menu	Summer Menu	Winter Menu
Grains, beans, nuts, and seeds					
Starchy foods	Corn, buckwheat, Jerusalem artichokes, oats, potatoes, quinoa, rice (white and whole), rye, wheat (refined and whole)	16	18	274.3	308.6
Pulses	Chickpeas, flageolet beans, lentils, red beans, split peas, white beans	2	2	34.3	34.3
Nuts and seeds	Almonds, cashew nuts, chia seeds, coconut, flax seeds, hazelnuts, macadamia nuts, peanuts, pecan nuts, pistachio nuts, sesame seeds, sunflower seeds, walnuts	0	1	0	2.9
Fruits, vegetables, spices, and herbs					
White	Apples, endive, mushrooms, quinces, parsnips, pears, salsify, turnips, white grapes	2	13	35.7	232.1
White/green	Celery, fennel, leek, shallots	2	3	35.7	53.6
Green	Avocados, asparagus, artichokes, courgettes, cress, cucumbers, flat beans, green beans, green bell peppers (capsicum), kiwifruit, lettuce, olives, peas, rocket, spinach	10	7.5	178.6	133.9
Yellow	Bananas, lemons, pineapple, yellow bell peppers (capsicum)	3	5	53.6	89.3
Orange	Carrots, mandarins, oranges, squash, yams	10	6	178.6	107.2
Red	Beetroot, cherries, cranberries, redcurrants, dates, figs, grapefruit, plums, raspberries, red bell peppers (capsicum), strawberries, tomatoes, watermelon	13	2	232.1	35.7
Purple	Plums, blackcurrants, blackberries, blueberries, eggplants, black grapes, red chicory	5	3	89.3	53.6
Cruciferous vegetables	Brussels sprouts, broccoli, cauliflower, green cabbage, kale, red cabbage, white cabbage	0	2	0	35.0
Radishes	Black radishes, red radishes	2	0	35.0	0
Allium spp.	Garlic, onions, chives	2	2	5.6	5.6
Herbs	Basil, coriander (cilantro), dill, mint, parsley, thyme	10	9	14.3	12.9
Beverages					
Coffee (filter)		3	3	85.7	85.7
Coffee (espresso)		7	7	60.0	60.0
Tea	Black tea, green tea	4	4	114.3	114.3
Wine	Red wine	2	2	34.3	34.3
Other	Sodas, energy drinks	1	1	28.0	28.0
Plant-derived sweets					
Chocolate	Dark chocolate (70–85% cocoa)	7	7	19.6	19.6

Table 3. Quantity of each phytochemical family (expressed in mg/day) provided by the menus, according to food category.

Food or Beverage Category	Phytochemical Content (Summer) [mg/Day]							Phytochemical Content (Winter) [mg/Day]						
	PA	F	A	T	Car	OS	Caf	PA	F	A	T	Car	OS	Caf
Grains, beans, nuts, and seeds														
Starchy foods	136.0	4.2	0.0	2.5	0.2	0.0	0.0	153.0	4.7	0.0	2.8	0.3	0.0	0.0
Pulses	14.8	0.8	0.8	61.9	0.0	0.0	0.0	14.8	0.8	0.8	61.9	0.0	0.0	0.0
Nuts and seeds	0.0	0.0	0.0	0.0	0.0	0.0	0.0	5.3	0.2	0.1	4.9	0.0	0.0	0.0
Fruits, vegetables, spices, and herbs														
White	21.0	1.7	0.2	12.2	0.0	0.0	0.0	136.6	11.2	1.1	79.0	0.1	0.0	0.0
White/green	0.2	18.2	0.0	0.0	0.4	0.0	0.0	0.3	27.3	0.0	0.0	0.6	0.0	0.0
Green	106.3	25.3	0.0	0.4	5.9	0.0	0.0	79.7	18.9	0.0	0.3	4.5	0.0	0.0
Yellow	17.2	1.5	0.0	0.5	0.0	0.0	0.0	5.7	22.8	0.0	0.2	0.3	0.0	0.0
Orange	98.1	6.7	0.8	25.7	5.3	0.0	0.0	100.0	1.5	0.2	3.2	8.9	0.0	0.0
Red	94.2	24.8	38.8	132.4	2.3	0.0	0.0	14.5	3.8	6.0	20.4	0.4	0.0	0.0
Purple	46.2	25.4	96.5	154.2	1.4	0.0	0.0	27.7	15.3	57.9	92.5	0.8	0.0	0.0
Cruciferous vegetables	0.0	0.0	0.0	0.0	0.0	0.0	0.0	2.9	2.8	10.5	24.5	0.7	28.7	0.0
Radishes	0.5	0.0	0.0	11.0	0.0	30.7	0.0	0.0	0.0	0.0	0.0	0.0	0.0	0.0
Allium spp.	0.1	0.8	0.0	0.0	0.0	39.0	0.0	0.1	0.8	0.0	0.0	0.0	39.0	0.0
Herbs	4.2	9.9	0.0	0.0	0.6	0.0	0.0	3.8	8.9	0.0	0.0	0.6	0.0	0.0
Beverages														
Coffee (filter)	181.8	0.0	0.0	0.0	0.0	0.0	44.0	181.8	0.0	0.0	0.0	0.0	0.0	44.0
Coffee (espresso)	60.8	0.0	0.0	0.0	0.0	0.0	42.8	60.8	0.0	0.0	0.0	0.0	0.0	42.8
Tea	17.9	110.6	0.0	4.5	0.0	0.0	18.3	17.9	110.6	0.0	4.5	0.0	0.0	18.3
Wine	4.2	16.6	7.5	7.7	0.0	0.0	0.0	4.2	16.6	7.5	7.7	0.0	0.0	0.0
Soda	0.0	0.0	0.0	0.0	0.0	0.0	6.6	0.0	0.0	0.0	0.0	0.0	0.0	6.6
Plant-derived sweets														
Chocolate (dark, 70–85% cocoa)	15.9	51.4	0.0	0.0	0.0	0.0	0.0	15.9	51.4	0.0	0.0	0.0	0.0	0.0
Total (mg)	802.8	247.0	155.7	401.9	16.4	69.8	111.6	809.0	246.2	83.9	301.9	17.1	67.7	111.6
Total polyphenols (PA + F + A + T)	1607.4							1441.0						

A, anthocyanins; Caf, caffeine; Car, carotenoids; F, flavonoids (except anthocyanins); OS, organosulfur compounds; PA, phenolic acids; T, tannins.

3.1. Polyphenols

The summer and winter menus were estimated to provide 1607.4 and 1441.0 mg/day, respectively, of polyphenols. Approximately 50% of the polyphenol content of each menu was accounted for by phenolic acids (800 mg/day), with no difference being observed between menus. Among individual foods and food categories, filter coffee and starchy foods (including cereal grains such as oats, rye, and wheat) were the most important sources of phenolic acids, accounting for approximately 22–23% and 17–19%, respectively, of estimated total phenolic acids intake. Fruits and vegetables were also found to be important sources of phenolic acids, providing around 350 mg/day.

Flavonoids (including anthocyanins) and tannins were each estimated to account for approximately 25% of total polyphenols (400 mg/day in summer and 300–330 mg/day in winter; Table 3). Seasonal differences were driven by greater consumption of red and purple fruits and vegetables during the warmer months of the year, leading to a higher intake of anthocyanins in summer than in winter. Red and purple fruits and vegetables provided 287 mg/day of tannins in summer (71% of total daily tannin consumption), but just 113 mg/day in winter (37% of total daily tannin consumption). Conversely, pulses and white fruits and vegetables accounted for a greater proportion of total tannin intake in winter than in summer (46.7% vs. 18.4%, respectively).

3.2. Carotenoids

As shown in Table 3, the carotenoid content of each menu was significantly lower than the polyphenol content on a milligram basis (by a factor of 100 in summer and 84 in winter). However, there was little difference between the daily carotenoid content of the summer menu (16.2 mg/day) and the winter menu (17.1 mg/day) due to the year-round availability of foods such as leafy greens, orange fruits and vegetables, and tomatoes. Virtually all of the carotenoid content of both menus was provided by fruits and vegetables, with very little coming from other sources.

3.3. Organosulfur Compounds

Estimated intakes of organosulfur compounds were comparable in summer and winter (approximately 70 mg/day), but sources varied between the seasons. In summer, radishes formed an important source of organosulfur compounds, with cruciferous vegetables being important in the winter. *Allium* spp., such as garlic and onions, were important sources of organosulfur compounds all year round.

3.4. Caffeine

Our menus provided 111.6 mg/day of caffeine in both winter and summer, the majority of which was from coffee.

4. Discussion

We used public domain data to estimate the daily amounts of phytochemicals, divided into seven families, that would be provided by two one-week seasonal menus that were considered to: (i) represent a healthy diet; and (ii) accurately reflect the seasonal availability of plant foods in France.

The estimated total polyphenol content, calculated as the sum of phenolic acids, flavonoids, anthocyanins, and tannins of each menu was 1607.4 and 1441.0 mg/day in summer and winter, respectively. These values are 20–35% higher than those found in the French SUVIMAX study [26], but comparable to those in a recent analysis of data from the US National Health and Nutrition Examination Survey (NHANES) [27]. In the latter study, participants had mean total polyphenol intakes of 1656.6 mg/day, although there were significant differences between subgroups defined by age, sex, educational level, and body mass index.

We found coffee and starchy foods to be the most important sources of phenolic acids in our sample diets. Regular coffee drinkers have been shown to have a reduced risk of type 2 diabetes and cardiovascular diseases compared with non-drinkers [28]. Although the benefits of coffee have been assumed to be a result of its caffeine content [28], decaffeinated coffee also appears to provide health benefits [29]. This could be due to the presence of chlorogenic acids, which are not removed by decaffeination; these compounds are responsible for the antioxidant and anti-inflammatory properties of coffee [28]. Starchy foods also contain phenolic acids in significant amounts, with cereal bran being a particularly rich source of ferulic acid [30]. Epidemiological studies have suggested that diets rich in wholegrain cereals have protective effects against cardiovascular disease, type 2 diabetes, and cancer, and are useful in weight management; the latter observation may be attributable to both dietary fiber and phenolic acid content [31]. Consumption of leafy green vegetables, which we also found contributed significantly to phenolic acid intake, has been associated with a significantly reduced risk of type 2 diabetes [32]. This reduction, however, could be due to the presence of other phytochemicals (for example, carotenoids) and dietary fiber.

Our menus provided approximately 400 mg/day of flavonoids (including anthocyanins), a level of intake that was associated in a recent meta-analysis with the maximal reduction in coronary heart disease risk [33]. Among flavonoid subtypes, flavonols and flavones were associated with reduced risks of coronary heart disease, but anthocyanins and flavan-3-ols were found to offer the greatest protection against cardiovascular disease overall [33].

In vitro and animal studies have shown that flavonoids have antioxidant and anti-inflammatory properties, and that they can inhibit mutagenesis and carcinogenesis [34]. The potential of anthocyanins to prevent a range of chronic diseases (including obesity, type 2 diabetes, cardiovascular disease, visual disorders, and neuropathies) has also been studied [35]. For example, a meta-analysis of 128 randomized controlled trials reported that the consumption of foods rich in anthocyanins was associated with favorable changes in blood pressure and total cholesterol in overweight or obese people [36].

As well as being rich in anthocyanins, red and purple fruits and vegetables are important dietary sources of tannins. The reduced availability (and hence consumption) of these foods in winter contributes to an approximately 25% reduction in tannin intake during the colder months. This may be particularly relevant to the health of people who are overweight or obese, in whom the consumption of foods rich in ellagitannins (for example, pomegranate, berries, and nuts) has been shown to lower total cholesterol, low-density lipoprotein (LDL)-cholesterol, and triglycerides levels, and to reduce diastolic blood pressure [36]. With respect to procyanidins, (condensed tannins), Wallace and colleagues have proposed an intake of 200 mg/day, with an upper limit of 800 mg/day [37]. Tannins have been described as antinutritional factors because of their potential to impair iron bioavailability, and tannin consumption has been linked to the high prevalence of iron deficiency [38].

Overall, however, a diet rich in a diverse range of polyphenols may be recommended as an effective nutritional strategy to improve the health of patients with metabolic syndrome, with potentially beneficial effects on body fat, blood pressure, dyslipidemia, and insulin resistance, and reductions in oxidative stress, inflammation, and vascular dysfunction [39].

The antioxidant (singlet oxygen quenching and free radical scavenging) and anti-inflammatory properties of carotenoids are mediated via nuclear factor kappa B (NF-κB) receptors, which modulate cytokine and chemokine production [40]. Higher intakes of carotenoids, particularly beta-carotene and lycopene, have been shown to be inversely associated with a lower incidence risk of coronary heart disease and stroke [41]; furthermore, blood concentrations of carotenoids and cryptoxanthin are inversely associated with the incidence of cardiovascular disease, total cancer, and all-cause mortality [41]. Additionally, consumption of carotenoid-rich foods may reduce the risk of metabolic syndrome [42]. In the eye, lutein (present in leafy green vegetables), zeaxanthin, and meso-zeaxanthin (present in corn (maize)) accumulate in the macula; their beneficial effects on vision and eye health are due to protective effects against the oxidative damage caused by ultraviolet light [43]. Daily intakes of 6 mg of lutein and 18 mg of lycopene have been recommended, with upper limits of 60 and 50 mg/day, respectively [37].

Cruciferous vegetables are a source of glucosinolates, which are converted in vivo to sulforaphane; this bioactive metabolite has been found, in in vitro and animal studies, to have anticarcinogenic effects [44]. Allium plant species (for example, onion and garlic) are a source of S-alk(en)yl-L-cysteine sulfoxides. *Allium* spp. may provide some protection against cancer, cardiovascular disease, metabolic disorders, and bone disease, due to their antioxidant, anti-inflammatory, and lipid-lowering properties [45,46].

Our menus delivered identical daily amounts of caffeine regardless of season. In France, tea and coffee are the two major dietary sources of caffeine. At one end of the scale, brewed black tea provides approximately 20 mg caffeine per 100 mL, while, at the other, espresso coffee provides approximately 75 mg caffeine per 100 mL [47]. However, the caffeine content of prepared coffee beverages is known to vary considerably (58–259 mg per 100 mL), with espresso coffees typically containing less caffeine than brewed coffees [48], and there is therefore likely to be wide inter- and intra-individual variation in caffeine intake among French people. It is also important to recognize that, in recent decades, energy drinks and sodas have become significant sources of caffeine.

Caffeine, among other properties, has been reported to increase energy expenditure [49], and its consumption may have measurable metabolic effects in at least some individuals. In a meta-analysis published in 2011, caffeine and catechins were found to synergistically augment fat oxidation [50]. Rigorous reviews have concluded that the consumption of up to 400 mg/day of caffeine is not associated with adverse effects in healthy adults [51–53]. An upper limit of 300 mg/day has been proposed for pregnant women [51].

There are limitations to the type of analysis that we have presented here. First, we only considered 116 food items. Second, a major consideration is that agronomic practices (for example, variety, irrigation, fertilization, and harvesting date) and methods of food storage and preparation can significantly modify the phytochemical content of plant foods [54–57]. A sensitivity study should be carried out in the future with the high, medium, and low values of phytochemicals. We did not take this into account, due to a lack of robust scientific data in the USDA and Phenol-Explorer databases on these effects. The extent to which processing affects nutrient content varies between foods, and it was therefore impossible to apply a universal multiplier or other factor to adjust for food preparation. Indeed, while cooking food generally results in the loss of water-soluble, oxidizable, and heat-sensitive phytochemicals, it can also lead to an improvement in the assimilation of others, such as carotenoids [58].

5. Conclusions

Our study estimates the levels of different phytochemicals that are present in a well-balanced French diet (i.e., one meeting current guidelines on macro- and micronutrient requirements) in adults. This estimation constitutes the first step to addressing, in the future, adequate intakes to support health benefits. Our findings indicate that consuming a diverse range of plant foods provides a broad spectrum of phytochemicals in both summer and winter, with estimated intakes of each phytochemical family being generally comparable between the seasons. Further research linking dietary phytochemical intake to health outcomes would allow existing approaches to PI calculation to be refined and improved. We believe our work will help dietitians and nutritionists to identify gaps between observed and target phytochemical intake in adults in France, and to recommend personalized nutritional strategies for maintaining good health. We plan to carry out further work to deliver personalized dietary solutions, taking into account individual specificities, such allergies, and food intolerances and preferences.

Supplementary Materials: The following are available online at https://www.mdpi.com/article/10.3390/nu13103628/s1: Table S1: Summer menu; Table S2: Winter menu.

Author Contributions: Conceptualization, M.-J.A., C.L. and S.R.; Methodology, M.-J.A., C.L. and S.R.; Formal Analysis, C.L. and S.R.; Validation, M.-J.A.; Writing—Original Draft Preparation, M.-J.A.; Writing—Review & Editing, M.-J.A., C.L., L.P. and S.R. All authors have read and agreed to the published version of the manuscript.

Funding: This research received no external funding.

Institutional Review Board Statement: Not applicable.

Informed Consent Statement: Not applicable.

Data Availability Statement: All scientific data calculated in the course of this study, and presented in this publication, are available from Christian Latgé and Sylvie Raynal upon reasonable request. All requests should be sent to: sylvie.raynal@pierre-fabre.com.

Acknowledgments: We would like to thank Richard Crampton of Springer Healthcare Communications who edited and formatted the manuscript for publication. This editorial assistance was funded by Pierre Fabre Laboratories, France. We are also grateful to Emilie Ondet, publication manager at Pierre Fabre, who ensured the follow-up of the paper's redaction and communication between the authors and the medical writer.

Conflicts of Interest: M-J. Amiot and L. Plumey have acted as consultants for, and as expert witnesses on behalf of, Pierre Fabre Laboratories, France. C. Latgé and S. Raynal are employees of Pierre Fabre Laboratories, France.

References

1. Nissensohn, M.; Román-Viñas, B.; Sánchez-Villegas, A.; Piscopo, S.; Serra-Majem, L. The Effect of the Mediterranean Diet on Hypertension: A Systematic Review and Meta-Analysis. *J. Nutr. Educ. Behav.* **2016**, *48*, 42–53. [CrossRef] [PubMed]
2. Korakas, E.; Dimitriadis, G.; Raptis, A.; Lambadiari, V. Dietary Composition and Cardiovascular Risk: A Mediator or a Bystander? *Nutrients* **2018**, *10*, 1912. [CrossRef]
3. Esposito, K.; Maiorino, M.I.; Bellastella, G.; Chiodini, P.; Panagiotakos, D.; Giugliano, D. A journey into a Mediterranean diet and type 2 diabetes: A systematic review with meta-analyses. *BMJ Open* **2015**, *5*, e008222. [CrossRef] [PubMed]
4. Jannasch, F.; Kröger, J.; Schulze, M.B. Dietary Patterns and Type 2 Diabetes: A Systematic Literature Review and Meta-Analysis of Prospective Studies. *J. Nutr.* **2017**, *147*, 1174–1182. [CrossRef]
5. Loughrey, D.G.; Lavecchia, S.; Brennan, S.; Lawlor, B.A.; Kelly, M.E. The Impact of the Mediterranean Diet on the Cognitive Functioning of Healthy Older Adults: A Systematic Review and Meta-Analysis. *Adv. Nutr.* **2017**, *8*, 571–586. [CrossRef] [PubMed]
6. Petersson, S.D.; Philippou, E. Mediterranean Diet, Cognitive Function, and Dementia: A Systematic Review of the Evidence. *Adv. Nutr.* **2016**, *7*, 889–904. [CrossRef] [PubMed]
7. Rosato, V.; Temple, N.J.; La Vecchia, C.; Castellan, G.; Tavani, A.; Guercio, V. Mediterranean diet and cardiovascular disease: A systematic review and meta-analysis of observational studies. *Eur. J. Nutr.* **2019**, *58*, 173–191. [CrossRef]
8. Schwingshackl, L.; Schwedhelm, C.; Galbete, C.; Hoffmann, G. Adherence to Mediterranean Diet and Risk of Cancer: An Updated Systematic Review and Meta-Analysis. *Nutrients* **2017**, *9*, 1063. [CrossRef]
9. Fraga, C.G.; Croft, K.D.; Kennedy, D.O.; Tomás-Barberán, F.A. The effects of polyphenols and other bioactives on human health. *Food Funct.* **2019**, *10*, 514–528. [CrossRef]
10. Serafini, M.; Peluso, I. Functional Foods for Health: The Interrelated Antioxidant and Anti-Inflammatory Role of Fruits, Vegetables, Herbs, Spices and Cocoa in Humans. *Curr. Pharm. Des.* **2016**, *22*, 6701–6715. [CrossRef]
11. Tolve, R.; Cela, N.; Condelli, N.; Di Cairano, M.; Caruso, M.C.; Galgano, F. Microencapsulation as a Tool for the Formulation of Functional Foods: The Phytosterols' Case Study. *Foods* **2020**, *9*, 470. [CrossRef]
12. Miękus, N.; Marszałek, K.; Podlacha, M.; Iqbal, A.; Puchalski, C.; Świergiel, A.H. Health Benefits of Plant-Derived Sulfur Compounds, Glucosinolates, and Organosulfur Compounds. *Molecules* **2020**, *25*, 3804. [CrossRef]
13. Kim, M.; Park, K. Association between phytochemical index and metabolic syndrome. *Nutr. Res. Pract.* **2020**, *14*, 252–261. [CrossRef]
14. Agence Nationale de Sécurité Sanitaire Alimentation. RAPPORT de l'Anses Relatif à l'Actualisation des Repères du PNNS: Étude des Relations Entre Consommation de Groupes d'Aliments et Risque de Maladies Chroniques Non Transmissibles. November 2016. Available online: https://www.researchgate.net/publication/312665902_Actualisation_des_reperes_du_PNNS_etude_des_relations_entre_consommation_de_groupes_d\T1\textquoterightaliments_et_risque_de_maladies_chroniques_non_transmissibles (accessed on 1 August 2021).
15. Estruch, R.; Ros, E.; Salas-Salvadó, J.; Covas, M.I.; Corella, D.; Arós, F.; Gómez-Gracia, E.; Ruiz-Gutiérrez, V.; Fiol, M.; Lapetra, J.; et al. Primary Prevention of Cardiovascular Disease with a Mediterranean Diet Supplemented with Extra-Virgin Olive Oil or Nuts. *N. Engl. J. Med.* **2018**, *378*, e34. [CrossRef]
16. Groupe d'Etude des Marches de Restauration Collective et Nutrition (GEM-RCN). Recommandation Nutrition. Available online: https://www.economie.gouv.fr/files/directions_services/daj/marches_publics/oeap/gem/nutrition/nutrition.pdf (accessed on 1 September 2021).
17. Chaltiel, D.; Adjibade, M.; Deschamps, V.; Touvier, M.; Hercberg, S.; Julia, C.; Kesse-Guyot, E. Programme National Nutrition Santé—Guidelines score 2 (PNNS-GS2): Development and validation of a diet quality score reflecting the 2017 French dietary guidelines. *Br. J. Nutr.* **2019**, *122*, 331–342. [CrossRef] [PubMed]
18. US Department of Agriculture (USDA). USDA Database for the Proanthocyanidin Content of Selected Foods, Release 2. 2015. Available online: https://data.nal.usda.gov/dataset/usda-database-proanthocyanidin-content-selected-foods-release-2-2015 (accessed on 1 September 2021).
19. US Department of Agriculture (USDA). USDA Database for the Flavonoid Content of Selected Foods. Release 3.2. November 2015. Available online: https://data.nal.usda.gov/dataset/usda-database-flavonoid-content-selected-foods-release-32-november-2015 (accessed on 1 September 2021).
20. US Department of Agriculture (USDA). USDA Branded Food Products Database. Available online: https://data.nal.usda.gov/dataset/usda-branded-food-products-database (accessed on 1 September 2021).
21. Rothwell, J.A.; Pérez-Jiménez, J.; Neveu, V.; Medina-Ramon, A.; M'Hiri, N.; Garcia Lobato, P.; Manach, C.; Knox, K.; Eisner, R.; Wishart, D.; et al. Phenol-Explorer 3.0: A major update of the Phenol-Explorer database to incorporate data on the effects of food processing on polyphenol content. *Database* **2013**, *2013*, bat070. [CrossRef] [PubMed]
22. Neveu, V.; Perez-Jiménez, J.; Vos, F.; Crespy, V.; du Chaffaut, L.; Mennen, L.; Knox, C.; Eisner, R.; Cruz, J.; Wishart, D.; et al. Phenol-Explorer: An online comprehensive database on polyphenol contents in foods. *Database* **2010**, *2010*, bap024. [CrossRef] [PubMed]
23. Phenol-Explorer. Database on Polyphenol Content in Foods. Available online: http://phenol-explorer.eu/foods (accessed on 1 September 2021).
24. McNaughton, S.A.; Marks, G.C. Development of a food composition database for the estimation of dietary intakes of glucosinolates, the biologically active constituents of cruciferous vegetables. *Br. J. Nutr.* **2003**, *90*, 687–697. [CrossRef]

25. Tennant, D.R.; Davidson, J.; Day, A.J. Phytonutrient intakes in relation to European fruit and vegetable consumption patterns observed in different food surveys. *Br. J. Nutr.* **2014**, *112*, 1214–1225. [CrossRef]
26. Pérez-Jiménez, J.; Fezeu, L.; Touvier, M.; Arnault, N.; Manach, C.; Hercberg, S.; Galan, P.; Scalbert, A. Dietary intake of 337 polyphenols in French adults. *Am. J. Clin. Nutr.* **2011**, *93*, 1220–1228. [CrossRef] [PubMed]
27. Huang, Q.; Braffett, B.H.; Simmens, S.J.; Young, H.A.; Ogden, C.L. Dietary Polyphenol Intake in US Adults and 10-Year Trends: 2007-2016. *J. Acad. Nutr. Diet.* **2020**, *120*, 1821–1833. [CrossRef]
28. O'Keefe, J.H.; Bhatti, S.K.; Patil, H.R.; DiNicolantonio, J.J.; Lucan, S.C.; Lavie, C.J. Effects of habitual coffee consumption on cardiometabolic disease, cardiovascular health, and all-cause mortality. *J. Am. Coll. Cardiol.* **2013**, *62*, 1043–1051. [CrossRef] [PubMed]
29. Sinha, R.; Cross, A.J.; Daniel, C.R.; Graubard, B.I.; Wu, J.W.; Hollenbeck, A.R.; Gunter, M.J.; Park, Y.; Freedman, N.D. Caffeinated and decaffeinated coffee and tea intakes and risk of colorectal cancer in a large prospective study. *Am. J. Clin. Nutr.* **2012**, *96*, 374–381. [CrossRef]
30. Călinoiu, L.F.; Vodnar, D.C. Whole Grains and Phenolic Acids: A Review on Bioactivity, Functionality, Health Benefits and Bioavailability. *Nutrients* **2018**, *10*, 1615. [CrossRef]
31. Seal, C.J.; Brownlee, I.A. Whole-grain foods and chronic disease: Evidence from epidemiological and intervention studies. *Proc. Nutr. Soc.* **2015**, *74*, 313–319. [CrossRef] [PubMed]
32. Li, M.; Fan, Y.; Zhang, X.; Hou, W.; Tang, Z. Fruit and vegetable intake and risk of type 2 diabetes mellitus: Meta-analysis of prospective cohort studies. *BMJ Open* **2014**, *4*, e005497. [CrossRef] [PubMed]
33. Micek, A.; Godos, J.; Del Rio, D.; Galvano, F.; Grosso, G. Dietary Flavonoids and Cardiovascular Disease: A Comprehensive Dose-Response Meta-Analysis. *Mol. Nutr. Food Res.* **2021**, *65*, e2001019. [CrossRef]
34. Panche, A.N.; Diwan, A.D.; Chandra, S.R. Flavonoids: An overview. *J. Nutr. Sci.* **2016**, *5*, e47. [CrossRef]
35. Khoo, H.E.; Azlan, A.; Tang, S.T.; Lim, S.M. Anthocyanidins and anthocyanins: Colored pigments as food, pharmaceutical ingredients, and the potential health benefits. *Food Nutr. Res.* **2017**, *61*, 1361779. [CrossRef]
36. García-Conesa, M.T.; Chambers, K.; Combet, E.; Pinto, P.; Garcia-Aloy, M.; Andrés-Lacueva, C.; de Pascual-Teresa, S.; Mena, P.; Konic Ristic, A.; Hollands, W.J.; et al. Meta-Analysis of the Effects of Foods and Derived Products Containing Ellagitannins and Anthocyanins on Cardiometabolic Biomarkers: Analysis of Factors Influencing Variability of the Individual Responses. *Int. J. Mol. Sci.* **2018**, *19*, 694. [CrossRef] [PubMed]
37. Wallace, T.C.; Bailey, R.L.; Blumberg, J.B.; Burton-Freeman, B.; Chen, C.O.; Crowe-White, K.M.; Drewnowski, A.; Hooshmand, S.; Johnson, E.; Lewis, R.; et al. Fruits, vegetables, and health: A comprehensive narrative, umbrella review of the science and recommendations for enhanced public policy to improve intake. *Crit. Rev. Food Sci. Nutr.* **2020**, *60*, 2174–2211. [CrossRef]
38. Delimont, N.M.; Haub, M.D.; Lindshield, B.L. The Impact of Tannin Consumption on Iron Bioavailability and Status: A Narrative Review. *Curr. Dev. Nutr.* **2017**, *1*, 1–12. [CrossRef]
39. Amiot, M.J.; Riva, C.; Vinet, A. Effects of dietary polyphenols on metabolic syndrome features in humans: A systematic review. *Obes. Rev.* **2016**, *17*, 573–586. [CrossRef]
40. Gouranton, E.; Thabuis, C.; Riollet, C.; Malezet-Desmoulins, C.; El Yazidi, C.; Amiot, M.J.; Borel, P.; Landrier, J.F. Lycopene inhibits proinflammatory cytokine and chemokine expression in adipose tissue. *J. Nutr. Biochem.* **2011**, *22*, 642–648. [CrossRef] [PubMed]
41. Aune, D.; Keum, N.; Giovannucci, E.; Fadnes, L.T.; Boffetta, P.; Greenwood, D.C.; Tonstad, S.; Vatten, L.J.; Riboli, E.; Norat, T. Dietary intake and blood concentrations of antioxidants and the risk of cardiovascular disease, total cancer, and all-cause mortality: A systematic review and dose-response meta-analysis of prospective studies. *Am. J. Clin. Nutr.* **2018**, *108*, 1069–1091. [CrossRef]
42. Goncalves, A.; Amiot, M.J. Fat-soluble micronutrients and metabolic syndrome. *Curr. Opin. Clin. Nutr. Metab. Care* **2017**, *20*, 492–497. [CrossRef] [PubMed]
43. Bernstein, P.S.; Li, B.; Vachali, P.P.; Gorusupudi, A.; Shyam, R.; Henriksen, B.S.; Nolan, J.M. Lutein, zeaxanthin, and mesozeaxanthin: The basic and clinical science underlying carotenoid-based nutritional interventions against ocular disease. *Prog. Retin. Eye Res.* **2016**, *50*, 34–66. [CrossRef] [PubMed]
44. Vanduchova, A.; Anzenbacher, P.; Anzenbacherova, E. Isothiocyanate from Broccoli, Sulforaphane, and Its Properties. *J. Med. Food* **2019**, *22*, 121–126. [CrossRef]
45. Ansary, J.; Forbes-Hernández, T.Y.; Gil, E.; Cianciosi, D.; Zhang, J.; Elexpuru-Zabaleta, M.; Simal-Gandara, J.; Giampieri, F.; Battino, M. Potential Health Benefit of Garlic Based on Human Intervention Studies: A Brief Overview. *Antioxidants* **2020**, *9*, 619. [CrossRef] [PubMed]
46. Wan, Q.; Li, N.; Du, L.; Zhao, R.; Yi, M.; Xu, Q.; Zhou, Y. Allium vegetable consumption and health: An umbrella review of meta-analyses of multiple health outcomes. *Food Sci. Nutr.* **2019**, *7*, 2451–2470. [CrossRef] [PubMed]
47. Reyes, C.M.; Cornelis, M.C. Caffeine in the Diet: Country-Level Consumption and Guidelines. *Nutrients* **2018**, *10*, 1772. [CrossRef] [PubMed]
48. McCusker, R.R.; Goldberger, B.A.; Cone, E.J. Caffeine content of specialty coffees. *J. Anal. Toxicol.* **2003**, *27*, 520–522. [CrossRef] [PubMed]
49. Gonzalez de Mejia, E.; Ramirez-Mares, M.V. Impact of caffeine and coffee on our health. *Trends Endocrinol. Metab.* **2014**, *25*, 489–492. [CrossRef] [PubMed]

50. Hursel, R.; Viechtbauer, W.; Dulloo, A.G.; Tremblay, A.; Tappy, L.; Rumpler, W.; Westerterp-Plantenga, M.S. The effects of catechin rich teas and caffeine on energy expenditure and fat oxidation: A meta-analysis. *Obes. Rev.* **2011**, *12*, e573–e581. [CrossRef] [PubMed]
51. Wikoff, D.; Welsh, B.T.; Henderson, R.; Brorby, G.P.; Britt, J.; Myers, E.; Goldberger, J.; Lieberman, H.R.; O'Brien, C.; Peck, J.; et al. Systematic review of the potential adverse effects of caffeine consumption in healthy adults, pregnant women, adolescents, and children. *Food Chem. Toxicol.* **2017**, *109*, 585–648. [CrossRef] [PubMed]
52. Nawrot, P.; Jordan, S.; Eastwood, J.; Rotstein, J.; Hugenholtz, A.; Feeley, M. Effects of caffeine on human health. *Food Addit. Contam.* **2003**, *20*, 1–30. [CrossRef] [PubMed]
53. EFSA. Scientific Opinion on the safety of caffeine. *EFSA J.* **2015**, *13*, 4102. Available online: https://www.efsa.europa.eu/en/efsajournal/pub/4102 (accessed on 1 September 2021).
54. Zhu, Q.; Wang, B.; Tan, J.; Liu, T.; Li, L.; Liu, Y.G. Plant Synthetic Metabolic Engineering for Enhancing Crop Nutritional Quality. *Plant Commun.* **2020**, *1*, 100017. [CrossRef]
55. Ceccanti, C.; Landi, M.; Benvenuti, S.; Pardossi, A.; Guidi, L. Mediterranean Wild Edible Plants: Weeds or "New Functional Crops"? *Molecules* **2018**, *23*, 2299. [CrossRef]
56. Björkman, M.; Klingen, I.; Birch, A.N.; Bones, A.M.; Bruce, T.J.; Johansen, T.J.; Meadow, R.; Mølmann, J.; Seljåsen, R.; Smart, L.E.; et al. Phytochemicals of Brassicaceae in plant protection and human health—Influences of climate, environment and agronomic practice. *Phytochemistry* **2011**, *72*, 538–556. [CrossRef]
57. Kesarwani, A.; Chiang, P.Y.; Chen, S.S. Distribution of phenolic compounds and antioxidative activities of rice kernel and their relationships with agronomic practice. *Sci. World J.* **2014**, *2014*, 620171. [CrossRef] [PubMed]
58. Palermo, M.; Pellegrini, N.; Fogliano, V. The effect of cooking on the phytochemical content of vegetables. *J. Sci. Food Agric.* **2014**, *94*, 1057–1070. [CrossRef] [PubMed]

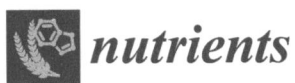

Article

Herbal Infusions as a Valuable Functional Food

Elżbieta Studzińska-Sroka [1,*], Agnieszka Galanty [2], Anna Gościniak [1], Mateusz Wieczorek [1], Magdalena Kłaput [3], Marlena Dudek-Makuch [1] and Judyta Cielecka-Piontek [1]

[1] Department of Pharmacognosy, Poznan University of Medical Sciences, Swiecickiego 4, 60-781 Poznań, Poland; annagos97@gmail.com (A.G.); mateuszwieczorek23@gmail.com (M.W.); dudum@poczta.onet.pl (M.D.-M.); jpiontek@ump.edu.pl (J.C.-P.)
[2] Department of Pharmacognosy, Faculty of Pharmacy, Jagiellonian University Medical College, Medyczna 9, 30-688 Kraków, Poland; agnieszka.galanty@uj.edu.pl
[3] Department of Pediatric Gastroenterology and Metabolic Diseases, Poznan University of Medical Sciences, 27/33 Szpitalna Str., 60-572 Poznań, Poland; magdalena.klaput@ump.edu.pl
* Correspondence: elastudzinska@ump.edu.pl

Abstract: Herbal infusions are an underestimated and easy to intake a source of biologically active natural compounds (polyphenols), which, in the dissolved form, are more easily absorbed. Therefore, this study aimed to assess the potential of herbal infusions as a functional food to reduce postprandial hyperglycemia (inhibition of α-amylase and α-glucosidase) and to reduce the effects of increased blood glucose level (antioxidant effect-DPPH, CUPRAC, and Fe^{2+} chelating assays, as well as anti-inflammatory activity-inhibition of collagenase). We showed that polyphenols are present in the examined aqueous herbal infusions (including chlorogenic and gallic acids). Subsequently, our research has shown that herbal infusions containing cinnamon bark, mulberry leaves, and blackberry fruits most strongly inhibit glucose release from complex carbohydrates, and that all herbal infusions can, to different degrees, reduce the effects of elevated blood sugar. In conclusion, infusions prepared from herbal blends could be recommended to prevent type II diabetes.

Keywords: antidiabetic activity; polyphenols; antioxidant activity; inhibition of α-glucosidase; inhibition of α-amylase; inhibition of collagenase

1. Introduction

Diabetes is a metabolic disease characterized by a chronic condition of hyperglycemia. According to the World Health Organization (WHO), it already affects 422 million adults worldwide [1]. As a result of diabetes development, the process of glycation of proteins, lipids, and nucleotides increases due to the persistence of high blood glucose levels. The reactive dicarbonyl molecules formed as a result of this glycation react with the amino groups of proteins, leading to the synthesis of advanced irreversible glycation products (AGEs). AGEs, by connecting to a specific receptor for advanced glycation end-products receptor found on the surface of e.g., lymphocytes, cardiomyocytes, or neurons of the central and peripheral nervous system, activate appropriate transcription factors, and induce the synthesis of reactive oxygen species. This intensifies the oxidation of glucose (glycoxidation) and lipids (lipoxidation), leading to the development and management of diabetes complications such as retinopathy, nephropathy, and diabetic neuropathy [2].

The development of diabetic complications also results from the insufficient effectiveness of pharmacotherapy of synthetic drugs [3]. Given the aging population, the trend of developing diabetes and the limited efficacy of synthetic drug therapy will be increasing. The strategy of combating type II diabetes involves also the change in the pharmacotherapy, from the use of old drug groups (e.g., sulfonylurea derivatives) that act directly in pancreatic cell membranes, and often produce side effects [4,5], to new therapeutic groups (e.g., dipeptidyl peptidase-4 inhibitors), based on the mechanisms of action in the intestine [6]. The compounds inhibiting α-glucosidase and α-amylase also have their mechanism in the intestine. Glucosidases are responsible for the reduction of dietary carbohydrates into simple sugars that are quickly absorbed by the small intestine [7]. The α-glucosidase and α-amylase inhibitors can reduce hyperglycemia, and decreased the side effects of hyperglycemic drugs.

Diet is an important factor in proper carbohydrate metabolism. Dietary ingredients not only affect the reduction of postprandial glucose, but also may even regulate blood sugar [8]. The most important mechanisms of natural compounds for lowering sugar into the blood include: inhibiting their absorption, increasing their metabolism by stimulating insulin secretion and degradation in peripheral cells, and accelerating sugar excretion by inducing increased renal diuresis [9,10]. Raw plant materials are often used to support type II diabetes as herbal drugs. According to the guidelines of the Committee on Herbal Medicinal Products, raw plant materials can be registered as herbal drugs as a result of their well-established use and traditional use procedure [11]. Therefore, the preventive or curative effects of herbal raw materials can be a significant support in combating diabetes, together with a proper diet or using appropriate functional food. The compounds most responsible for the antidiabetic activity of plant materials include: flavonoids, anthocyanins, phenolic acids, some polysaccharides such as inulin which are not degradable to monosaccharides, alkaloids (deoxynojirimycin, found in mulberry leaves), as well as tannins or ingredients of essential oils, including cinnamaldehyde, found in a large amount in the cinnamon bark [12].

Herbal infusions are an easy-to-apply form of the herbs, which is an important argument, especially for senior patients with swallowing problems. Plant infusions also provide a very good distribution of active compounds in the intestine, which results in their effectiveness. The significant availability of a variety of herbal blends (HBs) for infusions preparations in the markets of each country is also important. In the view of the "silent epidemic" of diabetes II, hypoglycemic infusions can be an important element in combating the development of this disease.

In this way, our study aimed to investigate the antidiabetic potential of HBs infusions dedicated as supportive treatment of diabetes.

2. Materials and Methods

2.1. Herbal Tea Blends

Seven HBs, often recommended to patients or people at risk of developing diabetes II, were included in the study. The tested HBs were all produced by Polish herb packaging companies, and were purchased in pharmacies and herbal stores in Poznan, Poland. The detailed compositions of the blends are presented in Table 1.

Table 1. Composition of the herbal tea blends.

Herbal Blend	Herbals Content of the Preparations
HB1	*Mori albi folium* 100%
HB2	*Mori albi folium* 25%, *Phaseoli pericarpium* 25%, *Fagopyrum esculentum squama* 25%, *Taraxaci radix* 12.5%, *Urticae folium* 12.5%
HB3	*Phaseoli pericarpium* 40%, *Urticae herba* 17%, *Mori albi folium* 15%, *Taraxaci herba* 15%, *Graminis rhizoma* 13%
HB4	*Phaseoli pericarpium* 40%, *Urticae herba vel Urticae folium* 30%, *Graminis rhizoma* 20%, *Taraxaci herba et radix* 10%
HB5	*Mori albi folium* 70%, *Cinnamomi cortex* 30%
HB6	*Mori albi folium* 95%, *Cinnamomi cortex* 5%
HB7	*Ribes nigrum fructus* 29%, *Aronia fructus* 29%, *Mali fructus* 26%, *Mori albi folium* 15,4%, *Fagopyrum esculentum squama* 0.3%, *Phaseoli pericarpium* 0.3%

2.2. Chemical Reagents

Ethanol, Folin–Ciocalteu reagent, (Merck, Darmstadt, Germany), 3,5-dinitrosalicylic acid, 2,2-diphenyl-1-picrylhydrazyl (DPPH), 4-nitrophenyl α-D-glucopyranoside (PNPG), α-glucosidase, α-amylase, acetonitrile, collagenase from *Clostridium histolyticum*, formic acid, iron (II) chloride tetrahydrate, ferrozine, N-[3-(2-Furyl)acryloyl]-Leu-Gly-Pro-Ala (FALGPA), neocuproine, tricine, (Sigma-Aldrich, St. Louis, MO USA); aluminum chloride anhydrous, ammonium acetate, calcium chloride, copper (II) chloride dihydrate, disodium hydrogen phosphate dodecahydrate, methanol, sodium carbonate anhydrous, sodium dihydrogen phosphate dehydrate, sodium chloride, sodium hydroxide, and sodium phosphate monobasic (Avantor Performance Materials Poland S.A., Gliwice, Poland), were used. Standards: gallic acid and acarbose, ethylenediaminetetraacetic acid (EDTA) (Sigma-Aldrich, St. Louis, MO USA), chlorogenic acid, protocatechuic acid, quercetin, and rutin (Carl Roth GmbH + Co. KG, Karlsruhe, Germany) were used.

2.3. Extracts Preparations

The infusions were prepared by pouring a 2-g fix sachet with 200 mL of boiling distilled water. For different weight sachets, the amount of water was proportional. Herbs were infused under a cover for 15 min. The resulting infusion was concentrated using a vacuum evaporator to a volume of 25 mL or 10 mL to obtain the initial test concentrations (weight of HB/mL).

2.4. Total Phenolic Content (TPC) and Total Flavonoid Content (TFC) Analysis

The TPC was determined by the modified Folin–Ciocalteu method [13]. Briefly, 25.0 µL of each extract or gallic acid solution at different concentrations were mixed with 200.0 µL distilled water and 15.0 µL of Folin–Ciocalteu reagent, and allowed to react at room temperature for 3 min. Finally, 60.0 µL of aqueous solution of sodium carbonate (20.0%, w/v) was added, and the mixture was incubated in 96 well plates at room temperature for 30 min. The absorbance was read at 760 nm (Multiskan GO 1510, Thermo Fisher Scientific, Vantaa, Finland). The blank sample contained water instead of the extract or gallic acid solution. The total phenolic concentration was calculated from a calibration curve $y = 0.0922x - 0.0199$ ($R^2 = 0.9999$), using gallic acid as a standard (0.52–8.33 µg/mL), and the obtained results were expressed as the gallic acid equivalents (GAE) (mg gallic acid per g of HB or plant material). The polyphenol content of the daily dose recommended by the manufacturer was also calculated.

The TFC was determined according to the aluminum chloride colorimetric method, in which 100.0 µL of the extract or quercetin solution at different concentrations were mixed with 100.0 µL 2% methanolic solution of aluminum chloride (complexing reagent), and incubated in 96 well plates at room temperature for 10 min. The absorbance was read at 415 nm (Multiskan GO 1510, Thermo Fisher Scientific, Vantaa, Finland). The blank contained methanol instead of aluminum chloride solution. The TFC was calculated from a calibration curve $y = 0.0262x - 0.0206$ ($R^2 = 0.9998$), using quercetin as a standard ($1.625–50.0 \times 10^{-3}$ mg/mL). The results were expressed as the quercetin equivalents (mg QE/g HB or plant material).

2.5. High-Performance Liquid Chromatography (HPLC) Analysis

Flavonoids and phenolic acids content was determined as described previously [14], using a Dionex HPLC system, with a PDA 100 detector, and a Hypersil Gold (C-18) column (5 µm, 250 × 4.6 mm, Thermo EC). The mobile phase consisted of 1% formic acid in water (A) and acetonitrile (B), in a gradient mode 5–60% B over 60 min. The compounds were identified by comparing their retention times and UV spectrum with the standards. Quantitative analysis was based on measuring the peak area regarding the appropriate standard curve prepared from five concentrations (0.0625–1 mg/mL). The results were expressed as the mg of compound/g HB or plant material.

2.6. Determination of Hypoglycemic Potential

2.6.1. α-Glucosidase Inhibitory Assay

Inhibition of α-glucosidase by the extracts was performed according to Studzińska-Sroka et al. [15], with some modifications. Briefly, 50.0 µL of sample solution (5–40 mg/mL), acarbose (5–40 mg/mL), chlorogenic acid, gallic acid, protocatechuic acid and rutin as a positive control, (0.5–20 mg/mL), 50.0 µL of 0.1 M phosphate buffer (pH 6.8) and 30.0 µL of α-glucosidase solution (0.5 U/mL) were pre-incubated in 96 well plates at 37 °C for 15 min. Next, 20.0 µL of 5 mM p-nitrophenyl-α-D-glucopyranoside (pNPG) solution in 0.1 M phosphate buffer (pH 6.8) was added and incubated at 37 °C for 20 min. The reaction was terminated by adding 100.0 µL of sodium carbonate (0.2 M) into the mixture. The absorbance of the liberated p-nitrophenol was measured after 2 min at 405 nm. The absorbance of enzyme solution without extracts/acarbose served as the control, with total enzyme activity. The absorbance in the absence of the enzyme was used as the blind control. The absorbance of extract/compound solution without enzyme was used as the blank for tested sample. The enzyme inhibition rate (presented for the final concentration of substance in enzymatic reaction) was expressed as a percentage of inhibition and calculated using the following formula:

$$\text{Inhibitory activity (\%)} = [(A_0 - A_1)/A_0] \times 100$$

where A_0 is the absorbance of the control (100% enzyme activity), and A_1 is the absorbance of the tested sample.

2.6.2. α-Amylase Inhibitory Assay

The α-amylase inhibitory activity of each herbal blends was determined by a spectrophotometric method. In the first step, 20 µL of α-amylase solution prepared by dissolving in phosphate buffer with pH = 6.9 (4.0 U/mL) and 20 µL of the test extract (80 mg/mL) or acarbose (0.008 mg/mL, used as a positive control) were preincubated in the 96-well plate at 37 °C. After 20 min, 20 µL of previously prepared in warm 0.1 M phosphate buffer (pH 6.9) and 0.5% starch solution was added to the wells and incubated again for 20 min at 37 °C. Then, 60 µL of color reagent was added to each well. Color reagent was containing 96 mM 3,5-dinitrosalicylic acid solution (20 mL), 5.31 M potassium sodium tartrate solution in 2 M sodium hydroxide (8 mL), and deionized water (12 mL). The plate was incubated at 85 °C for 15 min, then cooled to room temperature, and 80 µL of water was added. The measurement of absorbance was carried out at 540 nm (Multiskan GO 1510, Thermo Fisher Scientific, Vantaa, Finland). Absorbance of the enzyme solution without extracts/acarbose was used as a control for total enzyme activity. Individual blanks containing test herbal blends without the enzyme and starch solution were prepared for correcting the background absorbance. The rate of enzyme inhibition (presented for the final concentration of substance in enzymatic reaction) was expressed as a percentage of inhibition, and calculated using the following formula:

$$\text{Inhibitory activity (\%)} = [(A_0 - A_1)/A_0] \times 100$$

where A_0 is the absorbance of the control reduced by the sample background (100% enzyme activity), and A_1 is the absorbance of the tested sample reduced by the sample background.

2.7. Determination of the Preventive Potential for Type II Diabetes Complications

2.7.1. DPPH and CUPRAC Assays

The DPPH assay was effected according to [15] with slight modifications. Briefly, 25.0 µL of the extract at different concentrations were mixed with 175.0 µL of DPPH• solution; then, the reaction mixture was shaken and incubated in the dark at room temperature for 30 min. DPPH• solutions were freshly prepared for each analysis (3.9 mg DPPH in 50.0 mL of MeOH). Absorbance was measured at 517 nm. The control blank contained

25.0 µL of distilled water and 175.0 µL of DPPH• solution. The inhibition of the DPPH• radical by the sample was calculated according to the following formula:

$$\text{DPPH scavenging activity (\%)} = [(A_0 - A_1)/A_0] \times 100\%$$

where A_0 is the absorbance of the control, and A_1 is the absorbance of the sample. The IC_{50} values (expressed as final concentration in the sample), i.e., the amount of antioxidant necessary to half of the initial DPPH• concentration, were used to compare the quality of the antioxidant potency of the studied extracts. A lower absorbance of the reaction mixture indicated a higher free radical scavenging activity.

The CUPRAC (cupric ion reducing antioxidant capacity) assay was effected according to Studzińska-Sroka et al. [15]. The stock solutions of CUPRAC reagent included equal parts of acetate buffer (pH 7.0), 7.5 mM neocuproine solution in 96% ethanol, and 10.0 mM $CuCl_2 \cdot xH_2O$ solution. Briefly, 50.0 µL of the extract at different concentrations was mixed with 150.0 µL of CUPRAC solution, then shaken and incubated at room temperature for 30 min in the dark condition. The absorbance was measured at 450 nm against blank sample (water mixed with CUPRAC solution). The results were expressed as the $IC_{0.5}$, which corresponds to the concentration (expressed as final concentration in the sample) required to produce absorbance value equal 0.5. A higher absorbance of the reaction mixture indicated a higher antioxidant reducing capacity.

2.7.2. Determination of Fe^{2+} Chelating Activity

The binding of Fe^{2+} by the extracts was effectuated according to Dinis et al. [16], with some modifications. Briefly, 200.0 µL of sample solution or EDTA (as a positive control), at different concentrations, and 10.0 µL of $FeCl_2 \cdot 4H_2O$ (1 mM) were mixed and pre-incubated in 96 well plates at room temperature for 10 min. Afterward, 10 µL of ferrozine (2.5 mM) was added and incubated at room temperature for 30 min. The absorbance of the iron (II)-ferrozine complex was measured at 562 nm. The chelating activity (presented for the final concentration of samples) was expressed as a percentage using the following equation:

$$\text{Chelating activity (\%)} = [(A_0 - A_1)/A_0] \times 100\%$$

where A_0 is the absorbance of the control, and A_1 is the absorbance of the sample.

2.7.3. Determination of Anti-Collagenase Potential

The collagenase inhibitory activity of each HBs was determined in vitro according to Widodo et al. [17], with some modifications. Briefly, 15.0 µL of enzyme, 60 µL of tricine buffer (pH 7.5), and 30 µL of HB extracts (10 mg/mL) or epigallocatechin gallate (EGCG) (1.0 mg/mL and 0.1 mg/mL, positive control) were mixed and incubated at 37 °C for 20 min. Next, 20 µL of FALGPA (0.5 mM) was added, and they were measured immediately at 325 nm using the plate reader (Multiskan GO 1510, Thermo Fisher Scientific, Vantaa, Finland), following the addition of the substrate, and then again after 20 min of incubation at 37 °C. The collagenase inhibition rate (presented for the final concentration of substance in enzymatic reaction) expressed as a percentage of inhibition was calculated using the following formula:

$$\text{Inhibitory activity (\%)} = [(A_0 - A_1)/A_0] \times 100$$

where A_0 is the absorbance of the control (100% enzyme activity), and A_1 is the absorbance of the tested sample.

2.8. Statistical Analysis

Analyses of determination of total flavonoids and phenolic compounds, as well as biological activity, were performed in six replicates; HPLC analysis was performed in three replicates. Results were expressed as means ± SD.

3. Results

3.1. Phytochemical Characterization of Herbal Blends

The examined herbal tea blends have a diverse composition of plant ingredients (Table 1). Thus, they were characterized by diverse content of polyphenolic compounds. Our results showed that the examined herbal infusions are characterized by different total polyphenol and flavonoid contents (Table 2). The highest total polyphenol content, determined for HB5, HB1, and HB6 (16.06, 14.94, and 13.97 mg GAE/g HB, respectively), was correlated with a high content of flavonoids (2.23, 3.06, and 2.03 mg QE/g HB, respectively). Interestingly, although HB2 had also high total polyphenols content (15.30 mg GAE/g HB), no such correlation was noted in this case (Table 2).

Table 2. Content of polyphenols (TPC) and flavonoids (TFC) and their daily dose in the tested extracts from herbal tea blends.

Herbal Blend	Content of Active Substances		Content of Active Substances in the Daily Dose Recommended by the Manufacturer	
	TPC (mg GAE/g HB)	TFC (mg QE/g HB)	Polyphenols (mg/day)	Flavonoids (mg/day)
HB1	14.94 ± 0.24	3.06 ± 0.05	89.64	18.36
HB2	15.30 ± 0.30	1.30 ± 0.06	61.20	5.20
HB3	11.89 ± 0.36	1.43 ± 0.05	35.67	4.29
HB4	3.83 ± 0.17	0.56 ± 0.06	30.64	4.48
HB5	16.06 ± 0.63	2.23 ± 0.03	96.36	13.38
HB6	13.97 ± 0.53	2.03 ± 0.03	83.82	12.18
HB7	10.92 ± 0.42	1.08 ± 0.07	98.28	9.72

HB: herbal blend; GAE: gallic acid equivalents; QE: quercetin equivalents.

To complete the total compounds analysis results, we examined in the tested infusions some polyphenols' contents (chlorogenic acid, gallic acid, protocatechuic acid, rutin), considered essential for antidiabetic activity [18]. The obtained results showed that the amount of selected compounds is varied in the investigated HBs (Table 3), with predomination of chlorogenic and gallic acids. Both protocatechuic acid and rutin were present in the samples in smaller amounts.

Table 3. Content of selected polyphenolic compounds in herbal blends.

Herbal Blend	Content of Selected Polyphenolic Compounds (mg/g Herbal Blend)			
	Chlorogenic Acid	Gallic Acid	Protocatechuic Acid	Rutin
HB1	1.490 ± 0.057	0.275 ± 0.009	0.060 ± 0.010	0.236 ± 0.015
HB2	0.474 ± 0.026	0.079 ± 0.007	0.040 ± 0.010	0.071 ± 0.007
HB3	0.722 ± 0.040	0.046 ± 0.003	n.a.	0.058 ± 0.010
HB4	0.079 ± 0.009	n.a.	0.070 ± 0.010	0.043 ± 0.006
HB5	0.407 ± 0.028	0.462 ± 0.014	n.a.	0.029 ± 0.008
HB6	0.107 ± 0.015	0.363 ± 0.021	0.147 ± 0.015	n.a.
HB7	1.896 ± 0.143	0.066 ± 0.009	n.a.	0.100 ± 0.023

n.a.: not active.

3.2. Determination of Hypoglycemic Potential

α-glucosidase and α-amylase are some of the key enzymes involved in carbohydrate metabolism, which digest oligosaccharides (disaccharides and polysaccharides) or other complex carbohydrates into monosaccharides (glucose) [7]. By inhibiting the activity of these enzymes, the digestion of carbohydrates and the absorption of glucose in the small intestine are blocked.

We evaluated the α-glucosidase inhibition potential of HBs at four different concentrations (1.7, 3.3, 6.7, and 13.3 mg/mL). The results indicate that the activity of the tested extracts was dose dependent. HB1, HB5, HB6, and HB7 showed the strongest inhibition of the enzyme (Table 4). It is worth noting that in the lowest tested concentration (1.7 mg/mL), only HB5 and HB7 inhibited the enzyme comparable to acarbose used at the same concentration (93.65%, 86.97%, and 80.83%, respectively) (Table 4). Additionally, the inhibitory activity of compounds detected in the tested HBs (chlorogenic acid, gallic acid, as well as protocatechuic acid, and rutin), was tested. For the most active compounds (chlorogenic acid and rutin), the tested concentrations were lower than those for the infusions (0.17 mg/mL and 0.3 mg/mL). However, gallic and protocatechuic acids acted much weaker, and only the concentration of 6.7 mg/mL allowed to observe their inhibitory effect on the tested enzyme. The results are presented in Table 4.

Table 4. Inhibition of α-glucosidase activity by the infusions from herbal blends.

Herbal Blend	Inhibition of α-Glucosidase Activity [%]			
	Concentration			
	1.7 mg/mL	3.3 mg/mL	6.7 mg/mL	13.3 mg/mL
HB1	35.26 ± 1.11	83.02 ± 1.72	92.82 ± 0.52	98.84 ± 1.48
HB2	6.73 ± 1.23	12.43 ± 2.28	44.60 ± 1.03	68.49 ± 4.69
HB3	6.91 ± 0.80	17.86 ± 5.81	29.70 ± 1.12	57.30 ± 5.55
HB4	2.87 ± 0.95	8.83 ± 0.50	17.13 ± 2.00	37.38 ± 3.59
HB5	93.65 ± 1.11	98.06 ± 0.90	99.78 ± 0.24	100.00
HB6	48.66 ± 3.51	73.71 ± 0.55	81.81 ± 1.78	88.14 ± 1.14
HB7	86.97 ± 5.63	97.27 ± 0.37	99.82 ± 0.26	99.22 ± 0.94
Acarbose	80.83 ± 1.02	88.07 ± 0.77	91.98 ± 0.17	93.73 ± 0.03
Active Compound	Concentration			
	0.17 mg/mL	0.33 mg/mL	3.3 mg/mL	6.7 mg/mL
Chlorogenic acid	46.44 ± 1.02	81.35 ± 3.34	n.d.	n.d.
Gallic acid	n.d.	n.d.	18.00 ± 5.09	99.65 ± 2.34
Protocatechuic acid	n.d.	n.d.	0.46 ± 1.42	99.99 ± 0.13
Rutin	65.33 ± 3.42	97.07 ± 0.55	n.d.	n.d.

n.d.: not determined.

The α-amylase inhibition of HBs was performed at 27.6 mg/mL concentration. Our study demonstrated that the most potent inhibitor is HB7, and the weaker inhibitors are HB5, HB6, HB2, and HB1, respectively. HB3 and HB4 exhibit no inhibitory effect. However, the activity of tested HBs is significantly lower than that of acarbose. The results are presented in Table 5.

Table 5. Inhibition of α-amylase activity by the infusions from herbal blends.

Herbal Blend	Inhibition of α-Amylase Activity [%]	
	Concentration	
	26.7 mg/mL	0.00267 mg/mL
HB1	3.62 ± 4.95	n.d.
HB2	4.02 ± 3.96	n.d.
HB3	0.31 ± 0.77	n.d.
HB4	0.13 ± 0.31	n.d.
HB5	20.14 ± 5.94	n.d.
HB6	5.62 ± 7.32	n.d.
HB7	96.16 ± 6.00	n.d.
Acarbose	n.d.	28.11 ± 2.80

n.d.: not determined.

3.3. Determination of the Preventive Potential for Type II Diabetes Complications

3.3.1. In Vitro Antioxidant Activity

Oxidative stress is responsible for the development of diabetes complications. Therefore, antioxidant activity is of great importance in preventing adverse complications of this disease. To test the antioxidant activity of HBs' extracts two complementary methods were chosen: the DPPH• radical, characterizing the ability of the tested sample to scavenge free radicals, and the CUPRAC reagent, assessing the reducing properties of metal ions.

The results of the HBs infusions antioxidant activity analysis showed that among the tested preparations, the most active was HB1 (IC_{50} DPPH = 310.03 µg/mL, $IC_{0.5}$ CUPRAC = 368.15 µg/mL) and HB5 (IC_{50} DPPH = 350.52 µg/mL, $IC_{0.5}$ CUPRAC = 344.43 µg/mL) herbal infusions. However, the effect of both tested water extracts was weaker than that of vitamin C, used as a standard (IC_{50} DPPH = 7.62 µg/mL and $IC_{0.5}$ CUPRAC = 14.64 µg/mL). HB4 (bean pod, nettle herb or leaf, nettle rhizome, dandelion root) performed much weaker than others, which indicates its poor antioxidant properties. The scavenging capacity of DPPH free radicals or the reducing properties of other tested preparations ranged from IC_{50} DPPH = 361.17 µg/mL to IC_{50} DPPH = 744.74 µg/mL, and from $IC_{0.5}$ CUPRAC = 409.92 µg/mL to $IC_{0.5}$ CUPRAC = 686.43 µg/mL (Table 6). The scavenging capacity of DPPH free radicals or the reducing properties of HB2 and HB3 was presented as approximately 2-times lower to the highest active herbal infusions (Table 6). The HB4 was characterised by the worst activity.

Table 6. Antioxidant activity of tested herbal infusions.

Herbal Blend	Antioxidant Activity	
	DPPH• (IC_{50} µg/mL) [1]	CUPRAC ($IC_{0.5}$ µg/mL) [1]
HB1	310.03	368.15
HB2	715.58	686.43
HB3	744.74	680.14
HB4	1336.03	931.00
HB5	350.52	344.43
HB6	394.76	409.92
HB7	361.17	591.50
vitamin C	7.62	14.64

[1] Concentration was expressed as mg of herbal blend in the tested sample.

The relationship between the decompartmentalized metal ions and diabetic complications is the content of many scientific works [19]. To know the potential of herbal infusions in this area, we assessed the chelating properties of Fe^{2+} ions by HBs water extracts, using a ferrozine in vitro test. The obtained results indicate a dose-dependent, robust activity of the studied samples. The water extracts of HB3, HB4, and HB6 showed the most potent effect, showing > 50% of chelating activity at the lowest concentration tested (0.45 mg/mL), which was also 20 times lower than when taken in the form of an infusion. The chelating ability close to 90% was achieved by HB1-HB6 blends for the concentration four times lower (2.3 mg/mL) than the concentration of the ready-to-drink herbal infusion (Table 7). The only herbal blend that showed no activity (at low concentrations) or little activity at the highest concentrations tested was HB7 (Table 7). This result contrasted with HB7's high anti-radical activity, as well as very good α-glucosidase and α-amylase inhibition properties and collagenase inhibition.

Table 7. Chelating activity of tested herbal infusions.

Herbal Blend	Chelating Activity Fe^{2+} [%]				
	Concentration				
	0.45 mg/mL	0.9 mg/mL	2.3 mg/mL	4.6 mg/mL	9.1 mg/mL
HB1	43.92 ± 1.34	70.36 ± 7.02	92.01 ± 0.68	95.55 ± 0.63	99.34 ± 1.38
HB2	27.53 ± 3.05	51.16 ± 1.80	89.49 ± 2.45	89.85 ± 1.75	87.98 ± 0.10
HB3	56.38 ± 5.93	89.47 ± 1.74	96.58 ± 0.79	96.15 ± 1.23	97.11 ± 0.57
HB4	62.81 ± 1.72	88.31 ± 0.35	94.05 ± 0.48	94.35 ± 0.28	93.21 ± 0.53
HB5	34.15 ± 1.14	67.49 ± 1.90	94.11 ± 0.58	94.65 ± 0.42	97.15 ± 1.64
HB6	62.10 ± 3.16	91.10 ± 1.17	98.38 ± 0.54	98.41 ± 1.06	99.44 ± 2.99
HB7	n.a.	n.a.	5.91 ± 4.33	9.43 ± 4.72	9.33 ± 3.19
Reference	Concentration				
	0.01 mg/mL	0.023 mg/mL	0.045 mg/mL	-	-
EDTA	66.50 ± 2.20	99.59 ± 0.57	100.24 ± 0.20	-	-

n.a.: not active.

3.3.2. In Vitro Anti-Inflammatory Activity

Our research has shown that the mixtures used to prepare infusions taken in the early stages of diabetes can inhibit collagenase, and the activity was recorded at a concentration that is intended for direct consumption. The HB5 mixture most strongly inhibited the enzyme (28.79%). The other blends, with the exception of HB3, which did not show any activity at the tested concentration, were less effective (8.47–21.46%). Despite the reported activity, the action level of the most active mixture was three times lower than the standard's 10-fold lower concentration (EGCG) (Table 8).

Table 8. Inhibition of collagenase activity by the infusions from herbal blends.

Herbal Blend	Inhibition of Collagenase Activity [%]		
	Concentration		
	2.4 mg/mL	0.24 mg/mL	0.024 mg/mL
HB1	16.22 ± 3.22	n.d.	n.d.
HB2	21.46 ± 3.04	n.d.	n.d.
HB3	n.a.	n.d.	n.d.
HB4	8.47 ± 4.66	n.d.	n.d.
HB5	28.79 ± 2.65	n.d.	n.d.
HB6	13.68 ± 6.21	n.d.	n.d.
HB7	18.42 ± 7.68	n.d.	n.d.
EGCG	n.d.	84.30 ± 8.83	35.78 ± 5.52

n.a.: not active; n.d.: not determined; EGCG: epigallocatechin gallate.

3.4. Summary of Antidiabetic Potential of Tested Herbal Blends

Finally, to better visualize and compare the obtained results, we performed the data as a star diagram (Figure 1). According to the presented relationship, HB7 and HB5 have the highest antidiabetic potential. Both of them were characterized by high hypoglycemic properties, especially by inhibiting α-glucosidase, and also, but in a moderate way, α-amylase. HB5 is also characterized by preventive potential against diabetic complications, due to its highest antioxidant capacity and the best collagenase inhibition properties. Another HBs, whose biological properties (at least 2 out of 3 examined) suggest an interesting preventive potential, are HB6, HB1, and HB4, respectively, for which the chelating and antioxidant potential were noticeable.

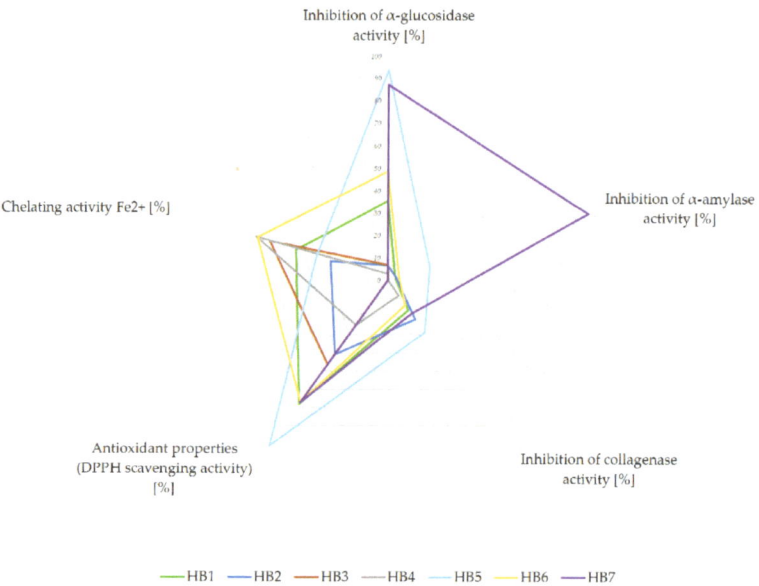

Figure 1. The antidiabetic potential of herbal blends 1–7 (HB 1–7), presented graphically, taking into account the measured biological properties expressed in %. The graph was made for the concentrations: inhibition of α-glucosidase activity 1.7 mg/mL; inhibition of α-amylase activity 26.7 mg/mL; inhibition of collagenase activity 2.4 mg/mL; antioxidant potential - DPPH assay 0.625 mg/mL; chelating activity 0.45 mg/mL.

4. Discussion

Diabetes is a metabolic disease that, if left untreated, leads to serious complications in the form of retinopathy, neuropathy, or nephropathy. Apart from the standard pharmacotherapy, the use of herbal drugs seems to be an interesting and complementary strategy to prevent or alleviate the symptoms of the disease. However, the effectiveness of multi-component HBs is often not scientifically proven and the mechanism of their activity also needs to be clarified.

Our in vitro study evaluated the antidiabetic potential of herbal infusions to prevent and support the treatment of early stages of type II diabetes. The key question is whether the extraction with hot water is effective enough to receive biological activity of the active ingredients. The products selected for our study contained pharmaceutical raw materials (according to the European Pharmacopoeia: dandelion root, dandelion herb with root, couch grass rhizome, nettle leaf, cinnamon) [20], or the components of dietary supplements (chokeberry fruit, blackcurrant fruit, apple fruit, buckwheat husk, mulberry leaf, bean pod).

The antidiabetic mechanisms of polyphenols include the possibility of inhibiting digestive enzymes (e.g., α-amylase or α-glucosidase), which are essential in limiting the absorption of sugars [21]. Polyphenols have also been reported as stimulants of intestinal peptides secretion that can stimulate insulin secretion in the pancreas [22]. The data confirm the ability of polyphenolic compounds to stimulate insulin production from β-cells of the pancreas, increasing glycolysis and reducing gluconeogenesis, [23,24], scavenging free radicals, and chelating metals, which translates into anti-inflammatory activity [25].

The mentioned antidiabetic potential of polyphenolic compounds prompted us to conduct phytochemical characterization of the studied herbal infusions. HBs containing mulberry leaves (HB1, HB2, HB5, HB6) had high polyphenols and total flavonoids content. The highest TFC value was for single-component HB1 with *Mori albi folium* (mulberry leaves) (Table 2). Some literature data confirm that flavonoids are the important fraction of natural substances in the mulberry leaves, responsible for its biological activity [26].

More detailed analysis showed that all the tested herbal infusions contained chlorogenic acid (Table 3), the compound of high importance in terms of regulating blood glucose level [27] and alleviating metabolic syndrome symptoms [26,28] in a number of in vitro and in vivo studies. The therapeutic efficacy of chlorogenic acid, both as a pure substance and in the form of an extract was also proven in some clinical studies [29]. The highest content of chlorogenic acid was determined for HB1, with mulberry leaves as the only ingredient (Table 3). Six out of the seven studied HBs contained gallic acid, whose antidiabetic potential has been supported by various studies [30,31]. The highest content of this phenolic compound was observed in the herbal infusions containing mulberry leaves (HB1, HB5, HB6), which is consistent with previous literature data [32]. Protocatechuic acid and rutin were presented in the tested HBs in small amounts (Table 3). The low concentration of rutin is due to the tested extracts' water nature, and the low solubility of the flavonoid in water [33,34].

The inhibition of α-glucosidase is a known mechanism of hypoglycemic activity. The chemical glucosidase inhibitors available on the pharmaceutical market are characterized by many side effects associated with gastrointestinal discomforts, such as abdominal distention, vomiting, and diarrhea [35], while some α-glucosidase inhibitors of plant origin can show hypoglycemic activity without the appearance of such side effects [36]. Therefore, we tested herbal infusions from HBs for their ability to inhibit α-glucosidase and α-amylase. Our study showed the α-glucosidase and α-amylase inhibitory potential of HBs. We noticed these properties are probably connected with the high quantity in all tested herbal infusions of phenolic compounds (total polyphenols and flavonoids, as well as individual phenolic acids: chlorogenic acid, gallic acid, protocatechuic acid, and rutin). We demonstrated significant inhibitory activity of examined pure substances for α-glucosidase, which is consistent with the results of other authors [18]. According to literature data, the active compounds we detected in the herbal infusions exhibit an inhibitory effect on α-amylase activity [37,38].

Subsequently we noticed that the potency of tested HBs in α-glucosidase and α-amylase inhibition is stronger with the increased amount of cinnamon in bark their composition, which was especially observed for HB5 and HB6 (Tables 4 and 5). We observed that HB5 containing 30% of cinnamon bark showed 98.06% of α-glucosidase inhibition at the concentration 3.3 mg/mL, while 5% of the bark in HB6 presented 73.71% of inhibitory activity at the same concentration. A similar effect was noticed for α-amylase inhibition, with HB5 showing 20.14% of enzyme inhibition in concentration 26.7 mg/mL, while HB6 presented 5.62% of enzyme inhibition in concentration 8.0 mg/mL. The strong ability to inhibit α-glucosidase and α-amylase by cinnamon bark has been described by other authors [39,40]. Moreover, an additive effect on the inhibition of intestinal enzymes (α-glucosidase and α-amylase) was demonstrated for cinnamon bark combined with acarbose [40]. The cinnamon bark phenolic acids' synergism with metformin was also observed [41]. The studies shown that the antidiabetic potential of cinnamon bark was highly correlated with their proanthocyanidin and condensed tannin [42]. Moreover the presence of flavonoids in mulberry leaves as the constituent of HB5 and HB6 water herbal infusions favors inhibiting the enzyme activity [43]. However, this issue needs further studies to explain the mutual relationships between the components of the herbal blends and the observed activity.

The HB7, containing anthocyanins-rich plants in, indicated high potential to inhibit the α-glucosidase and α-amylase enzymes. Sui et al. [44] demonstrated in vitro inhibitory effects of anthocyanins against pancreatic α-amylase verified, also by an in silico molecular docking study. Barik et al. [45] suggest anthocyanins regulate postprandial hyperglycemia not solely by inhibiting α-glucosidase, but also as a result of modulating glucose uptake and sugar transporters. Moreover, Boath et al. [46] show that the blackcurrant, constituting the important part of HB7, has strong ability to inhibit α-glucosidase. What is more, it synergistic effect with acarbose was also observed [46]. It is also known that both chokeberry and blackcurrant fruit contain active flavonoids and tannins, which affect the antidiabetic potential by different mechanisms, including inhibition of the enzymes [12].

Cells' oxidative stress contributes to the development of insulin resistance and also causes changes in the walls of blood vessels, which, in the conditions of increased hyperglycemia, leads to complications of diabetes [47]. Conducted experiments show that herbal infusions can exhibit antioxidant properties that can prevent diabetes complications and protect, among others, before the oxidation of unsaturated lipids and promoting oxidative damage at different levels.

In our study, high antioxidant activity (however, weaker than vitamin C used as a standard) was noted for most of the herbal infusions prepared from tested HBs (Table 6). What is more, these results correlated with the high total polyphenols or total flavonoid contents (Table 2), as well as with high content of chlorogenic and gallic acid, compared to other tested infusions (Table 3). Moreover, the anthocyanins and condensed proanthocyanidins, compounds of blackcurrant or chokeberry fruits [48] (the components of HB7), could explain the antioxidant potential of HB7. The HB5 and HB6, in addition to mulberry leaves, also contained cinnamon bark, a valuable source of antioxidant and hypoglycemic compounds [49]. Our research indicated no relationship between the increased content of cinnamon bark in the two-component blends (mulberry leaf and cinnamon bark) and their antioxidant properties.

The ability to chelate metal ions increases total antioxidant potential [50] which may result in a reduction in the concentration of the catalyzing transition metal in lipid peroxidation. This approach determined the emergence of therapies in which the use of substances can chelate transition metals aided in the treatment of chronic hyperglycemia [51]. The chelating abilities of metals are mainly due to polyphenol compounds [52], including chlorogenic, gallic, or protocatechuic acids and flavonoids [42,52,53]. For HB1, HB5, and HB6, the dominant component was the polyphenol-rich mulberry leaves, which can influence high chelating abilities. The chelating properties of cinnamon bark (a component of HB5 and HB6) have been proven for cinnamaldehyde present in the raw material in large amounts [54]. Our research shows that quite possibly not only polyphenols have an impact on the assessed activity. The composition of the chelating active HB3 and HB4 blends suggests that the large amounts of *Phaseoli pericarpium* (among others sources of amino acids, chromium salts, guanidine derivatives, triterpenes, condensed tannins, sterols, and small quantities of polyphenols) [55,56] and aerial parts from *Urtica dioica* (besides polyphenols, the source of amines, amino acids, terpenes, organic acids, sterols) [57,58] can affect the increase of the ability of chelation. Carrasco-Castilla et al. [59] state that peptide fractions isolated from *Phaseolus vulgaris* showed the ability to chelate iron ions in vitro. According to Drużyńska et al. [56], *Phaseoli pericarpium*'s condensed tannins increase the chelation of transition metal ions. The high capacity of aqueous extracts from aerial parts of *Urtica dioica* to chelate iron ions was demonstrated by Gülçin et al. [60].

The results of the analysis concerning HB7, active in other trials, but with the weakest chelating ability among the tested HBs, seem interesting. This may be explained by the substantial amounts of dried chokeberry and blackcurrant fruits, rich in anthocyanins, the reduced chelating ability of which is related to the presence of one- or two-metal binding sites, when compared the other polyphenols, with three or four metal-binding sites [52].

Collagenase, belonging to the group of metalloproteinases, is an enzyme whose activity in tissues increases significantly in diabetic disease [61,62], that results in the development of complications related to the disturbance of collagen metabolism in periodontal diseases [61], vascular complications [63–65], or inflammation of the gastrointestinal tract [62]. The compounds of plant origin, both as pure substances and in the form of plant extracts, can effectively inhibit metalloproteinases [66,67], which was especially proven for flavonoids (including rutin and potent inhibitor of collagenase EGCG [68]), phenolic acids (in chlorogenic acid and gallic acid), anthocyanins (including from blackcurrant (delphinidin derivatives)) or procyanidins [69]. Moreover, collagenase-inhibiting properties were noted for extracts from nettle [70], and black chokeberries [71], present in the examined

HBs. Our results indicated moderate anti-collagenase activity of all the tested HBs, with the exception of HB3. Therefore, it seems that the regular consumption of herbal infusions may help in the likely consequences of hyperglycemia, such as inflammation of the oral cavity or further digestive tract sections. Moreover, it should be noted that the absorption capacity of the active substances present in HBs also provides the possibility of systemic action, which increases the effectiveness of the prevention of diabetic complications. However, this requires further research.

5. Conclusions

We have proven that the extraction with hot water during the preparation of herbal infusions allows for the achievement of adequate concentrations of phenolic acids, flavonoids, and other probably synergistic compounds to provide the potential for hypoglycemic action. The examined herbal blends demonstrated a multidirectional mechanism of action, and are helpful in the prevention or treatment of early stages not only of diabetes, but also other metabolic diseases leading to several complications. With the obtained results, we can recommend herbal infusions containing mulberry leaves, especially those containing cinnamon bark or anthocyanins, to support the treatment of diabetes type II and to prevent its grave implications.

Author Contributions: Conceptualization, E.S.-S.; methodology, E.S.-S. and A.G. (Agnieszka Galanty); formal analysis, M.W., E.S.-S., A.G. (Agnieszka Galanty), A.G. (Anna Gościniak); investigation, E.S.-S., M.W., A.G. (Agnieszka Galanty), A.G. (Anna Gościniak); resources, J.C.-P., A.G. (Agnieszka Galanty) and E.S.-S.; data curation, M.W., A.G. (Agnieszka Galanty), A.G. (Anna Gościniak), E.S.-S.; writing—original draft preparation, M.W., E.S.-S., J.C.-P.; writing—review and editing, E.S.-S., J.C.-P., A.G. (Agnieszka Galanty), A.G. (Anna Gościniak), M.D.-M. and M.K.; visualization E.S.-S. and J.C.-P.; supervision, E.S.-S. and J.C.-P.; project administration, E.S.-S.; funding acquisition, E.S.-S., J.C.-P. All authors have read and agreed to the published version of the manuscript.

Funding: This research was funded by the grant from Minister of Education and Science, Poland: SKN/SP/496064/2021.

Institutional Review Board Statement: Not applicable.

Informed Consent Statement: Not applicable.

Data Availability Statement: The data supporting reported results were be found in: Department of Pharmacognosy, Poznan University of Medical Sciences and Department of Pharmacognosy, Faculty of Pharmacy, Jagiellonian University Medical College.

Conflicts of Interest: The authors declare no conflict of interest.

References

1. World Health Organization. Diabetes. Available online: https://www.who.int/news-room/fact-sheets/detail/diabetes (accessed on 4 November 2021).
2. Wierusz-Wysocka, B.; Araszkiewicz, A.; Schlaffke, J. Końcowe produkty glikacji—Nowy biomarker cukrzycy i jej powikłań? *Clin. Diabetol.* **2013**, *2*, 96–103.
3. Abdulmalik, H.; Tadiwos, Y.; Legese, N. Assessment of drug-related problems among type 2 diabetic patients on follow up at Hiwot Fana Specialized University Hospital, Harar, Eastern Ethiopia. *BMC Res. Notes* **2019**, *12*, 771. [CrossRef] [PubMed]
4. Latek, D.; Rutkowska, E.; Niewieczerzal, S.; Cielecka-Piontek, J. Drug-induced diabetes type 2: In silico study involving class B GPCRs. *PLoS ONE* **2019**, *14*, e0208892. [CrossRef]
5. Pasznik, P.; Rutkowska, E.; Niewieczerzal, S.; Cielecka-Piontek, J.; Latek, D. Potential off-target effects of beta-blockers on gut hormone receptors: In silico study including GUT-DOCK—A web service for small-molecule docking. *PLoS ONE* **2019**, *14*, e0210705. [CrossRef] [PubMed]
6. Deacon, C.F.; Lebovitz, H.E. Comparative review of dipeptidyl peptidase-4 inhibitors and sulphonylureas. *Diabetes Obes. Metab.* **2016**, *18*, 333–347. [CrossRef]
7. Sonia, T.A.; Sharma, C.P. *Oral Delivery of Insulin*; Elsevier: Cambridge, UK, 2014; ISBN 1908818689.
8. Stamataki, N.S.; Yanni, A.E.; Karathanos, V.T. Bread making technology influences postprandial glucose response: A review of the clinical evidence. *Br. J. Nutr.* **2017**, *117*, 1001–1012. [CrossRef] [PubMed]
9. Babu, P.V.A.; Liu, D.; Gilbert, E.R. Recent advances in understanding the anti-diabetic actions of dietary flavonoids. *J. Nutr. Biochem.* **2013**, *24*, 1777–1789. [CrossRef]

10. Purohit, P.; Mishra, B. Systematic review on interaction studies of synthetic antidiabetic drugs and herbal therapies. *J. Pharm. Res.* **2017**, *16*, 86–94. [CrossRef]
11. EMA. European Medicines Agency. Committee on Herbal Medicinal Products (HMPC). Available online: https://www.ema.europa.eu/en/committees/committee-herbal-medicinal-products-hmpc (accessed on 30 April 2021).
12. Vinayagam, R.; Xu, B. Antidiabetic properties of dietary flavonoids: A cellular mechanism review. *Nutr. Metab.* **2015**, *12*, 1–20. [CrossRef]
13. Studzińska-Sroka, E.; Dudek-Makuch, M.; Chanaj-Kaczmarek, J.; Czepulis, N.; Korybalska, K.; Rutkowski, R.; Łuczak, J.; Grabowska, K.; Bylka, W.; Witowski, J. Anti-inflammatory Activity and Phytochemical Profile of Galinsoga Parviflora Cav. *Molecules* **2018**, *23*, 2133. [CrossRef]
14. Makowska-Wąs, J.; Galanty, A.; Gdula-Argasińska, J.; Tyszka-Czochara, M.; Szewczyk, A.; Nunes, R.; Carvalho, I.S.; Michalik, M.; Paśko, P. Identification of predominant phytochemical compounds and cytotoxic activity of wild olive leaves (Olea europaea L. ssp. sylvestris) harvested in south Portugal. *Chem. Biodivers.* **2017**, *14*, e1600331. [CrossRef] [PubMed]
15. Studzińska-Sroka, E.; Czapska, I.; Bylka, W. Biological Activity and Polyphenol Content in Selected Herbal Tea Blends Used in Diabetes. *Acta Pol. Pharm. Res.* **2019**, *76*, 1037–1042.
16. Dinis, T.C.P.; Madeira, V.M.C.; Almeida, L.M. Action of phenolic derivatives (acetaminophen, salicylate, and 5-aminosalicylate) as inhibitors of membrane lipid peroxidation and as peroxyl radical scavengers. *Arch. Biochem. Biophys.* **1994**, *315*, 161–169. [CrossRef]
17. Widodo, W.S.; Widowati, W.; Ginting, C.N.; Lister, I.; Armansyah, A.; Girsang, E. Comparison of antioxidant and anti-collagenase activity of genistein and epicatechin. *Pharm. Sci. Res.* **2019**, *6*, 6.
18. Hunyadi, A.; Martins, A.; Hsieh, T.J.; Seres, A.; Zupkó, I. Chlorogenic Acid and Rutin Play a Major Role in the In Vivo Anti-Diabetic Activity of Morus alba Leaf Extract on Type II Diabetic Rats. *PLoS ONE* **2012**, *7*, e50619. [CrossRef]
19. Frizzell, N.; Baynes, J.W. Chelation therapy for the management of diabetic complications: A hypothesis and a proposal for clinical laboratory assessment of metal ion homeostasis in plasma. *Clin. Chem. Lab. Med.* **2014**, *52*, 69–75. [CrossRef]
20. *European Pharmacopoeia*, 10th ed.; Council of Europe: Strasbourg, France, 2019; p. 1390, 1407–1409, 1551.
21. Brown, A.; Anderson, D.; Racicot, K.; Pilkenton, S.J.; Apostolidis, E. Evaluation of Phenolic Phytochemical Enriched Commercial Plant Extracts on the In Vitro Inhibition of α-Glucosidase. *Front. Nutr.* **2017**, *4*, 56. [CrossRef] [PubMed]
22. Domínguez Avila, J.A.; Rodrigo García, J.; González Aguilar, G.A.; de la Rosa, L.A. The Antidiabetic Mechanisms of Polyphenols Related to Increased Glucagon-Like Peptide-1 (GLP1) and Insulin Signaling. *Molecules* **2017**, *22*, 903. [CrossRef]
23. Guo, H.; Xia, M.; Zou, T.; Ling, W.; Zhong, R.; Zhang, W. Cyanidin 3-glucoside attenuates obesity-associated insulin resistance and hepatic steatosis in high-fat diet-fed and db/db mice via the transcription factor FoxO1. *J. Nutr. Biochem.* **2012**, *23*, 349–360. [CrossRef] [PubMed]
24. Kawser Hossain, M.; Abdal Dayem, A.; Han, J.; Yin, Y.; Kim, K.; Kumar Saha, S.; Yang, G.-M.; Choi, H.Y.; Cho, S.-G. Molecular Mechanisms of the Anti-Obesity and Anti-Diabetic Properties of Flavonoids. *Int. J. Mol. Sci.* **2016**, *17*, 569. [CrossRef] [PubMed]
25. Kopustinskiene, D.M.; Jakstas, V.; Savickas, A.; Bernatoniene, J. Flavonoids as Anticancer Agents. *Nutrients* **2020**, *12*, 457. [CrossRef]
26. Peng, C.-H.; Lin, H.-T.; Chung, D.-J.; Huang, C.-N.; Wang, C.-J. Mulberry leaf extracts prevent obesity-induced NAFLD with regulating adipocytokines, inflammation and oxidative stress. *J. Food Drug Anal.* **2018**, *26*, 778–787. [CrossRef]
27. Yan, Y.; Zhou, X.; Guo, K.; Zhou, F.; Yang, H. Use of Chlorogenic Acid against Diabetes Mellitus and Its Complications. *J. Immunol. Res.* **2020**, *2020*, 9680508. [CrossRef]
28. Naveed, M.; Hejazi, V.; Abbas, M.; Kamboh, A.A.; Khan, G.J.; Shumzaid, M.; Ahmad, F.; Babazadeh, D.; FangFang, X.; Modarresi-Ghazani, F.; et al. Chlorogenic acid (CGA): A pharmacological review and call for further research. *Biomed. Pharmacother.* **2018**, *97*, 67–74. [CrossRef]
29. Zuñiga, L.Y.; Aceves-de la Mora, M.C.A.; González-Ortiz, M.; Ramos-Nuñez, J.L.; Martínez Abundis, E. Effect of Chlorogenic Acid Administration on Glycemic Control, Insulin Secretion, and Insulin Sensitivity in Patients with Impaired Glucose Tolerance. *J. Med. Food* **2018**, *21*, 469–473. [CrossRef]
30. Adefegha, S.A.; Oboh, G.; Ejakpovi, I.I.; Oyeleye, S.I. Antioxidant and antidiabetic effects of gallic and protocatechuic acids: A structure–function perspective. *Comp. Clin. Pathol.* **2015**, *24*, 1579–1585. [CrossRef]
31. Patel, S.S.; Goyal, R.K. Cardioprotective effects of gallic acid in diabetes-induced myocardial dysfunction in rats. *Pharmacogn. Res.* **2011**, *3*, 239–245. [CrossRef]
32. Polumackanycz, M.; Wesolowski, M.; Viapiana, A. Morus alba L. and Morus nigra L. Leaves as a Promising Food Source of Phenolic Compounds with Antioxidant Activity. *Plant Foods Hum. Nutr.* **2021**, 1–8. [CrossRef] [PubMed]
33. Miyake, K.; Arima, H.; Hirayama, F.; Yamamoto, M.; Horikawa, T.; Sumiyoshi, H.; Noda, S.; Uekama, K. Improvement of solubility and oral bioavailability of rutin by complexation with 2-hydroxypropyl-beta-cyclodextrin. *Pharm. Dev. Technol.* **2000**, *5*, 399–407. [CrossRef]
34. Kim, G.-N.; Jang, H.-D. Flavonol content in the water extract of the mulberry (*Morus alba* L.) leaf and their antioxidant capacities. *J. Food Sci.* **2011**, *76*, C869–C873. [CrossRef] [PubMed]
35. Hwang, S.H.; Li, H.M.; Lim, S.S.; Wang, Z.; Hong, J.-S.; Huang, B. Evaluation of a standardized extract from morus alba against α-glucosidase inhibitory effect and postprandial antihyperglycemic in patients with impaired glucose tolerance: A randomized double-blind clinical trial. *Evid. Based Complementary Altern. Med.* **2016**, *2016*, 8983232. [CrossRef]

36. Dabur, R.; Sharma, B.; Mittal, A. Mechanistic approach of anti-diabetic compounds identified from natural sources. *Chem. Biol. Lett.* **2018**, *5*, 63–99.
37. Zheng, Y.; Yang, W.; Sun, W.; Chen, S.; Liu, D.; Kong, X.; Tian, J.; Ye, X. Inhibition of porcine pancreatic α-amylase activity by chlorogenic acid. *J. Funct. Foods* **2020**, *64*, 103587. [CrossRef]
38. Dubey, S.; Ganeshpurkar, A.; Ganeshpurkar, A.; Bansal, D.; Dubey, N. Glycolytic enzyme inhibitory and antiglycation potential of rutin. *Future J. Pharm. Sci.* **2017**, *3*, 158–162. [CrossRef]
39. Ranilla, L.G.; Kwon, Y.-I.; Apostolidis, E.; Shetty, K. Phenolic compounds, antioxidant activity and in vitro inhibitory potential against key enzymes relevant for hyperglycemia and hypertension of commonly used medicinal plants, herbs and spices in Latin America. *Bioresour. Technol.* **2010**, *101*, 4676–4689. [CrossRef] [PubMed]
40. Adisakwattana, S.; Lerdsuwankij, O.; Poputtachai, U.; Minipun, A.; Suparpprom, C. Inhibitory activity of cinnamon bark species and their combination effect with acarbose against intestinal α-glucosidase and pancreatic α-amylase. *Plant Foods Hum. Nutr.* **2011**, *66*, 143–148. [CrossRef]
41. Adisakwattana, S. Cinnamic Acid and Its Derivatives: Mechanisms for Prevention and Management of Diabetes and Its Complications. *Nutrients* **2017**, *9*, 163. [CrossRef]
42. Lin, G.-M.; Chen, Y.-H.; Yen, P.-L.; Chang, S.-T. Antihyperglycemic and antioxidant activities of twig extract from Cinnamomum osmophloeum. *J. Tradit. Complementary Med.* **2016**, *6*, 281–288. [CrossRef]
43. Tao, Y.; Zhang, Y.; Cheng, Y.; Wang, Y. Rapid screening and identification of α-glucosidase inhibitors from mulberry leaves using enzyme-immobilized magnetic beads coupled with HPLC/MS and NMR. *Biomed. Chromatogr.* **2013**, *27*, 148–155. [CrossRef] [PubMed]
44. Sui, X.; Zhang, Y.; Zhou, W. In vitro and in silico studies of the inhibition activity of anthocyanins against porcine pancreatic α-amylase. *J. Funct. Foods* **2016**, *21*, 50–57. [CrossRef]
45. Barik, S.K.; Russell, W.R.; Moar, K.M.; Cruickshank, M.; Scobbie, L.; Duncan, G.; Hoggard, N. The anthocyanins in black currants regulate postprandial hyperglycaemia primarily by inhibiting α-glucosidase while other phenolics modulate salivary α-amylase, glucose uptake and sugar transporters. *J. Nutr. Biochem.* **2020**, *78*, 108325. [CrossRef]
46. Boath, A.S.; Stewart, D.; McDougall, G.J. Berry components inhibit α-glucosidase in vitro: Synergies between acarbose and polyphenols from black currant and rowanberry. *Food Chem.* **2012**, *135*, 929–936. [CrossRef] [PubMed]
47. Chokki, M.; Cudălbeanu, M.; Zongo, C.; Dah-Nouvlessounon, D.; Ghinea, I.O.; Furdui, B.; Raclea, R.; Savadogo, A.; Baba-Moussa, L.; Avamescu, S.M. Exploring antioxidant and enzymes (A-amylase and B-Glucosidase) inhibitory activity of Morinda lucida and Momordica charantia leaves from Benin. *Foods* **2020**, *9*, 434. [CrossRef]
48. Castro-Acosta, M.L.; Smith, L.; Miller, R.J.; McCarthy, D.I.; Farrimond, J.A.; Hall, W.L. Drinks containing anthocyanin-rich blackcurrant extract decrease postprandial blood glucose, insulin and incretin concentrations. *J. Nutr. Biochem.* **2016**, *38*, 154–161. [CrossRef]
49. Tsui, P.-F.; Lin, C.-S.; Ho, L.-J.; Lai, J.-H. Spices and atherosclerosis. *Nutrients* **2018**, *10*, 1724. [CrossRef]
50. Jin, Q.; Yang, J.; Ma, L.; Wen, D.; Chen, F.; Li, J. Identification of polyphenols in mulberry (genus Morus) cultivars by liquid chromatography with time-of-flight mass spectrometer. *J. Food Compos. Anal.* **2017**, *63*, 55–64. [CrossRef]
51. Ouyang, P.; Gottlieb, S.H.; Culotta, V.L.; Navas-Acien, A. EDTA chelation therapy to reduce cardiovascular events in persons with diabetes. *Curr. Cardiol. Rep.* **2015**, *17*, 1–9. [CrossRef]
52. Lakey-Beitia, J.; Burillo, A.M.; La Penna, G.; Hegde, M.L.; Rao, K.S. Polyphenols as Potential Metal Chelation Compounds Against Alzheimer's Disease. *J. Alzheimer's Dis.* **2021**, *82*, S335–S357. [CrossRef] [PubMed]
53. Santana-Gálvez, J.; Cisneros-Zevallos, L.; Jacobo-Velázquez, D.A. Chlorogenic Acid: Recent Advances on Its Dual Role as a Food Additive and a Nutraceutical against Metabolic Syndrome. *Molecules* **2017**, *22*, 358. [CrossRef] [PubMed]
54. Sharma, U.K.; Sharma, A.K.; Pandey, A.K. Medicinal attributes of major phenylpropanoids present in cinnamon. *BMC Complementary Altern. Med.* **2016**, *16*, 156. [CrossRef] [PubMed]
55. Łabuda, H.; Buczkowska, H.; Papliński, R.; Najda, A. Secondary metabolites of Phaseoli pericarpium. *Acta Sci. Pol. Hortorum Cultus* **2017**, *16*, 187–200. [CrossRef]
56. Druzynska, B.; Klepacka, M. Wlasciwosci przeciwutleniajace preparatow polifenoli otrzymanych z okrywy nasiennej fasoli czarnej, rozowej i bialej [Phaseolus]. *Żywność Nauka Technol. Jakość* **2004**, *11*, 69–78.
57. Adhikari, B.M.; Bajracharya, A.; Shrestha, A.K. Comparison of nutritional properties of Stinging nettle (Urtica dioica) flour with wheat and barley flours. *Food Sci. Nutr.* **2016**, *4*, 119–124. [CrossRef]
58. Otles, S.; Yalcin, B. Phenolic compounds analysis of root, stalk, and leaves of nettle. *Sci. World J.* **2012**, *2012*, 564367. [CrossRef]
59. Carrasco-Castilla, J.; Hernández-Álvarez, A.J.; Jiménez-Martínez, C.; Jacinto-Hernández, C.; Alaiz, M.; Girón-Calle, J.; Vioque, J.; Dávila-Ortiz, G. Antioxidant and metal chelating activities of peptide fractions from phaseolin and bean protein hydrolysates. *Food Chem.* **2012**, *135*, 1789–1795. [CrossRef]
60. Gülçin, I.; Küfrevioglu, O.I.; Oktay, M.; Büyükokuroglu, M.E. Antioxidant, antimicrobial, antiulcer and analgesic activities of nettle (Urtica dioica L.). *J. Ethnopharmacol.* **2004**, *90*, 205–215. [CrossRef] [PubMed]
61. Balci Yuce, H.; Karatas, Ö.; Tulu, F.; Altan, A.; Gevrek, F. Effect of diabetes on collagen metabolism and hypoxia in human gingival tissue: A stereological, histopathological, and immunohistochemical study. *Biotech. Histochem.* **2019**, *94*, 65–73. [CrossRef]
62. Pradeepkumar Singh, L.; Vivek Sharma, A.; Swarnakar, S. Upregulation of collagenase-1 and -3 in indomethacin-induced gastric ulcer in diabetic rats: Role of melatonin. *J. Pineal Res.* **2011**, *51*, 61–74. [CrossRef] [PubMed]

63. Thrailkill, K.M.; Bunn, R.C.; Moreau, C.S.; Cockrell, G.E.; Simpson, P.M.; Coleman, H.N.; Frindik, J.P.; Kemp, S.F.; Fowlkes, J.L. Matrix metalloproteinase-2 dysregulation in type 1 diabetes. *Diabetes Care* **2007**, *30*, 2321–2326. [CrossRef]
64. Drankowska, J.; Kos, M.; Kościuk, A.; Marzęda, P.; Boguszewska-Czubara, A.; Tylus, M.; Święch-Zubilewicz, A. MMP targeting in the battle for vision: Recent developments and future prospects in the treatment of diabetic retinopathy. *Life Sci.* **2019**, *229*, 149–156. [CrossRef]
65. Kozakova, M.; Morizzo, C.; Goncalves, I.; Natali, A.; Nilsson, J.; Palombo, C. Cardiovascular organ damage in type 2 diabetes mellitus: The role of lipids and inflammation. *Cardiovasc. Diabetol.* **2019**, *18*, 1–11. [CrossRef]
66. Anuar, N.N.M.; Zulkafali, N.I.N.; Ugusman, A. Modulation of Matrix Metalloproteinases by Plant-derived Products. *Curr. Cancer Drug Targets* **2021**, *21*, 91–106. [CrossRef] [PubMed]
67. Shukri, S.M.; Pardi, F.; Sidik, N.J. In Vitro anti-collagenase activity and total phenolic content of five selected herbs: A review. *Sci. Lett.* **2021**, *15*, 117–127. [CrossRef]
68. Thring, T.S.A.; Hili, P.; Naughton, D.P. Anti-collagenase, anti-elastase and anti-oxidant activities of extracts from 21 plants. *BMC Complementary Altern. Med.* **2009**, *9*, 27. [CrossRef]
69. Wittenauer, J.; Mäckle, S.; Sußmann, D.; Schweiggert-Weisz, U.; Carle, R. Inhibitory effects of polyphenols from grape pomace extract on collagenase and elastase activity. *Fitoterapia* **2015**, *101*, 179–187. [CrossRef] [PubMed]
70. Salam, M.A.; Al-Zhrani, G.; Kosa, S.A. Simultaneous removal of copper(II), lead(II), zinc(II) and cadmium(II) from aqueous solutions by multi-walled carbon nanotubes. *C. R. Chim.* **2012**, *15*, 398–408. [CrossRef]
71. Choi, E.-Y.; Kim, E.-H.; Lee, J.-B.; Do, E.-J.; Kim, S.-J.; Kim, S.-H.; Park, J.-Y.; Lee, J.-T. Mechanisms for anti-wrinkle activities from fractions of Black Chokeberries. *J. Life Sci.* **2016**, *26*, 34–41. [CrossRef]

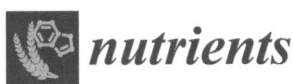

Article

Microbial and Chemical Profiles of Commercial Kombucha Products

Jieping Yang [1], Venu Lagishetty [1,2], Patrick Kurnia [1], Susanne M. Henning [1], Aaron I. Ahdoot [1,2] and Jonathan P. Jacobs [1,2,3,*]

[1] Department of Medicine, David Geffen School of Medicine at UCLA, Los Angeles, CA 90095, USA; jiepingyang@mednet.ucla.edu (J.Y.); vlagishetty@gmail.com (V.L.); patrickt75@g.ucla.edu (P.K.); shenning@mednet.ucla.edu (S.M.H.); aaronahdoot@ucla.edu (A.I.A.)
[2] The Vatche and Tamar Manoukian Division of Digestive Diseases, David Geffen School of Medicine at UCLA, Los Angeles, CA 90095, USA
[3] Division of Gastroenterology, Hepatology and Parenteral Nutrition, Veterans Affairs Greater Los Angeles Healthcare System, Los Angeles, CA 90073, USA
* Correspondence: jjacobs@mednet.ucla.edu

Abstract: Kombucha is an increasingly popular functional beverage that has gained attention for its unique combination of phytochemicals, metabolites, and microbes. Previous chemical and microbial composition analyses of kombucha have mainly focused on understanding their changes during fermentation. Very limited information is available regarding nutrient profiles of final kombucha products in the market. In this study, we compared the major chemicals (tea polyphenols, caffeine), antioxidant properties, microbial and metabolomic profiles of nine commercial kombucha products using shotgun metagenomics, internal transcribed spacer sequencing, untargeted metabolomics, and targeted chemical assays. All of the nine kombucha products showed similar acidity but great differences in chemicals, metabolites, microbes, and antioxidant activities. Most kombucha products are dominated by the probiotic *Bacillus coagulans* or bacteria capable of fermentation including *Lactobacillus nagelii*, *Gluconacetobacter*, *Gluconobacter*, and *Komagataeibacter* species. We found that all nine kombuchas also contained varying levels of enteric bacteria including *Bacteroides thetaiotamicron*, *Escherischia coli*, *Enterococcus faecalis*, *Bacteroides fragilis*, *Enterobacter cloacae* complex, and *Akkermansia muciniphila*. The fungal composition of kombucha products was characterized by predominance of fermenting yeast including *Brettanomyces* species and *Cyberlindnera jadinii*. Kombucha varied widely in chemical content assessed by global untargeted metabolomics, with metabolomic variation being significantly associated with metagenomic profiles. Variation in tea bases, bacteria/yeast starter cultures, and duration of fermentation may all contribute to the observed large differences in the microbial and chemical profiles of final kombucha products.

Keywords: kombucha; bacteria; yeast; metagenome; metabolome; tea polyphenols; antioxidants

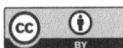

1. Introduction

Kombucha is a fermented tea drink commonly consumed for its potential health benefits [1]. The fermentation occurs by providing Symbiotic Culture of Bacteria and Yeasts (SCOBY), a biofilm of cellulose containing the bacteria and yeasts, as a starter to sugary tea [2,3]. Kombucha yeast have been reported to include members of the *Zygosaccharomyces* and *Brettanomyces* genera [4]. Bacteria reported in kombucha cultures include acetic acid bacteria (*Gluconacetobacter* and *Acetobacter*) and lactic acid bacteria (*Lactobacillus*) [3,5]. The extensive interactions between bacteria and yeasts feeding on sugar, tea base as well as other added substrates lead to the production of a wide range of bioactive metabolites including vitamins, amino acids, and ethanol [5].

The most commonly used teas for fermentation are black tea, white tea and green tea [6]. The chemical composition of tea has been well documented and a variety of factors, such as storage and manufacturing process, determine the tea chemical composition [7].

Tea polyphenols constitute up to 30% of the green tea dry weight and are known for their health benefits [8–10]. Catechins are the characteristic components of tea polyphenols, including catechin (C), epicatechin (EC), epigallocatechin (EGC), and epigallocatechin gallate (EGCG) [11]. During the production of black tea, about 75% of catechins undergo enzymatic transformation consisting of oxidation and partial polymerization into thearubigins [9,12]. The unique chemical profiles of each tea base are likely to be reflected in the final chemical composition of kombucha and may lead to different biological activities [13–15].

There has been great interest in fermented food products, including kombucha, as a source of probiotics (i.e., live microbes with beneficial effects on health). Potential beneficial properties of probiotics including inhibition of pathogenic bacteria, promotion of health-associated gut microbial communities, interaction with the intestinal epithelium, metabolism of certain nutrients, and modulation of signaling within the immune system [16]. Many existing purported probiotics belong to the *Lactobacillus* genus, which are often present in kombucha [17]. To satisfy the claim of probiotics, several probiotics are often added to commercial kombucha products. *Bacillus coagulans*, a lactic acid-producing bacteria resistant to high temperature, has been one of the most common [18]. Other probiotics that are added to commercial kombucha products include *Bacillus subtilis*, *Saccharomyces boulardii*, and *Lactobacillus rhamnosus* [1].

The complex interactions among the different combination of yeast/bacteria, tea base, manufacturing process, and probiotic addition create the potential for a wide diversity of bacterial and fungal compositions, tea polyphenol levels, and metabolite contents of kombucha products [3,19,20]. Such variation could greatly impact the overall health benefits of kombucha. In this study, we investigated heterogeneity among a sample of commercial kombucha products from a multi-omics perspective. For this purpose, we employed chemical, metabolomics and metagenomics analyses to understand the diversity of kombucha by profiling nine commercial kombucha products.

2. Materials and Methods

2.1. Kombucha Samples

Nine different commercial kombucha products (n = 3 samples per product), either in original or ginger flavor to minimize differences in added ingredients, were purchased from three supermarkets in the Los Angeles metropolitan area on 2/2/21: GT's Synergy Gingerade (A1), GT's Classic Original (A2), Better Booch Ginger Boost (B), Bottled Brew Dr. Ginger Lemon (C1), Canned Brew Dr. Ginger Lemon (C2), Health Ade Ginger Lemon (D), Humm Kombucha Ginger (E1), Humm Zero Kombucha Ginger Lemonade (E2), and Kevita Master Brew Ginger Kombucha (F). These kombucha products were selected based upon the high market share of these six manufacturers, which together represent an estimated 86% of commercial kombucha sales in the United States in 2021 [21]. As samples for each kombucha product came from the same batch, this analysis could not assess for differences across batches of the same kombucha product. Ingredient labels and nutritional information provided by each manufacturer are shown in Table 1. The kombucha product labels indicated a range of energy values from 3 to 17 kcal/100 g; use of black tea, green tee, or both; additional probiotic cultures in some products; and various flavoring ingredients. Within three days of purchase, the contents of each bottle or can were carefully mixed so that no visible sediment remained. The mixed kombucha products were then aliquoted into 50 mL conical tubes and centrifuged at 1300× g for 10 min. The supernatant was separated from the pellets and both were kept frozen at −80 °C until assays were performed.

Table 1. List of kombucha products.

Product	Ingredients Label	Nutrition (per 100 mL)	Expiration
A1	**Probiotics**: kombucha culture, Bacillus Coagulans GBI-306086 (4 billion organisms), *S. Boulardii* (4 billion organisms), *Lactobacillus bacteria* (4 billion) **Tea**: black tea, green tea **Flavors**: kiwi juice, ginger juice	Calories: 10.6 Carbohydrate: 2.54 g, Added Sugar: 0 g Sodium: 2.11 mg Lactic acid: 21.1 mg, Acetic acid: 15.9 mg, Glucuronic acid: 296.0 mg, Gluconic acid: 137.4 mg	5/6/2021
A2	**Probiotics**: kombucha culture, *Lactobacillus bacteria* (4 billion organisms), *S. Boulardii* (4 billion organisms) **Tea**: black tea, green tea **Sugar**: cane sugar	Calories: 12.5 Carbohydrate: 3.33 g, Added Sugar: 2.08 g Sodium: 2.08 g Lactic acid: 20.83 mg, Acetic acid: 15.6 mg, Glucuronic acid: 291.7 mg, Gluconic acid: 135.4 mg Polyphenols: 2.1 mg	4/14/2021
B	**Probiotics**: kombucha culture **Tea**: black tea **Sugar**: cane sugar **Flavors**: ginger, lemongrass, orange peel, spearmint, peppermint	Calories: 12.7 Carbohydrate: 2.56 g, Added Sugar: 1.83 g Sodium: 3.67 mg	8/12/2021
C1	**Probiotics**: kombucha culture **Tea**: green tea **Sugar**: cane sugar **Flavors**: dried lemon, lemon verbena, ginger juice, ginger extract	Calories: 16.9 Carbohydrate: 4.10 g, Added Sugar: 3.14 g Sodium: 0 mg	5/22/2021
C2	**Probiotics**: kombucha culture **Tea**: green tea **Sugar**: cane sugar **Flavors**: dried lemon, lemon verbena, ginger juice, ginger extract	Calories: 16.9 Carbohydrate: 3.94 g, Added Sugar: 3.38 g Sodium: 0 mg	3/9/2021
D	**Probiotics**: kombucha culture **Sugar**: cane sugar **Flavors**: ginger juice, black tea, green tea, lemon juice	Calories: 14.8 Carbohydrate: 2.96 g, Added Sugar: 1.69 g Sodium: 0 mg	7/21/2021
E1	**Probiotics**: kombucha culture, Bacillus subtilis, vitamin B12 **Tea**: green tea, black tea **Sugar**: cane sugar **Flavors**: white grape juice, apple juice, ginger juice, lemon juice	Calories: 9.6 Carbohydrate: 2.41 g, Added Sugar: 0 g Sodium: 0 mg	8/4/2021
E2	**Probiotics**: kombucha culture, Bacillus subtilis, Vitamin B12, Bacillus coagulans **Tea**: green tea, black tea **Flavors**: white grape juice, cane sugar, allulose syrup, monk fruit, ginger juice, natural flavors	Calories: 3.03 Carbohydrate: 3.03 g Added Sugar: 0 g Sodium: 0 mg	8/24/2021
F	**Probiotics**: kombucha culture, Bacillus coagulans MTCC 5856 **Tea**: black tea, green tea, black tea extract, green tea extract, black tea essence, green coffee bean extract (caffeine) **Sugar**: cane sugar **Flavors**: ginger extract, stevia leaf extract, sparkling water, natural flavor	Calories: 13.3 Carbohydrate: 3.56 g Added Sugar: 3.33 g Sodium: 3.33 mg Gluconic and acetic acid: 112.7 mg	6/3/2021

Products were labelled by manufacturer (e.g., A, B). Numbers indicate distinct products from the same manufacturer (e.g., 1, 2).

2.2. Levels of Tea Catechins and Caffeine Analyzed by High Performance Liquid Chromatography (HPLC)

The kombucha supernatant samples were centrifuged at 14,000 rpm for 10 min and the supernatants were used for the analysis. Analysis was performed on a Waters 2690 HPLC equipped with photodiode array detector. Chromatographic separation was achieved on a Zorbax SB-C18 (4.6 × 250 mm 5 um Agilent, Santa Clara, CA, USA) column and the column temperature was held at 35 C. Eluent A consisted of 0.1% phosphoric acid in water and eluent B consisted of 0.1% phosphoric acid in acetonitrile. Gradient elution was performed with the 95% A to 70% A in 40 min with flow rate of 0.75 mL/min. Catechins and caffeine concentration were determined at 280 nm.

2.3. Gallic Acid Equivalent (GAE) Assay

GAE assay was performed as previously described using the Folin–Ciocalteau reagent [22]. The reading was performed at 755 nm in a ThermoMax microplate reader (Molecular Devices, Sunnyvale, CA, USA) at room temperature. Standard curves were used to convert the average absorbance of each sample into mg/g GAE.

2.4. Trolox Equivalent Antioxidant Capacity (TEAC) Assay

TEAC was performed as previously described [23]. Kombucha supernatant samples were centrifuged at 4000 rpm for 15 min at 4 °C and the supernatants were transferred into a clean tube and diluted in Na/K buffer (pH 7.0). The Kombucha sample absorbance readings (750 nm) were in the linear range of Trolox standard curve. Total antioxidant activity was calculated using a Trolox (Sigma-Aldrich, St. Louis, MO, USA) standard curve with a concentration range of 0 to 300 µM and was expressed in Trolox equivalents. All samples were performed in triplicate and final TEAC result was calculated as Trolox equivalents (mg) per L.

2.5. Ethanol Content ANALYZED by Gas Chromatography (GC)

The kombucha supernatant samples were centrifuged at 14,000 rpm for 10 min and the supernatants were diluted with Milipore water (1:1). The ethanol content in diluted kombucha supernatants was quantified by GC FID (Agilent 7890A) and RTX-Stabilwax capillary column (Restek, Bellefonte, PA, USA). Ethanol concentration was determined by comparing the peak area and retention with the ethanol standard peak area and retention time.

2.6. pH Measurements

The pH of each product was measured using a Cole-Parmer P200 pH meter. Each measurement was replicated three times.

2.7. Shotgun Metagenomics Analysis

Microbial DNA was extracted from frozen pellets using the Qiagen Powersoil Pro kit with bead beating according to the manufacturer's protocol. DNA libraries were then prepared using the Celero PCR Workflow with Enzymatic Fragmentation DNA-Seq library preparation kit (Cat # 9363; NuGEN Technologies, Inc., San Carlos, CA, USA) according to the manufacturer's protocol. Briefly, 200 ng of extracted DNA was enzymatically fragmented followed by adapter ligation, amplification and purification. Library concentrations were measured by Qubit and size distribution was assessed by Bioanalyzer. Purified libraries were diluted to 10 nM and pooled for 2 × 150 paired-end sequencing using the Illumina Novaseq 6000 sequencing system (S4 flowcell). Mean sequence depth for the kombucha samples was 24.8 million paired-end reads per sample (range 9.7–68.1 million). Read-level quality control was performed using KneadData with default settings [24]. Taxonomic annotations were made using MetaPhlAn 3.0, which uses clade-specific markers to identify microbial species present in a sample and their relative abundances. Alpha diversity was assessed using the Shannon index implemented in the R phyloseq package [25]. Beta diversity was calculated using Bray–Curtis dissimilarity and visualized by principal coordinates analysis using the vegan package in R. Functional annotation was performed using HUMAnN 3.0 with the UniRef90 database. Microbial gene abundances were collapsed into functional pathways defined by MetaCyc annotations.

2.8. ITS Sequencing

The fungal internal transcribed spacer (ITS) region was amplified from extracted DNA samples using the ITS1f and ITS2 primers according to a published protocol [26]. Amplified product was then pooled and sequenced using an Illumina MiSeq (250 × 2 bp sequencing, v2 kit). DADA2 was used to perform primer trimming, quality-filtering, inference of amplicon sequence variants (ASV), chimera removal, and taxonomy assignment based on the UNITE database [27]. Mean sequence depth after processing was 312,677 paired-end sequences per sample (range 23,664–472,429). Alpha and beta diversity were assessed as was described for shotgun metagenomics data.

2.9. Metabolomics

Metabolomics analysis of kombucha supernatant samples was performed by The Metabolomics Innovation Center (Edmonton, Canada). The workflow included sample pre-treatment and normalization, chemical isotope labeling (CIL), LC-MS analysis, data processing and metabolite identification. In the CIL LC-MS metabolome analysis, the whole metabolome was analyzed by targeting four submetabolomes or channels: amine/phenol-, carboxyl-, hydroxyl- and carbonyl-submetabolome.[1] The combined results from four channels could provide comprehensive profile of the entire metabolome, e.g., about 86% to 96% of the chemical space in various metabolome databases.[1] In each channel, after sample pre-treatment step (e.g., protein precipitation, metabolite extraction, etc.), all samples were first derivatized with a pair of isotopic labeling reagents (i.e., ^{12}C-/^{13}C-reagents) prior to LC-MS analysis. Individual samples were labeled with ^{12}C-reagents and a pooled sample, which was generated by mixing an aliquot from each individual sample, was labeled with ^{13}C-reagents. After labeling, the ^{12}C-labeled individual sample was mixed with the same amount of the ^{13}C-labeled pool, followed by LC-MS analysis. In the mass spectra, each metabolite was detected as a peak pair, i.e., the light peak from the ^{12}C-labeled individual sample and the heavy peak from the ^{13}C-labeled pool. The peak intensity ratio between ^{12}C-peak and ^{13}C-peak represents the relative quantification result for a specific metabolite in an individual sample. Since the same ^{13}C-labeled pooled sample was spiked into all the ^{12}C-labeled individual samples, the ^{12}C-/^{13}C-peak ratio values of a specific metabolite in all the individual samples reflected the concentration differences of the metabolite in these samples. The ^{13}C-labeled pooled sample served as an internal reference for analyzing all individual samples to correct for matrix and ion suppression effects as well as any instrument sensitivity drifts for accurate and precise quantification. All LC-MS analysis were carried out on using Agilent 1290 LC linked to Bruker Impact II QTOF Mass Spectrometer. The column used was Agilent eclipse plus reversed-phase C18 column (150 × 2.1 mm, 1.8 μm particle size) and the column oven temperature was 40 °C. Mobile phase A was 0.1% (v/v) formic acid in water and mobile phase B was 0.1% (v/v) formic acid in acetonitrile. The gradient setting was: t = 0 min, 25% B; t = 10 min, 99% B; t = 15 min, 99% B; t = 15.1 min, 25% B; t = 18 min, 25% B. The flow rate was 400 μL/min. Mass spectral acquisition rate was 1 Hz, with an m/z range from 220 to 1000.

Peaks were annotated using a three-tier approach. In tier 1, peak pairs were searched against a labeled metabolite library (CIL Library, contains more than 1500 entries) based on accurate mass and retention time. 251 peak pairs were positively identified in this manner. In tier 2, linked identity library (LI Library) was used for putative identification of the remaining peak pairs. The LI Library includes over 9000 pathway-related metabolites, providing high-confidence putative identification results based on accurate mass and predicted retention time matches. 1090 peak pairs were putatively identified by this approach. In tier 3, the remaining peak pairs were searched, based on accurate mass match, against the MyCompoundID (MCID) library composed of 8021 known human endogenous metabolites (zero-reaction library), their predicted metabolic products from one metabolic reaction (375,809 compounds) (one-reaction library) and two metabolic reactions (10,583,901 compounds) (two-reaction library). 1197, 2976 and 748 peak pairs were matched in the zero-, one- and two-reaction libraries, respectively. In total, 7459 unique peak pairs were detected, of which 1341 were identified with high-confidence (tiers 1 and 2) and the majority of the remaining peaks had putative annotations.

Global differences in metabolomics profiles were visualized by performing principal coordinates analysis of Euclidean distances. Sparse partial least-squares discriminant analysis (sPLS-DA) implemented in the mixOmics package in R was used to select a limited number of annotated metabolites that differentiate kombucha samples [28]. A tuning process was performed to select the optimal number of metabolites for each of two components (X-variates) to minimize the balanced error rate in 5-fold validation.

2.10. Statistical Analysis

Data distributions were summarized by both mean and SD as well as by median, minimum, and maximum (Supplementary Table S1). Normality of distribution was assessed by the Shapiro–Wilk test. Significance of differences across samples in measured chemicals and alpha diversity was assessed by ANOVA in R using the built-in aov function. Upon finding significant differences across all products, we used Tukey's Post-hoc Test to perform pairwise comparisons between each kombucha product. For measures in which one or two out of the nine groups showed a significant p-value by the Shapiro–Wilk test, we generated additional figures showing distributions as boxplots with significance determined by Kruskal–Wallis with post-hoc Dunn's test (Supplementary Figure S1).

Significance of global differences across kombucha products (beta diversity) in bacterial composition, fungal composition, microbial gene abundances, and metabolomics profiles was determined using multivariate Adonis in the R package vegan. Metagenomics data (UniRef genes) and metabolomics data were superimposed using Procrustes and significance was assessed using the Mantel test implemented in the vegan package in R. MetaCyc pathways and metabolites that were differentially abundant across kombucha products were identified using Kruskal–Wallis. p-values for differential abundance were adjusted using the Benjamini–Hochberg method to correct for multiple hypothesis testing ($p < 0.05$ for significance). Partial Spearman correlations adjusting for kombucha product were calculated for all pairwise combinations of differentially abundant pathways and metabolites using the PResiduals package in R. Correlations were adjusted by the Benjamini–Hochberg method to control false discovery rate (FDR) at <0.1.

3. Results

3.1. Microbial Composition

Shotgun metagenomics sequencing was performed of three samples each from nine commercial kombucha products shown in Table 1. The initial analysis focused on bacterial composition at the species level based on annotation of shotgun reads against a reference database. Most kombucha products were found to have low bacterial diversity due to dominance by a single bacterium, among which A2 showed significantly higher diversity compared to all other products and F showed significantly lower diversity (Figure 1A). Bacterial composition was strongly associated with kombucha product ($p < 10^{-5}$). In all cases, the three samples from each product tightly clustered with one another (Figure 1B). The nine kombucha products formed three groups according to their dominant bacteria (Figure 1B,C). The first group (E1, E2, A1, F) was characterized by predominance of *Bacillus coagulans* and/or *Gluconacetobacter liquefaciens*. The second group (C1, C2, D) was characterized by predominance of *Lactobacillus nagelii*. One of the remaining kombucha products (B) was characterized by high abundance of *Lactobacillus mali* and presence of *Gluconobacter* species while the other (A2) included both fermenting bacteria in the *Komagataeibacter* genus (primarily *K. rhaeticus*) as well as large populations of gut-derived bacteria. *E. coli* and *Bacteroides thetaiotamicron* together represented the majority of bacteria detected in all three samples of A2. Given the high abundances of enteric bacteria found in this kombucha product, we assessed whether these bacteria could also be detected in the other eight kombucha products. All were found to contain enteric bacteria, especially *Bacteroides thetaiotamicron*, *E. coli*, and *Enterococcus faecalis*, as well as less commonly other species including *Enterobacter cloacae complex*, *Bacteroides fragilis* and *Akkermansia muciniphila* (Figure 2). A2 had significantly higher levels of *E. coli* and *B. thetaiotamicron* than the other products while F had significantly lower levels of these microbes.

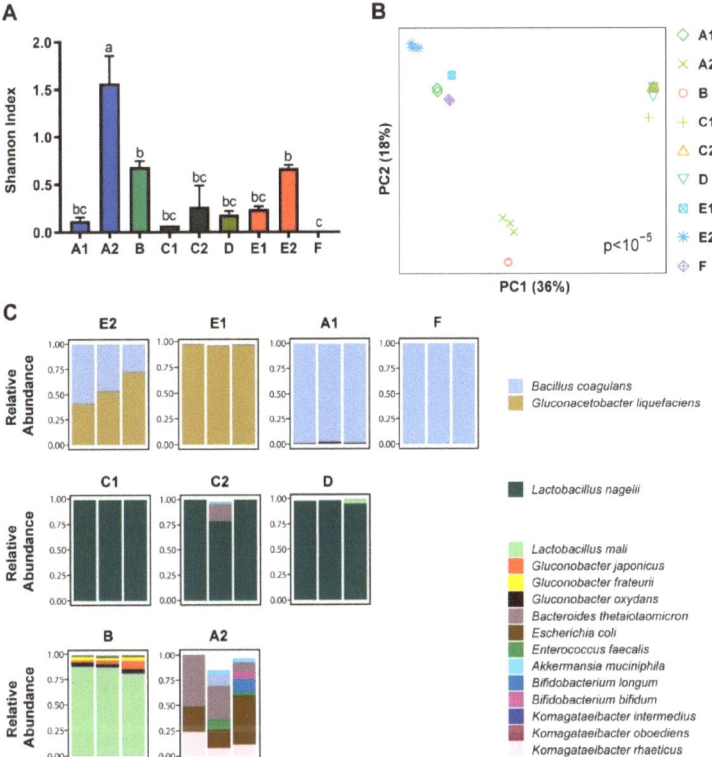

Figure 1. Kombucha products vary greatly in microbial composition and diversity. (**A**) Microbial alpha diversity as measured by the Shannon index of richness and evenness is shown for each sample, grouped by kombucha product. Means in a column without a common letter differ; $p < 0.05$. Product C2 had $p < 0.05$ by the Shapiro–Wilk test of normality. (**B**) Principal coordinates analysis plot visualizing microbial beta diversity by Bray–Curtis dissimilarity. Each symbol represents a sample; kombucha product is indicated by symbol color and shape. Significance of differences across products was assessed by Adonis. (**C**) Taxa summary plots showing the relative abundances of the 16 most abundant bacterial species across the samples. Each bar represents one sample; samples are grouped by kombucha product. Color indicates species. The bars do not necessarily add to 1 as lower abundance microbes are not shown.

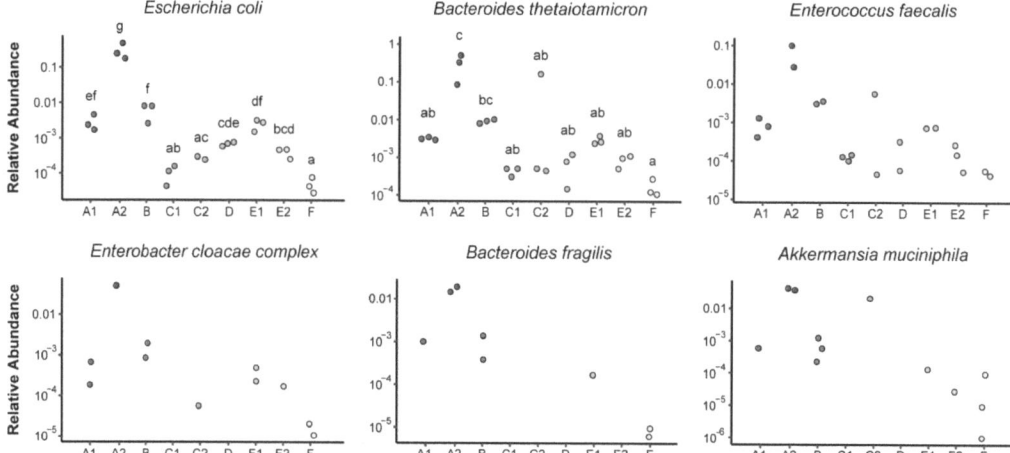

Figure 2. Relative abundances of enteric bacteria detected in kombucha. Each dot represents one sample with detectable levels of the indicated enteric bacteria. Significance of differences in two widely detected enteric bacteria, *E. coli* and *B. thetaiotamicron*, was determined by ANOVA with post-hoc Tukey. Means in a column without a common letter differ; $p < 0.05$.

The reference database used to annotate shotgun metagenomics sequence data contained over 500 fungal genomes, but of these, only *Saccharomyces cerevisiae* was detected in the kombucha samples. Given the paucity of detected kombucha yeast genomes, we assessed the fungal composition of kombucha by ITS sequencing. Kombucha products varied in fungal diversity with a pattern that differed from that of bacterial diversity (Figure 3A). For instance, the kombucha product with lowest bacterial diversity (F) had the highest fungal diversity. Fungal composition was strongly associated with kombucha product ($p < 10^{-5}$) (Figure 3B). The nine kombucha products had similar yeast composition across the three samples of each product with the exception of a single product (D). Most kombucha products showed predominance of one or two yeast species and grouped together based on manufacturer and the dominant yeast (Figure 3B,C). The largest group (A1, A2, C1, C2, and two samples of D) showed predominance of an uncharacterized species of *Brettanomyces* (a yeast genus associated with wine fermentation) and a related yeast, *Dekkera anomala* (a member of the *Brettanomyces* genus). A second group (B, F, and one sample of D) was characterized by predominance of *Cyberlindnera jadinii*. The remaining two kombucha products (E1, E2) grouped together and were characterized by predominance of *Trigonopsis variabilis* or *Issatchenkia orientalis*.

3.2. Metabolomics and Metagenomics Profiles

We then used the shotgun metagenomics data to assess the functional potential of kombucha microbes based on UniRef90 annotation. Gene content was strongly associated with kombucha product ($p < 10^{-5}$), with the three samples of each product clustering together (Figure 4A). When summarized at the pathway level, 62 MetaCyc pathways were found to be differentially abundant across kombucha products. Global untargeted metabolomics was then performed to compare chemical composition of the nine kombucha products. Metabolite profiles were strongly associated with kombucha product ($p < 10^{-5}$) and differential abundance testing demonstrated 1257 positively or putatively identified metabolites that significantly differed across kombucha products (Figure 4B). Sparse partial least squares discriminant (sPLS-DA)—a method for feature selection and classification—was used to identify 14 of these metabolites that formed two derived axes that could differentiate the kombucha products (Figure 4C). The first axis (X-variate 1) consisted of nine dipeptides and separated four products (E1, E2, B, D) from the others (Figure 4D). Dipeptides have been reported to rise markedly during fermentation of black tea and may represent a marker of the black tea base of kombucha products and/or their breakdown during kombucha fermentation [29]. The second axis (X-variate 2) consisted of 5 chemicals that are associated with black tea fermentation (5-O-Caffeoylshikimic acid), rooibos tea (nothofagin), and plants (7-hydroxy-8-methoxycoumarin and viburtinal) [30–32]. This axis, which may reflect the properties of the tea base, separated three products from the others (E1, E2, A2).

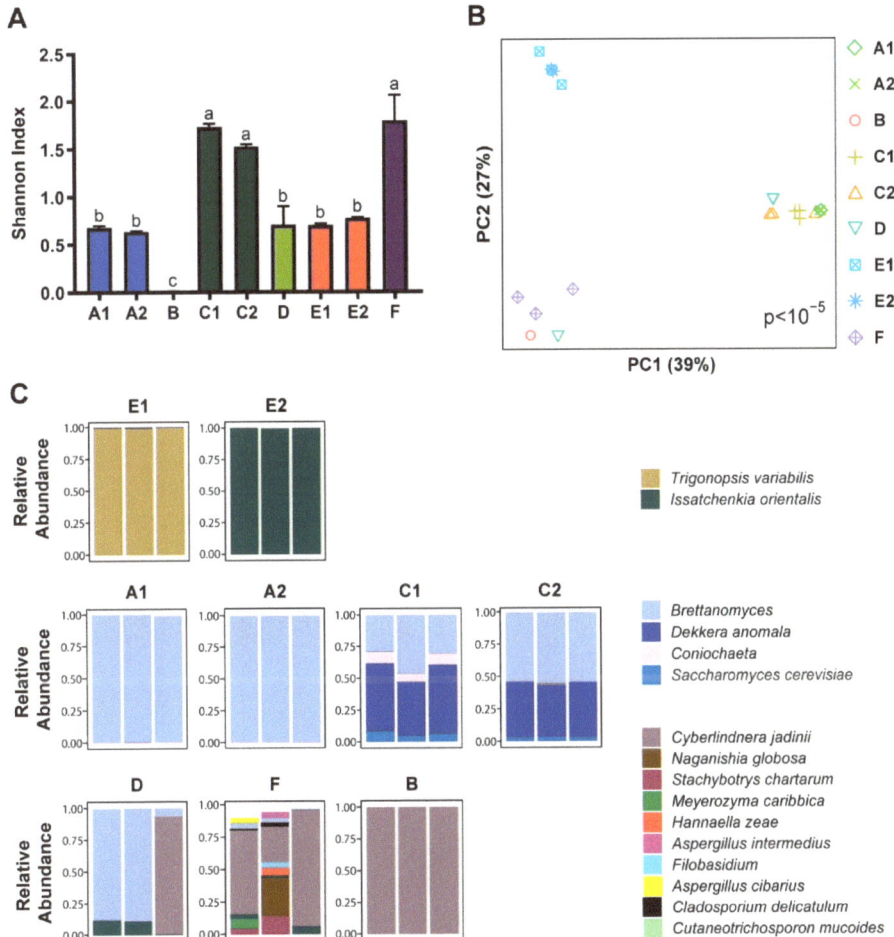

Figure 3. Fungal diversity and composition vary across kombucha products. (**A**) Fungal alpha diversity as measured by the Shannon index of richness and evenness is shown for each sample, grouped by kombucha product. Means in a column without a common letter differ; $p < 0.05$. Product D had $p < 0.05$ by the Shapiro–Wilk test of normality. (**B**) Principal coordinates analysis plot visualizing fungal beta diversity by Bray–Curtis dissimilarity. Each symbol represents a sample; kombucha product is indicated by symbol color and shape. Significance of differences across products was assessed by Adonis. (**C**) Taxa summary plots showing the relative abundances of the 16 most abundant fungal species across the samples. Each bar represents one sample; samples are grouped by kombucha product. Color indicates species. In some cases, the species was uncharacterized, in which case only the genus name is shown. The bars do not necessarily add to 1 as lower abundance fungi are not shown.

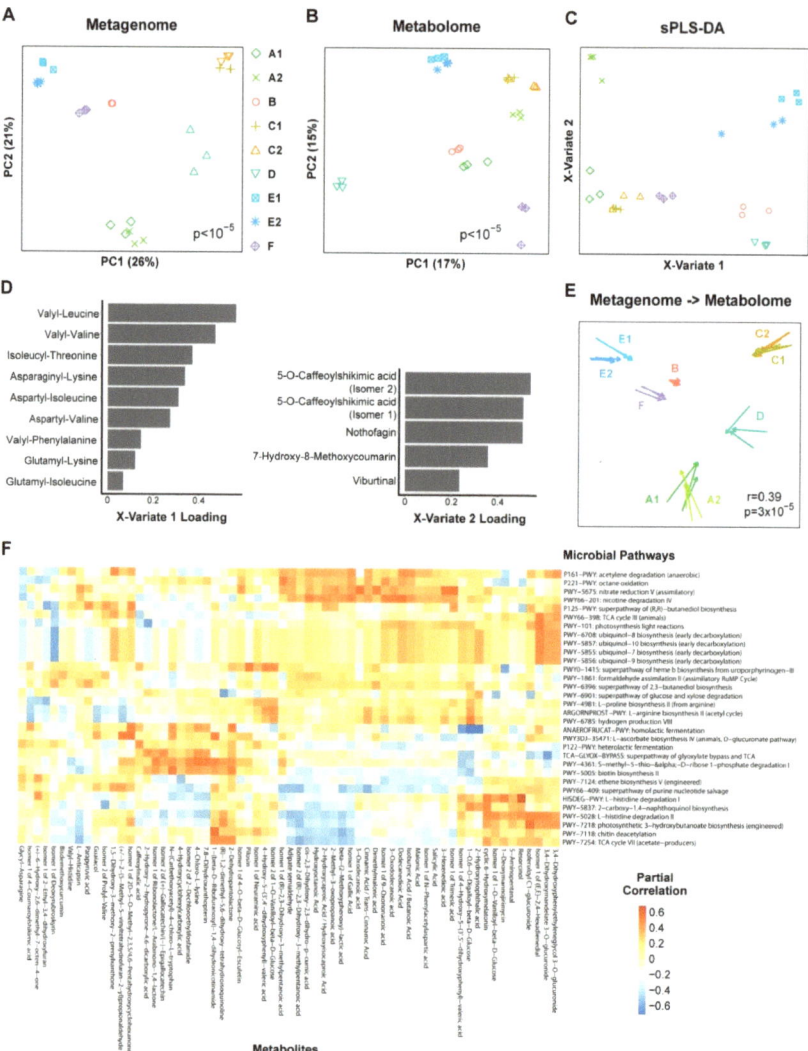

Figure 4. Differences in metabolites and microbial gene content across kombucha products. (**A**,**B**) Principal coordinates analysis plots representing (**A**) microbial gene content ("metagenome") and (**B**) metabolomics profiles across the kombucha samples, with symbol/color indicating kombucha product. Significance of differences across products was assessed by Adonis. (**C**) Sparse partial least squares discriminant analysis (sPLS-DA) was used to visualize kombucha products in a supervised manner based upon two derived axes (X-variates 1 and 2) containing 9 and 5 metabolites, respectively. (**D**) Loadings of the metabolites contributing to X-variates 1 and 2 derived from sPLS-DA. (**E**) Procrustes analysis superimposing microbial gene abundances and metabolomics profiles. Arrows in the Procrustes plot point from the gene content data ("Metagenome") to the metabolomics data ("Metabolome"). Significance of correlations between the two data sets was determined by the Mantel test with 100,000 permutations. (**F**) Heat map depicting partial correlations between MetaCyc pathways and metabolites that were differentially abundant across kombucha products. Correlations were adjusted for kombucha product and are only shown for pathways and metabolites that had at least one partial correlation with FDR <0.1.

Procrustes analysis was performed to assess for a relationship between variation in microbial gene content and metabolites across kombucha products. Differences in microbial gene content across kombucha products were significantly associated with the differences in metabolomics profiles ($p = 3 \times 10^{-5}$) (Figure 4E). Partial correlation analysis was performed to identify specific microbe-metabolite correlations underlying this global association after controlling for kombucha product. There were 83 microbe-metabolite correlations with false discovery rate less than 0.1, representing 32 MetaCyc pathways and 62 metabolites (Figure 4F).

3.3. Ethanol, Acidity, and Caffeine Content of Kombucha

Fermentation of kombucha decreases pH due to production of organic acids [5]. The nine kombucha products had small variations in acidity with pH range from 3–3.2 (Figure 5A). One major product of fermentation is ethanol, which was detected in eight out of nine kombocha products. Ethanol content of these nine kombucha products showed large variation, ranging from 0% (F) to 1.29% (A2) (Figure 5B). The kombucha products also varied greatly in concentrations of tea catechins (C, EC, EGCG and ECG) and caffeine (Figure 6). Levels of C, EC, EGCG and ECG among these nine kombucha products were highly correlated, with correlation coefficients ranges from 0.599–0.952 (Supplementary Table S2). Ranking of total tea catechins (μg/mL) in the nine kombucha products was E1 (88.6(34.8)) > C2 (82.5(13)) > C1 (76.5(6.9)) > E2 (75.4(6.3)) > A1 (49.1(2.2)) > D (27(1.4)) > A2 (19.6(1.1)) > B (15.9(0.4)) > F (15.3(1.3)). Ranking of caffeine (μg/mL) was F (112.6(5.8)) > A2 (42.5(1.6)) > A1 (42.2(1.8)) > E1 (37.7(2.4)) > C2 (29.2(4.9)) > C1 (27.7(2.7)) > E (227.4(2.3)) > D (24.7(1.3)) > B (15.1(0.3)).

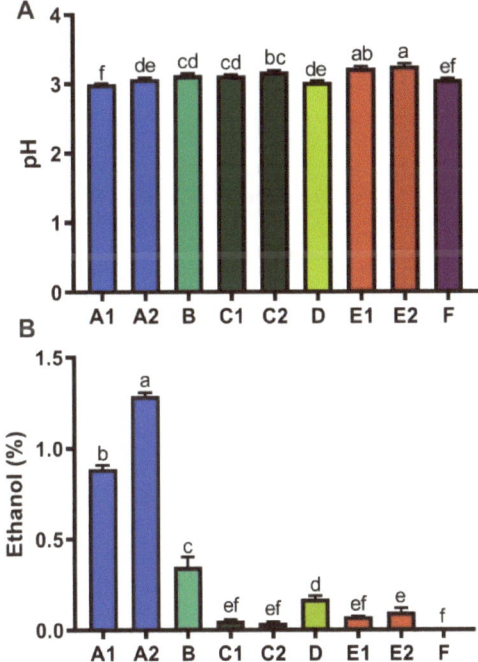

Figure 5. Variation in ethanol content and pH across kombucha products. pH (**A**) and ethanol (**B**) are shown for the kombucha products. Data presented as mean ± SEM ($n = 3$). Means in a column without a common letter differ; $p < 0.05$. Ethanol measurements for Product C1 had $p < 0.05$ by the Shapiro–Wilk test of normality.

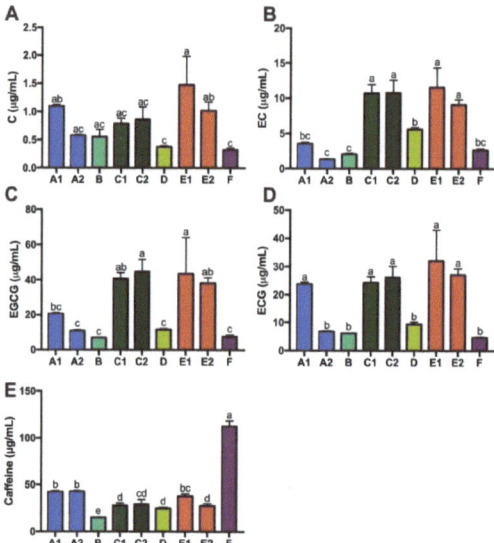

Figure 6. Tea catechin levels and caffeine content vary across kombucha products. Green tea catechins (**A**) C, (**B**) EC, (**C**) EGCG, (**D**) ECG, and (**E**) caffeine were measured in the nine kombucha products. Data are presented as mean ± SEM (n = 3). Means in a column without a common letter differ; $p < 0.05$. Products A1 (C, caffeine), A2 (EC), B (ECG), D (EC), and F (C, caffeine) had $p < 0.05$ by the Shapiro–Wilk test of normality for the indicated catechin or caffeine.

3.4. Tea Catechins, Antioxidant Capacity and Total Tea Polyphenols of Kombucha Products

TEAC and GAE assays were conducted to determine the antioxidant properties and total tea polyphenols of the nine kombucha products. Results from TEAC (antioxidant capacity) and GAE (total tea polyphenols) showed a significant correlation (Pearson correlation 0.81, $p = 0.00$) between these two assays. In both assays, F had significantly lower antioxidant capacity compared to all other kombucha products with only 306.2 mg/L TEAC and 121.6 mg/L GAE. Product B was consistently highest for both assays with 842.0 mg/L TEAC and 380 mg/L GAE, showing almost a three-fold higher TEAC compared with F (Figure 7).

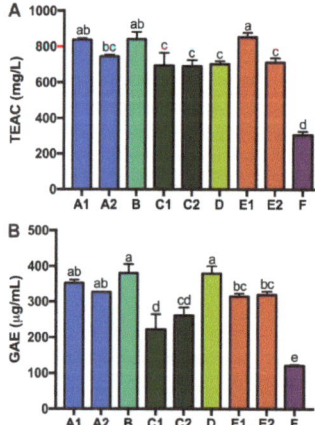

Figure 7. Antioxidant capacity differs across kombucha products. TEAC (**A**) and GAE (**B**) are shown as mean ± SEM (n = 3). Means in a column without a common letter differ; $p < 0.05$.

4. Discussion

Kombucha as a functional food represents a quickly growing sector of the food and beverage industry. Many beverage companies are entering the market and generating new kombucha products with variable fermentation processes and starter ingredients, potentially impacting the chemical and microbial profiles of the final products and thereby their health effects. Here, we selected nine commercial kombucha products and analyzed their microbial and chemical profiles. These nine kombucha products were prepared from green tea (C1, C2), black tea (B) or a mixture of green/black tea (A1, A2, D, E1, E2, K) (Table 1). In addition to different tea bases, these products varied in the addition of probiotics to the kombucha. Our microbial composition analysis demonstrated that in some cases (A1 and F; E2 to a lesser extent) the final kombucha products were dominated by one of these probiotics, *Bacillus coagulans*. *Bacillus coagulans* has many known effects on health and has been commonly added to foods due to its heat resistance [18]. Many studies have reported that acetic acid bacteria were more commonly found in kombucha products than lactic bacteria, with a study of over 100 commercial kombucha starter cultures reporting that *Komagataeibacter* was most prevalent and abundant [1,33–35]. Lactic acid bacteria (primarily *Lactobacillus*) are less commonly used in kombucha fermentation to enhance its biological function or added as probiotics [36]. Our results showed that four out of nine commercial kombucha products (B, C1, C2 and D) were dominated by *Lactobacillus*.

The high abundance of gut-derived microbes such as *E. coli* and *B. thetaiotamicron* in some kombucha samples was surprising given the literature on antimicrobial activities of kombucha, including against *E. coli* [37,38]. However, it has been reported that *E. coli* can survive the kombucha fermentation process in some settings, supporting the possibility that gut microbes could establish a place in kombucha cultures under certain conditions [39]. Our findings that enteric microbes were present in all kombucha products is consistent with at least one previous study which found low levels of gut microbes in kombucha batches after 14 days of fermentation, including *Akkermansiaceae, Bifidobacteriaceae, Enterobacteriaceae*, and *Bacteroidaceae* [40]. The potential for these microbes to have benefit for consumers is exemplified by the high abundance of *Akkermansia muciniphila*, up to 4.3% in one sample of A2. This microbe has been reported in many human and animal model studies to be associated with improved metabolic health, including one randomized clinical trial, and to our knowledge has not been previously shown to exist in any food product [41]. However, since we do not know the absolute count of these enteric bacteria or what fraction remain viable, further investigation is required to determine whether the presence of these enteric bacteria has any health impact. Another limitation is the possibility that there was contamination during the extraction and/or sequencing steps which introduced a signal for enteric bacteria. We did not find evidence of this based upon absence of detected enteric bacteria in a blank extraction control as well as in a sample of unfermented tea base provided by a kombucha manufacturer (other than *B. thetaiotamicron*). In contrast, we observed low abundances of enteric microbes in a sample of unfermented tea base with kombucha starter culture (data not shown).

Consistent with prior studies, we found that *Brettanomyces* was the predominant yeast in five of the kombucha products [35,42]. However, the three other common yeast genera present in kombucha cultures (*Zygosaccharomyces, Lachancea* and *Starmerella*) were largely undetected in the nine kombucha products [35]. Instead, two products and one sample of a third product showed predominance of *Cyberlindnera jadinii*. This yeast is also known as torula and is commonly used in food products. It has been reported once in the literature to be present in kombucha [3]. The remaining two kombucha products had predominance of *Trigonopsis variabilis* or *Issatchenkia orientalis*; the latter has previously been reported in at least one kombucha sample [42].

We further identified large differences in chemical composition across kombucha products both at a global level with untargeted metabolomics and in concentrations of tea polyphenols and antioxidants. The kombucha products could be differentiated by dipeptides and tea-derived chemicals that may reflect differences in the tea base used across the products. We observed significant correlation of global metabolomics profiles with microbial gene content, suggesting that variability in the chemical composition of kombucha products may also be partially attributable to the distinct metabolic capabilities of the microbes present in various kombucha products. This was supported by the associations of many bacterial pathways with specific metabolites in kombucha. One limitation is that the kombucha products varied in their ingredients, energy content, and use of green vs. black tea base which would contribute to the observed differences. The relationships of microbes with chemical composition are likely to be greatly impacted by differences in the fermentation process and tea base across the kombucha products and would require further information on these factors to elucidate. As the samples of each kombucha product were obtained at the same time and were likely manufactured in the same batch, it is also unclear how much variability exists between batches of the same commercial kombucha product.

Antioxidant potential (TEAC) is of great interest to consumers and was found to vary across the nine kombucha products, highly correlated with variation in total tea polyphenols (GAE). However, the tea catechins, known for their antioxidant capability, did not correlate with antioxidant potential and total tea polyphenols. The four tea catechins measured in this study, C, EC, ECG and EGCG, are mainly green tea catechins, which oxidize to theaflavins during black tea production. Theaflavins and catechins provide equal antioxidant potential [43]. It is therefore possible that other tea polyphenols we did not measure, such as theoflavines, theobromines and gallates [44], are important contributors to the total antioxidant capacity. Storage conditions after initial production may have also affected the observed profiles, as it has been recently demonstrated that refrigeration of homemade kombucha for longer than 4 months results in reduced polyphenol content and antioxidant properties [45].

5. Conclusions

Our results demonstrate that commercial kombucha products differ from each other on multiple levels that interest the consumer and are potentially relevant for their health effects, including tea polyphenols, chemical profiles, and microbes.

Supplementary Materials: The following supporting information can be downloaded at: https://www.mdpi.com/article/10.3390/nu14030670/s1, Table S1: Data distributions, Table S2: Spearman correlation between tea catechins, Figure S1: Data distributions shown as boxplots.

Author Contributions: Conceptualization, J.Y. and J.P.J.; methodology, J.Y., V.L., S.M.H., A.I.A., and J.P.J.; formal analysis, J.Y., V.L., P.K. and J.P.J.; investigation, J.Y., V.L., P.K., S.M.H., A.I.A. and J.P.J.; resources, J.P.J.; data curation, J.Y., V.L. and J.P.J.; writing—original draft preparation, J.Y. and J.P.J.; writing—review and editing, J.Y., V.L., P.K., S.M.H., A.I.A. and J.P.J.; visualization, J.Y. and J.P.J.; supervision, J.P.J.; project administration, J.P.J.; funding acquisition, J.P.J. All authors have read and agreed to the published version of the manuscript.

Funding: This research was supported by an unrestricted educational grant provided by GT's Living Foods, Los Angeles, California.

Institutional Review Board Statement: Not applicable.

Informed Consent Statement: Not applicable.

Data Availability Statement: The data presented in this study are available on request from the corresponding author.

Conflicts of Interest: J.P.J. is a member of the Scientific Advisory Board for GT's Living Foods, Los Angeles, California. J.Y., V.L., P.K., S.M.H., and A.I.A. declare no conflict of interest. The funders had no role in the design of the study; in the collection, analyses, or interpretation of data; in the writing of the manuscript, or in the decision to publish the results.

References

1. Kim, J.; Adhikari, K. Current Trends in Kombucha: Marketing Perspectives and the Need for Improved Sensory Research. *Beverages* **2020**, *6*, 15. [CrossRef]
2. Chakravorty, S.; Bhattacharya, S.; Chatzinotas, A.; Chakraborty, W.; Bhattacharya, D.; Gachhui, R. Kombucha tea fermentation: Microbial and biochemical dynamics. *Int. J. Food Microbiol.* **2016**, *220*, 63–72. [CrossRef] [PubMed]
3. Jayabalan, R.; Malbaša, R.V.; Lončar, E.S.; Vitas, J.S.; Sathishkumar, M. A Review on Kombucha Tea—Microbiology, Composition, Fermentation, Beneficial Effects, Toxicity, and Tea Fungus. *Compr. Rev. Food Sci. Food Saf.* **2014**, *13*, 538–550. [CrossRef]
4. Vina, I.; Semjonovs, P.; Linde, R.; Denina, I. Current Evidence on Physiological Activity and Expected Health Effects of Kombucha Fermented Beverage. *J. Med. Food* **2014**, *17*, 179–188. [CrossRef]
5. Mousavi, S.M.; Hashemi, S.A.; Zarei, M.; Gholami, A.; Lai, C.W.; Chiang, W.H.; Omidifar, N.; Bahrani, S.; Mazraedoost, S. Recent Progress in Chemical Composition, Production, and Pharmaceutical Effects of Kombucha Beverage: A Complementary and Alternative Medicine. *Evid.-Based Complement. Altern. Med.* **2020**, *2020*, 4397543. [CrossRef]
6. Yang, D.-J.; Hwang, L.S.; Lin, J.-T. Effects of different steeping methods and storage on caffeine, catechins and gallic acid in bag tea infusions. *J. Chromatogr. A* **2007**, *1156*, 312–320. [CrossRef] [PubMed]
7. Lin, Y.S.; Tsai, Y.J.; Tsay, J.S.; Lin, J.K. Factors affecting the levels of tea polyphenols and caffeine in tea leaves. *J. Agric. Food Chem.* **2003**, *51*, 1864–1873. [CrossRef]
8. Graham, H.N. Green tea composition, consumption, and polyphenol chemistry. *Prev. Med.* **1992**, *21*, 334–350. [CrossRef]
9. Khan, N.; Mukhtar, H. Tea polyphenols for health promotion. *Life Sci.* **2007**, *81*, 519–533. [CrossRef] [PubMed]
10. Khan, N.; Mukhtar, H. Tea Polyphenols in Promotion of Human Health. *Nutrients* **2018**, *11*, 39. [CrossRef] [PubMed]
11. Dufresne, C.; Farnworth, E. Tea, Kombucha, and health: A review. *Food Res. Int.* **2000**, *33*, 409–421. [CrossRef]
12. Lee, K.W.; Lee, H.J.; Lee, C.Y. Antioxidant activity of black tea vs. green tea. *J. Nutr.* **2002**, *132*, 786. [CrossRef] [PubMed]
13. Gramza-Michalowska, A. Caffeine in Tea Camellia Sinensis—Content, Absorption, Benefits and Risks of Consumption. *J. Nutr. Health Aging* **2014**, *18*, 143–149. [CrossRef] [PubMed]
14. Heber, D.; Zhang, Y.J.; Yang, J.P.; Ma, J.E.; Henning, S.M.; Li, Z.P. Green Tea, Black Tea, and Oolong Tea Polyphenols Reduce Visceral Fat and Inflammation in Mice Fed High-Fat, High-Sucrose Obesogenic Diets. *J. Nutr.* **2014**, *144*, 1385–1393. [CrossRef] [PubMed]
15. Chan, E.W.C.; Soh, E.Y.; Tie, P.P.; Law, Y.P. Antioxidant and antibacterial properties of green, black, and herbal teas of Camellia sinensis. *Pharm. Res.* **2011**, *3*, 266–272. [CrossRef]
16. Sengun, I.; Kirmizigul, A. Probiotic Potential of Kombucha. *J. Clin. Gastroenterol.* **2020**, *54*, S28.
17. Vargas, B.K.; Fabricio, M.F.; Ayub, M.A.Z. Health effects and probiotic and prebiotic potential of Kombucha: A bibliometric and systematic review. *Food Biosci.* **2021**, *44*, 101332.
18. Konuray, G.; Erginkaya, Z. Potential Use of Bacillus coagulans in the Food Industry. *Foods* **2018**, *7*, 92. [CrossRef] [PubMed]
19. Blanc, P.J. Characterization of the tea fungus metabolites. *Biotechnol. Lett.* **1996**, *18*, 139–142. [CrossRef]
20. Villarreal-Soto, S.A.; Beaufort, S.; Bouajila, J.; Souchard, J.-P.; Taillandier, P. Understanding Kombucha Tea Fermentation: A Review. *J. Food Sci.* **2018**, *83*, 580–588. [CrossRef] [PubMed]
21. SPINS TOTAL US $ SALES (MULO, CONVENIENCE, NATURAL) L52W ENDING 12.27.20. Available online: https://www.spins.com (accessed on 1 December 2021).
22. Singleton, V.L.; Esau, P. Phenolic substances in grapes and wine, and their significance. *Adv. Food Res. Suppl.* **1969**, *1*, 1–261. [PubMed]
23. Henning, S.M.; Zhang, Y.; Seeram, N.P.; Lee, R.P.; Wang, P.; Bowerman, S.; Heber, D. Antioxidant capacity and phytochemical content of herbs and spices in dry, fresh and blended herb paste form. *Int. J. Food Sci. Nutr.* **2011**, *62*, 219–225. [CrossRef] [PubMed]
24. Beghini, F.; McIver, L.J.; Blanco-Miguez, A.; Dubois, L.; Asnicar, F.; Maharjan, S.; Mailyan, A.; Manghi, P.; Scholz, M.; Thomas, A.M.; et al. Integrating taxonomic, functional, and strain-level profiling of diverse microbial communities with bioBakery 3. *Elife* **2021**, *10*, e65589. [CrossRef] [PubMed]
25. McMurdie, P.J.; Holmes, S. phyloseq: An R package for reproducible interactive analysis and graphics of microbiome census data. *PLoS ONE* **2013**, *8*, e61217. [CrossRef]
26. Walters, W.; Hyde, E.R.; Berg-Lyons, D.; Ackermann, G.; Humphrey, G.; Parada, A.; Gilbert, J.A.; Jansson, J.K.; Caporaso, J.G.; Fuhrman, J.A.; et al. Improved Bacterial 16S rRNA Gene (V4 and V4-5) and Fungal Internal Transcribed Spacer Marker Gene Primers for Microbial Community Surveys. *mSystems* **2016**, *1*, e00009-15. [CrossRef] [PubMed]
27. Nilsson, R.H.; Larsson, K.H.; Taylor, A.F.S.; Bengtsson-Palme, J.; Jeppesen, T.S.; Schigel, D.; Kennedy, P.; Picard, K.; Glockner, F.O.; Tedersoo, L.; et al. The UNITE database for molecular identification of fungi: Handling dark taxa and parallel taxonomic classifications. *Nucleic Acids Res.* **2019**, *47*, D259–D264. [CrossRef] [PubMed]
28. Le Cao, K.A.; Boitard, S.; Besse, P. Sparse PLS discriminant analysis: Biologically relevant feature selection and graphical displays for multiclass problems. *BMC Bioinform.* **2011**, *12*, 253. [CrossRef]
29. Xue, J.; Liu, P.; Guo, G.; Wang, W.; Zhang, J.; Wang, W.; Le, T.; Yin, J.; Ni, D.; Jiang, H. Profiling of dynamic changes in non-volatile metabolites of shaken black tea during the manufacturing process using targeted and non-targeted metabolomics analysis. *LWT* **2022**, *156*, 113010. [CrossRef]

30. Joubert, E. HPLC quantification of the dihydrochalcones, aspalathin and nothofagin in rooibos tea (Aspalathus linearis) as affected by processing. *Food Chem.* **1996**, *55*, 403–411. [CrossRef]
31. Godeau R., P.; Rossi J., C.; Fouraste, I. Methyl-4-formyl-7 cyclopenta(c)pyrane isolated by acid hydrolysis from Viburnum tinus. *Phytochemistry* **1977**, *16*, 604–605. [CrossRef]
32. Barua, N.; Sharma, R.P.; Madhusudanan, K.P.; Thyagarajan, G.; Herz, W. Coumarins in Artemisia Caruifolia. *Phytochemistry* **1980**, *9*, 2.
33. De Roos, J.; De Vuyst, L. Acetic acid bacteria in fermented foods and beverages. *Curr. Opin. Biotechnol.* **2018**, *49*, 115–119. [CrossRef] [PubMed]
34. May, A.; Narayanan, S.; Alcock, J.; Varsani, A.; Maley, C.; Aktipis, A. Kombucha: A novel model system for cooperation and conflict in a complex multi-species microbial ecosystem. *PeerJ* **2019**, *7*, e7565. [CrossRef] [PubMed]
35. Harrison, K.; Curtin, C. Microbial Composition of SCOBY Starter Cultures Used by Commercial Kombucha Brewers in North America. *Microorganisms* **2021**, *9*, 1060. [CrossRef]
36. Nguyen, N.K.; Dong, N.T.; Nguyen, H.T.; Le, P.H. Lactic acid bacteria: Promising supplements for enhancing the biological activities of kombucha. *Springerplus* **2015**, *4*, 91. [CrossRef]
37. Sreeramulu, G.; Zhu, Y.; Knol, W. Kombucha fermentation and its antimicrobial activity. *J. Agric. Food Chem.* **2000**, *48*, 2589–2594. [CrossRef]
38. Bhattacharya, D.; Bhattacharya, S.; Patra, M.M.; Chakravorty, S.; Sarkar, S.; Chakraborty, W.; Koley, H.; Gachhui, R. Antibacterial Activity of Polyphenolic Fraction of Kombucha against Enteric Bacterial Pathogens. *Curr. Microbiol.* **2016**, *73*, 885–896. [CrossRef]
39. Brewer, S.S.; Lowe, C.A.; Beuchat, L.R.; Ortega, Y.R. Survival of Salmonella and Shiga Toxin-Producing Escherichia coli and Changes in Indigenous Microbiota during Fermentation of Home-Brewed Kombucha. *J. Food Prot.* **2021**, *84*, 1366–1373. [CrossRef]
40. Gaggìa, F.; Baffoni, L.; Galiano, M.; Nielsen, D.; Jakobsen, R.; Castro-Mejía, J.; Bosi, S.; Truzzi, F.; Musumeci, F.; Dinelli, G.; et al. Kombucha Beverage from Green, Black and Rooibos Teas: A Comparative Study Looking at Microbiology, Chemistry and Antioxidant Activity. *Nutrients* **2018**, *11*, 1. [CrossRef]
41. Depommier, C.; Everard, A.; Druart, C.; Plovier, H.; Van Hul, M.; Vieira-Silva, S.; Falony, G.; Raes, J.; Maiter, D.; Delzenne, N.M.; et al. Supplementation with Akkermansia muciniphila in overweight and obese human volunteers: A proof-of-concept exploratory study. *Nat. Med.* **2019**, *25*, 1096–1103. [CrossRef]
42. Mayser, P.; Fromme, S.; Leitzmann, C.; Grunder, K. The yeast spectrum of the 'tea fungus Kombucha'. *Mycoses* **1995**, *38*, 289–295. [CrossRef] [PubMed]
43. Leung, L.K.; Su, Y.; Chen, R.; Zhang, Z.; Huang, Y.; Chen, Z.Y. Theaflavins in black tea and catechins in green tea are equally effective antioxidants. *J. Nutr.* **2001**, *131*, 2248–2251. [CrossRef] [PubMed]
44. Dutta, H.; Paul, S.K. *Kombucha Drink: Production, Quality, and Safety Aspects*; Elsevier: Amsterdam, The Netherlands, 2019; pp. 259–288. [CrossRef]
45. La Torre, C.; Fazio, A.; Caputo, P.; Plastina, P.; Caroleo, M.C.; Cannataro, R.; Cione, E. Effects of Long-Term Storage on Radical Scavenging Properties and Phenolic Content of Kombucha from Black Tea. *Molecules* **2021**, *26*, 5474. [CrossRef] [PubMed]

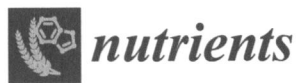

Review

A Review of the Health Benefits of Food Enriched with Kynurenic Acid

Monika Turska [1,*], Piotr Paluszkiewicz [2], Waldemar A. Turski [3] and Jolanta Parada-Turska [4]

1. Department of Molecular Biology, The John Paul II Catholic University of Lublin, 20-708 Lublin, Poland
2. Department of General, Oncological and Metabolic Surgery, Institute of Hematology and Transfusion Medicine, 02-778 Warsaw, Poland
3. Department of Experimental and Clinical Pharmacology, Medical University of Lublin, 20-090 Lublin, Poland
4. Department of Rheumatology and Connective Tissue Diseases, Medical University of Lublin, 20-090 Lublin, Poland
* Correspondence: turskamk@gmail.com

Abstract: Kynurenic acid (KYNA), a metabolite of tryptophan, is an endogenous substance produced intracellularly by various human cells. In addition, KYNA can be synthesized by the gut microbiome and delivered in food. However, its content in food is very low and the total alimentary supply with food accounts for only 1–3% of daily KYNA excretion. The only known exception is chestnut honey, which has a higher KYNA content than other foods by at least two orders of magnitude. KYNA is readily absorbed from the gastrointestinal tract; it is not metabolized and is excreted mainly in urine. It possesses well-defined molecular targets, which allows the study and elucidation of KYNA's role in various pathological conditions. Following a period of fascination with KYNA's importance for the central nervous system, research into its role in the peripheral system has been expanding rapidly in recent years, bringing some exciting discoveries. KYNA does not penetrate from the peripheral circulation into the brain; hence, the following review summarizes knowledge on the peripheral consequences of KYNA administration, presents data on KYNA content in food products, in the context of its daily supply in diets, and systematizes the available pharmacokinetic data. Finally, it provides an analysis of the rationale behind enriching foods with KYNA for health-promoting effects.

Keywords: food; food analysis; food ingredients; infant formula; kynurenic acid; nutrition

1. Introduction

In 2013, we published a review paper describing the potential role of kynurenic acid (KYNA) in the digestive system. It summarized the presence of KYNA in the lumen of the gastrointestinal tract, and its beneficial health effects in digestive diseases, as well as its presence in food, were summarized. At that time, we pointed out many gaps in the knowledge and understanding of KYNA's effects outside the central nervous system. However, even then, we assumed that KYNA administration might have some therapeutic potential and, despite many knowledge gaps, we envisaged the relevance of its supplementation [1]. KYNA is a metabolite of tryptophan. It is synthesized endogenously in human and animal bodies and/or absorbed from the digestive system. Although KYNA's deficiency symptoms have not been described to date, it is reasonable to investigate the benefits of its supplementation. Nowadays, after 10 years of unprecedented progress in the research on KYNA, we can deliberate whether it is legitimate to supplement our diet with KYNA. The current review focuses on the presence of KYNA in food, including estimations of the daily dietary intake of KYNA, its absorption, distribution, and excretion, and it summarizes the scientifically approved health benefits of KYNA administered via the alimentary route, which are not limited to the digestive system.

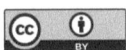

2. Molecular Targets of Kynurenic Acid

Over 40 years of research, several molecular targets on which KYNA acts have been identified (Figure 1). Further research is ongoing and it was recently proposed that KYNA may be a ligand for the hydroxycarboxylic acid receptor 3 (HCAR3) and adrenoceptor alpha-2B (ADRA2B) [2]. However, no direct evidence is available yet to support this hypothesis.

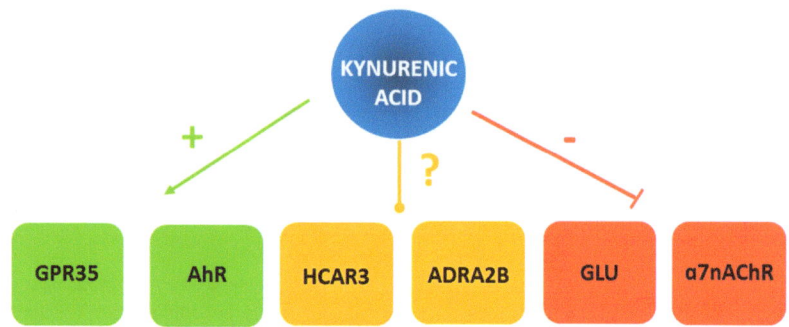

Figure 1. Graphical presentation of molecular targets of kynurenic acid. ADRA2B—adrenoceptor alpha 2B; AhR—aryl hydrocarbon receptor; GPR35—G protein-coupled receptor 35; GLU—glutamate receptor group; HCAR3—hydroxycarboxylic acid receptor 3; α7nAChR—alpha-7 nicotinic acetylcholine receptor; (+)—agonist; (−) antagonist; (?)—putative ligand.

Glutamatergic receptors occur preferentially in the brain, and since KYNA does not cross the blood–brain barrier, their importance is not discussed in the context of alimentary supplementation. Data on this subject can be found in recent review publications [3]. Whether and how KYNA acts on the alpha-7 nicotinic receptor (α7nAChR) is still a matter of scientific debate [4]. Therefore, the effect of KYNA on the aryl hydrocarbon receptor (AhR) and the G protein-coupled receptor 35 (GPR35), which are abundant in peripheral tissues, is of greatest concern. It should, however, be noted that AhR is an intracellular receptor, and so far, no uptake of KYNA has been demonstrated. Thus, it is uncertain whether exogenously administered KYNA can effectively influence these receptors. In this context, studies on KYNA's peripheral activity have focused mostly on its agonistic action on GPR35. It is worth noting that these receptors are particularly densely represented on both the immune cells and cells of the gastrointestinal tract mucosa [5,6].

GPR35 is a rhodopsin-like, 7-transmembrane class A G-protein coupled receptor firstly described in 1998 by O'Dowd et al. [7]. GPR35 gene transcript in humans can be alternatively spliced into variants GPR35a and GPR35b containing 309 and 340 aminoacids, respectively. The differences between these two variants were limited to GPR35 extracellular domain [8]. Six of seventy described single nucleotide polymorphisms in GPR35 gene were indicated as risk variants for inflammatory bowel disease, ankylosing spondylitis, psoriasis, lupus erythematosus, and primary sclerosing cholangitis [9].

Activation of GPR35 by endogenous ligands such as KYNA, lysophosphatidic acid (LPA), or mucosal chemokine CXCL17 resulted in internalization of GPR35 and activation of ERK and Rho phosphorylation signaling pathway. A basal activity of GPR35 was connected with Na/K-ATPase pump and induction of Src signaling in epithelial cells responsible for cell proliferation and neovascularization. Moreover, the presence and high expression of GPR35 in intestine together with high concentration of KYNA in its lumen, GPR35 coexpression with both cholecystokinin GPR65 receptor suggest that GPR35 may be a part of the gut-brain signal axis regulating energy balance [10].

3. Absorption of Kynurenic Acid from the Digestive Tract

3.1. Human Studies

The absorption of KYNA from the digestive tract in humans was demonstrated by Kaihara et al. (1956) and by Turska et al. (2019) [11,12]. In the study by Kaihara et al. (1956), synthetic KYNA was suspended in water and ingested by three human subjects. Different doses of KYNA were administered, i.e., 164, 410, and 820 µmole (equivalent to 31, 77.5, and 155 mg, respectively). The urinary excretion of KYNA was measured the day before and on days 1, 2, and 3 after KYNA ingestion. It was found that KYNA administration resulted in its enhanced excretion, especially on the first days after administration [12], which proves that KYNA is absorbed from the digestive tract after its oral ingestion. In the study by Turska et al. (2019), chestnut honey containing KYNA in an amount of 600 µg/g [13] was used. Honey was dissolved in water with a ratio of 1:1 (w:v). Then, 200 mL of the obtained solution was consumed over a 5 min period by both male and female healthy volunteers. All study participants refrained from eating any food and drank only mineral water for 6 h before the study. Venous blood samples were drawn from a peripheral venous catheter at specified times after the administration of the honey beverage: baseline (0), 15, 30, 60, 90, and 120 min. It was found that the mean KYNA concentration in the serum before the administration of chestnut honey was 0.052 ± 0.004 µM and 0.051 ± 0.014 µM in men and women, respectively. Thirty minutes after the ingestion of chestnut honey dissolved in water, the content of KYNA reached its maximum value of 237% and 308% vs. control in men and women, respectively, which proves that KYNA is absorbed from the digestive tract after its oral administration in food. Notably, after 2 h, the level of KYNA was almost back to normal [11].

3.2. Animal Studies

The absorption of KYNA from the digestive tract in animals was demonstrated by Kaihara et al. (1956) and by Turska et al. (2018) [12,14]. In the study by Kaihara et al. (1956), KYNA was suspended in water and administered to rats by a stomach tube at the dose of 164 µmole (equivalent to 31 mg). The measurement of the urinary excretion of KYNA was performed on the day before and on days 1, 2, and 3 after KYNA application. It was found that intragastric KYNA administration resulted in its enhanced excretion [12], which proves that KYNA is absorbed from the digestive tract after its alimentary administration in rats. In the study by Turska et al. (2018), labeled 5,7-^{3}H-KYNA was dissolved in saline (1 mCi/mL) and administered intragastrically by oral gavage in a volume of 1 mL per 100 g of adult male Swiss mice body weight. Urine, blood, and tissue samples were collected 1, 3, 6, 12, and 24 h after KYNA administration. It was found that labeled KYNA was present in the blood, the spleen, and the liver, as well as in urine [14], proving that KYNA is absorbed from the digestive tract after its intragastric administration in mice.

KYNA administered orally or intragastrically is rapidly absorbed and is present in peripheral blood plasma several minutes after ingestion. The absorption dynamics suggest simple transmission of KYNA in the upper gastrointestinal tract.

4. Distribution of Kynurenic Acid

4.1. Human Studies

KYNA content in human tissues is shown in Figure 2, presented in Tables S1 and S2 in the Supplementary Materials, and described separately in the respective subsections below.

4.1.1. Serum

The presence of KYNA in human blood serum has been repeatedly reported (Table S1). The content of KYNA in the serum obtained from adult healthy humans ranges from 0.016 to 0.071 µM and is within the same limits in the serum obtained from children [15–25].

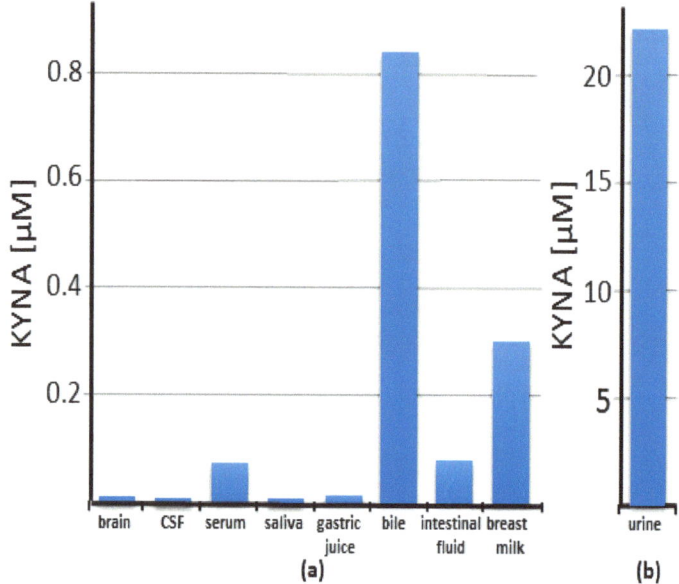

Figure 2. Content of kynurenic acid (KYNA) in human brain and body fluids. Note that the scale on panel (**b**) is 25 times larger than on panel (**a**). CSF—cerebrospinal fluid.

4.1.2. Saliva

The presence of KYNA in human saliva was disclosed by Kuc et al. (2006). In this study, the unstimulated saliva was collected from male adults who refrained from eating, drinking, smoking, and oral hygiene for 2 h before the collection. The presence of KYNA was evidenced in all these saliva samples. The mean concentration of KYNA in the saliva obtained from healthy subjects was 0.0034 μM [26] (Figure 2a).

4.1.3. Gastric Juice

The presence of KYNA in human gastric juice was reported by Paluszkiewicz et al. (2009). Included in this study were 23 adults (15 women and 8 men, mean age: 58 years) who were candidates for nonsteroid anti-inflammatory drugs therapy due to complaints of pain in the course of discopathia and arthrosis. Patients with signs of chronic gastrointestinal disorders or who had proton pump inhibitors were excluded. Upper gastrointestinal endoscopy was performed after 12 h of fasting. Gastric juice was aspirated via the suction channel. The presence of KYNA was determined in all these gastric juice samples. The mean KYNA content was 0.0099 μM. The level of KYNA was neither gender- nor age-dependent [27] (Figure 2a).

4.1.4. Bile

The presence of KYNA in human bile was disclosed by Paluszkiewicz et al. (2009). In this study, bile was obtained from patients with uncomplicated cholecystolithiasis. The group of 18 patients (12 women and 6 men, mean age: 55 years) underwent elective cholecystectomy due to bile stones localized in the gallbladder with uneventful outcomes. The bile samples were obtained extracorporally from the removed gallbladder. The presence of KYNA was determined in all these gallbladder and hepatic bile samples. The mean concentrations of KYNA in the bile obtained from patients with uncomplicated cholecystolithiasis and obstructive jaundice were 0.833 and 0.307 μM, respectively [27] (Figure 2a).

4.1.5. Intestinal Fluid

The presence of KYNA in the human intestinal fluid was reported by Walczak et al. (2011). In this study, 30 ambulatory adult patients scheduled for elective colonoscopy were enrolled. All patients underwent endoscopy after standard bowel cleansing with macrogol. The participants received a single dose of atropine sulphate immediately before the colonoscopy. The colonoscopies were performed under sedation using propofol. The samples (1–2 mL of mucus) were aspirated from the cecum or from the proximal part of the ascending colon. KYNA was detected in all samples obtained from the group of patients without pathological changes in the intestine. Its mean concentration was 0.0822 µM [28] (Figure 2a).

4.1.6. Synovial Fluid

Under physiological conditions, the amount of synovial fluid is too small to be collected for reliable testing. Therefore, the presence of KYNA was detected in the samples of synovial fluid obtained from patients with rheumatoid arthritis, inflammatory spondyloarthropathies, and osteoarthritis, with mean values of 0.0189, 0.0215, and 0.0305 µM, respectively [29].

4.1.7. Sweat

KYNA was detected in sweat samples. Since the density of sweat is very variable, the content of KYNA in sweat was expressed in relation to the sodium content. Two sampling methods were used: an absorbent patch was fixed to the skin for the entire exercise period, or sweat was absorbed at the end of this period by cotton ear tips. In nontrained subjects, the content of KYNA was 14.80 and 8.16 fmol/µg Na, respectively [30].

4.1.8. Cerebrospinal Fluid

The presence of KYNA in human cerebrospinal fluid has been repeatedly reported (Table S2). The content of KYNA in cerebrospinal fluid obtained from adult healthy humans ranges from 0.0009 to 0.005 µM [16,20,21,31–37]. The content of KYNA in cerebrospinal fluid obtained from children is within the same limits [38].

4.1.9. Brain

The presence of KYNA in human brain tissue was unequivocally proved by Turski and Schwarcz (1988) [39]. Shortly thereafter, this finding was supported by Moroni et al. (1988), by Connick et al. (1989), and by Swartz et al. (1990) [37,40,41]. In the study by Turski and Schwarcz (1988), human brain tissue was obtained *post mortem* from male subjects (age range: 50–71 years). KYNA was found in all studied brain samples. In this study, the content of KYNA in the human brain varied from 0.14 to 1.58 pmol/mg wet weight tissue (approximately 0.00014–0.00158 µM) in the cerebellum and the caudate nucleus, respectively [39]. Moroni et al. (1988) reported KYNA concentration in human cortex amounting to 0.15 pmol/mg wet weight tissue (approximately 0.00015 µM) [41]. In the study by Swartz et al. (1990), the content of KYNA in human cerebral cortex expressed per proteins amounted to 2.07 pmol/mg protein in the cerebral cortex, and to 3.38 pmol/mg protein in the putamen [37]. A similar range of KYNA content was reported by Baran et al. (2000) in the frontal cortex and the cerebellum, by Schwarcz et al. (2001) in the Brodmann area 9, 10, and 19, and by Baran et al. (2012) in the control frontal cortex and the cerebellum [42–44].

4.1.10. Other Organs

There are no data on the content of KYNA in human tissues other than the brain. Our previous review paper presented the content of KYNA in various tissues and organs of rats [1].

4.1.11. Breast Milk

The presence of KYNA in human milk was reported by O'Rourke et al. (2018) and by Milart et al. (2021) [45,46] (Figure 2a). In the paper by O'Rourke et al. (2018), 12 lactating mothers with term babies (>38 weeks) successfully completed the study. Two specimens of hindmilk were collected from all mothers postpartum, on day 7 and day 14 from their homes. The milk samples were manually expressed into sterile polypropylene containers and kept in the fridge until their collection by the researcher. At the laboratory, all samples were stored initially at $-20\ °C$ and then at $-80\ °C$ until assayed. It was found that the KYNA levels in breast milk were 0.057 and 0.221 μM on day 7 and day 14, respectively [45]. In the study by Milart et al. (2021), breast milk was obtained from 25 healthy breastfeeding women during the first 6 months after labor. The milk samples were collected six times: on day 3 and day 7, at week 2, and in the 1st, 3rd, 4th, 5th, and 6th months after the delivery. The women were instructed on how to collect their breast milk. The samples of human breast hindmilk, after the first breastfeeding of the day, were collected by means of breast pumps, in the amount of 5 mL, to plastic containers and stored in a fridge for no longer than 3 h. Then, placed in human tissue transport boxes, they were delivered to the laboratory, and transferred to glass sterile probes and stored. KYNA was found in all tested samples of human breast milk. The concentration of KYNA increased gradually from 0.021 μM on day 3 to 0.299 μM in the 6th month of breastfeeding [46].

4.1.12. Urine

The presence of KYNA in human urine obtained from adults and children has been repeatedly reported [47–62] (Figure 2b) (Table S3). The urine concentration of KYNA ranges between 4.04 and 22.18 μM in adults. Its concentration in children's urine, as reported by Uberos et al., is 74.07 and 93.12 μM at night- and daytime, respectively [59].

4.2. Animal Studies

4.2.1. Distribution of Kynurenic Acid Administered via the Alimentary Route

The detailed distribution pattern of KYNA after its administration via the alimentary route came from an animal study by Turska et al. (2018). In this study, labeled 5,7-^{3}H-KYNA was used. Adult male mice were fasted for 12 h before KYNA administration. KYNA dissolved in saline was applied intragastrically by oral gavage in a volume of 1 mL per 100 g of body weight. Urine, blood, and tissue samples were collected 1, 3, 6, 12, and 24 h after KYNA administration and radioactivity was analyzed. It was found that labeled KYNA was present in various parts of the digestive tract: the highest amounts were found in the stomach and the ileum, and lower in the cecum. An unexpectedly high amount of radioactivity was recorded in the intestinal content of the cecum, whereas no accumulation of KYNA was found in internal organs. As can be expected, as early as 1 h after labeled KYNA administration, a very high amount of radioactivity was found in urine [14].

4.2.2. Blood–Brain Barrier

There is a consensus that KYNA does not cross, or only poorly crosses, the blood–brain barrier under normal conditions [63–65]. Thus, it is not expected that KYNA administered orally can be distributed into the brain.

4.2.3. Blood–Placental Barrier

KYNA does not cross the placental barrier between the mother and the fetus, as evidenced in the pregnant mice by Goeden et al. [66]. KYNA (10 mg/kg) was administered orally on embryonic day 18. Although a slight but nonsignificant elevation of KYNA was noted, the final conclusion of the study was as follows: "no increase in KYNA levels was observed in the fetal plasma and brain after KYNA itself was given maternally, indicating that peripherally applied KYNA does not cross the placenta". According to this statement, it is not to be expected that KYNA administered orally can be distributed into the fetus. Independently of the placental barrier function, the concentration of KYNA as high as

1.13 µM in last-trimester amniotic fluid was reported [23]. Amniotic fluid surrounded the fetus and filled the fetal respiratory and digestive lumen during pregnancy. This phenomenon indicated that fetal production of KYNA was initiated independently of the mother's plasma concentration.

The tissue distribution of KYNA is organ- and system-selective. After peak concentration in blood plasma after ingestion, the highest concentration of KYNA was observed in bile, pancreatic juice, and intestinal lumen, gradually increasing along the intestine. Moreover, the elevation of KYNA administered by digestive route was not recorded in central nervous system and fetus. These findings indicate tight blood–brain and blood–placental barriers for KYNA administered by digestive route in normal conditions. It is thought-provoking that KYNA concentration in milk obtained from breastfeeding mothers gradually increases along breastfeeding time after delivery. This phenomenon suggests specific regulation of KYNA synthesis or excretion in breast tissue; however, data describing such mechanisms were not available to date.

5. Metabolism of Kynurenic Acid

5.1. Human Studies

Despite some previous research indicating that KYNA might be metabolized to quinaldic acid, it is widely accepted that KYNA is excreted unmetabolized. In 1955, Brown and Price reported the presence of quinaldic acid in amounts of 4.6–6.9 µmol/day in human urine. Moreover, it was found that after the ingestion of tryptophan (39.2 mmol), the content of urine quinaldic acid rose to 45 µmol/day in humans [67]. In 1956, Kaihara et al. showed that the ingestion of KYNA (164–820 µmol) resulted in a 4–8-fold increase in the quinaldic acid content in human urine [12].

5.2. Animal Studies

In 1955, Brown and Price reported the presence of quinaldic acid in amounts of 19 µmol in dog urine. Importantly, it was found that after tryptophan (9.8 mmole) ingestion, the content of urine quinaldic acid rose to 96 µmole in dogs. In cats and rats, the content of quinaldic acid was not confirmed [67]. In the study by Kaihara et al. (1956), KYNA was suspended in water and administered to rats by a stomach tube at the dose of 164 µmol (equivalent to 31 mg). It was found that KYNA administration resulted in enhanced excretion of quinaldic acid, which suggests that KYNA is metabolized to quinaldic acid after its alimentary administration [12]. On the other hand, in the study performed by Turski and Schwarcz (1988), labeled ^{3}H-KYNA was used. Male adult rats were chronically implanted with a unilateral guide cannula, directed towards the dorsal hippocampus. Seven days after the surgery, intrahippocampal injections of the labeled KYNA were made in unanesthetized rats via an injection cannula. Brain and urine samples were obtained from the same animals. Urine was collected over a period of 30 or 120 min after completion of the intrahippocampal injection. A careful chromatographic analysis failed to reveal the presence of any metabolic product of KYNA, including quinolinic acid, in either the hippocampus or urine [68].

It is generally accepted that KYNA, despite its biologically receptor-related activity, is not metabolized and is described as an end product in tryptophan kynurenine pathway. To date, any metabolic route of KYNA inactivation in studied biological systems has not been identified.

6. Excretion of Kynurenic Acid

6.1. Human Studies

6.1.1. Urine

The excretion of KYNA in human urine has been repeatedly reported [47–62] (Table S3). It can be concluded that the excretion of KYNA in urine ranges from 1.14 to 6.29 mg/day/adult person. According to Uberos et al. (2010), in children, the urinary excretion of KYNA is even higher, ranging from 14.0–17.6 mg/day/person [59]. In another study performed by Molina-Carballo et al. (2021) on children aged 5–14 years, KYNA was found to be 5–7 μg per mg creatinine [60]. After mathematical conversion, the amount of the excreted KYNA can be estimated at the level of 2.64–3.30 mg/day/child. However, it must be considered that these are only two reports and that more detailed studies involving children of different ages are needed before any final conclusions can be drawn.

6.1.2. Feces

The presence of KYNA in the feces of adult humans was evidenced by Dong et al. (2020). In this study, the median and mean content of KYNA was 7.39 and 9.74 nmol/g, respectively. The range was wide, from 0.42 to 29.24 nmol/g [69]. A similar concentration of KYNA, 12.4 nmol/g, was reported in the feces of children by Shestopalov et al. (2020) [25]. Based on these results and an assumption that humans excrete an average of 128 g of fresh feces per person per day [70], it can be calculated that the excretion of KYNA in feces is approximately 0.18–0.23 mg/day/person (Table 1).

Table 1. Estimation of daily excretion of kynurenic acid (KYNA) by adult human.

	KYNA Excretion	
	Minimal Level (mg/day)	Maximal Level (mg/day)
Urine	1.14	6.29
Feces	0.010	0.707
Sweat	0.00069	0.00503
Total	1.15	7.00

See body text for references. Calculations of mean KYNA excretion in urine based on data presented in detail in Table S3.

6.1.3. Sweat

Saran et al. (2021) reported that the content of KYNA in sweat ranged between 8.16 and 14.80 fmol/μg Na^+ [30]. Based on these data and an assumption that humans produce 0.5–2 L of sweat/day [71] and excrete Na^+ in the amount of 0.9 g/L [72], we calculated that the excretion of KYNA in sweat approximated 0.00069–0.00503 mg (Table 1).

6.1.4. Total Daily Excretion of Kynurenic Acid

The loss of KYNA in urine, feces, and sweat was taken into account in the estimation of the total excretion of KYNA (Table 1). The amount of KYNA excreted into the intestinal lumen as gastric juice, bile, and intestinal fluid was not considered separately, because KYNA can be absorbed from the gastrointestinal tract and, even if not all, the unabsorbed KYNA is excreted in the feces. All calculations were performed based on data from publications cited in appropriate sections of the paper. The results of our analyses are presented in Table 1. It can be concluded that the total estimated excretion of KYNA amounts to 1.15–7.0 mg/day/adult person. Most of that, 90–99% is excreted in urine. Feces account for 0.9–10% of KYNA excretion. The amount of KYNA removed in sweat is marginal, less than 0.1% (Table 1).

All available data indicate that KYNA is eliminated in unchanged form by bile, pancreatic juice, and urine. The elimination is observed rapidly after digestive absorption, which confirms that KYNA is only temporarily stored in tissues without any evidence of its accumulation.

7. Kynurenic Acid in Food

7.1. Human Food

It has been repeatedly shown that KYNA is a natural component of food. Its content in food and food products varies within a wide range of concentrations, from trace amounts up to 2 mg/gram of chestnut honey [73–80] (Figure 3; Table S4).

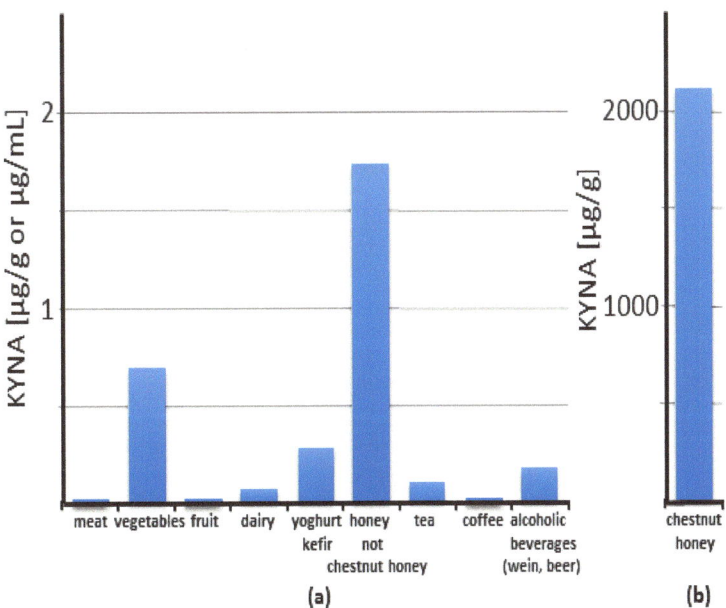

Figure 3. Content of kynurenic acid (KYNA) in food categories: an overview. The columns reflect the value of the highest reported content of KYNA in each category. Note that the scale on panel (**b**) is 1000 times larger than on panel (**a**).

7.1.1. Meat

It can be stated that the content of KYNA in meat is low: 0.0014, 0.0031, and 0.0037 µg/g wet weight in beef, pork, and fish, respectively. Even pig liver contains only slightly more KYNA—0.0091 µg/g wet weight. Since KYNA is rapidly excreted from the animal's body (see Chapter 6), it does not seem possible to easily increase its amount in meat.

7.1.2. Vegetables

Vegetables are a richer source of KYNA (Figure 3; Table S4). Cauliflower, potato, and broccoli are some of the richest sources, containing KYNA in amounts of 0.0473, 0.1301, and 0.4184 µg/g wet weight, respectively [73]. However, it should be noted that large differences between varieties exist. The comparison of 16 different edible potato varieties grown under similar soil and climatic conditions showed up to 10-fold differences in KYNA content, from 0.04 to 0.65 µg/g wet weight [76]. Similarly, the comparison of yellow- and purple-fleshed potato cultivar Ismena and Provita revealed a threefold difference in KYNA content, 0.226 and 0.683 µg/g wet weight, respectively [81]. The origin of KYNA in plants is poorly understood. Both its synthesis from kynurenine and the absorption of KYNA from the soil were presented [82]. Since KYNA is found in the soil in varying amounts, and in extraordinary large amounts in manure [82], its content in the plant may depend on the site and cultivation method. This may also be the reason for significant differences in KYNA content even in the same type of vegetable. At the same time, it provides an opportunity to increase KYNA content in the plant by appropriate fertilization.

7.1.3. Fruit

The only fruit that has been studied is the apple, which contained 0.0023 µg of KYNA/g wet weight (Table S4) [73].

7.1.4. Spices and Herbs for Cooking

KYNA content in spices and herbs for cooking was determined in 19 different products (Table S4). The highest amount of KYNA was found in basil and thyme, 14.08 and 8.87 µg/g wet weight, respectively [77]. The numbers seem to be relatively high in comparison to plants. However, it must be stressed that, generally, commercially marketable spices are dried. Therefore, it is hard to accurately compare the concentration of KYNA in spices and fresh plants.

7.1.5. Honey

Unexpectedly, honey and other bee products contain relatively large amounts of KYNA (Figure 3; Table S4). An extremely high amount of KYNA was found in chestnut honey, up to 2114.9 µg/g [74]. Interestingly, this applies to chestnut honey obtained from different locations in Europe and Korea [13,74,80]. This is a phenomenon even among other types of honey. KYNA content in popular honey such as sunflower, multiflorous, buckwheat, acacia, and linden honey is 1.73, 0.877, 0.33, 0.181, and 0.179 µg/g, respectively. A high level of KYNA in chestnut honey seems to be related to the high KYNA content in male flowers of the chestnut tree [13].

7.1.6. Dairy

In commercially available dairy products, the content of KYNA is as follows: cow's milk: 0.017 µg/mL, kefir: 0.2417 µg/mL, yoghurt: 0.2868 µg/mL, white cheese: 0.0766 µg/g, and hard cheese: 0.0084 [42,49] (Figure 3; Table S4) [73,78].

7.1.7. Fermented Food and Beverages

A relatively high KYNA content was found in fermented food products (Figure 3; Table S4). It was found in kefir and yoghurt in amounts of up to 0.242 and 0.287 µg/mL, respectively [73,78]. In addition, cocoa powder contains KYNA in the amount of 4.486 µg/g [78]. Interestingly, the alcoholic beverages wine and beer contain KYNA in a broad range of concentrations, up to 0.179 and 0.051 µg/mL, respectively [11,78,79]. These results indicate that the fermenting microorganisms produce KYNA and that this process may significantly increase the KYNA content in food and beverages.

7.1.8. Medicinal Herbs and Supplements

The presence of KYNA has been demonstrated in medicinal herbs and supplements (Table S5). The highest content expressed on a dry weight basis of the herbs was found in leaves of peppermint, nettle, birch, and horsetail, ranging from 2.27 to 3.82 µg/g dry weight [83]. The intake of KYNA in herbal infusions prepared according to manufacturer's instructions were found to vary from 1.08 µg/day in the nettle root infusion to 32.5 and 32.6 µg/day in the nettle leaf and St. John's wort infusion, respectively. Herbal supplements in the form of tablets also contain KYNA. KYNA delivery calculated in a maximum recommended dose of the supplement equals from 0.41 to 30.38 µg/g in chamomile and St. John's wort tablets, respectively [82].

7.1.9. Baby Food

KYNA was found in human milk [45,46,73] (Table S6). Interestingly, the content of KYNA in human milk increases more than 14 times during the time of breastfeeding, starting from 0.004 µg/mL on day 3 after labor and reaching a value of 0.057 µg/mL in the 6th month of feeding [46]. KYNA was also found in all 46 artificial baby milk formulas studied. However, in comparison with human milk, in which its content naturally changed over time, the concentration of KYNA in artificial formulas was substantially lower and did not follow its physiological dynamics of changes [46]. In first-food formulas, KYNA content is clearly higher in products containing vegetables (0.0056–0.0148 µg/g) than in meat-based food (0.01 µg/g). In fruit and vegetable juice, its concentration is 0.0019 µg/g [73]. It should be noted that this estimation is based on single measurement results only, which are insufficient to draw definite conclusions.

7.2. Animal Food

The presence of KYNA was studied in animal feed for livestock, cats, dogs, and fish. It was shown that KYNA is present in animal feed in varying concentrations. The highest concentration of KYNA was found in feed for livestock, where it varied from 0.198 µg/g fresh weight to 0.414 µg/g fresh weight. Based on the measurement of KYNA content in feed ingredients, the authors concluded that the concentration of KYNA in animal feed was not controlled and deliberately set, but its final content depended on the ingredients used [84].

8. Kynurenic Acid Supplementation
8.1. Health Effects of Kynurenic Acid Supplementation

Since KYNA is formed endogenously in the body and can also be supplied in food, the question about the relevance of its supplementation is legitimate. No human studies devoted to health effects of exogenously administered KYNA have been conducted to date. An exception is a study in which a solution of chestnut honey was administered to young volunteers and pharmacokinetic parameters of KYNA were determined afterwards. No side effects were reported in this study [11]. Indirectly, the lack of KYNA toxicity can be inferred from studies in which tryptophan was administered to humans. It was found that tryptophan load resulted in an increase in kynurenines, including KYNA, in the blood. Very recently, Sathyasaikumar et al. (2022) reported no serious adverse events and no long-term changes in behavior and health in tryptophan-treated humans who had plasma KYNA levels that increased as much as 145-fold compared to pre-tryptophan values [85].

Further conclusions should be drawn based on the data obtained from studies on rodents. The data search performed showed that there are few publications describing KYNA administration via the alimentary route for the period lasting from 3 days to 2 months (Table 2).

Table 2. Consequences of kynurenic acid (KYNA) dietary supplementation in rodents.

Species	KYNA Treatment (Dose, Schedule)	Effect/Properties	Reference
Adult animals			
Rats, mice	25 or 250 mg/L in drinking water for 3–21 days	• Body weight gain/no effect. • Body composition/no effect.	[86]
Mice	2.5, 25, or 250 mg/L in drinking water for 3, 7, 14, 28 days	Activity of peripheral blood leukocytes in vitro/immunomodulation; antioxidant properties.	[87]
Mice	2.5, 25, or 250 mg/L in drinking water for 7–14 days	• Hematological parameters/no effect. • Splenocytes in vitro/immunomodulatory effect on cytokine production.	[88]
Spontaneously hypertensive rats	25 mg/kg/day in drinking water for 3 weeks	• Heart rate/decrease. • Mean arterial pressure/no effect.	[89]

Table 2. *Cont.*

Species	KYNA Treatment (Dose, Schedule)	Effect/Properties	Reference
Mice	5 mg/kg/day, intragastric; once a day for 8 weeks	High-fat diet induced: • Increase of body weight gain/reduction. • Increase of daily energy intake/reduction. • Increase of serum triglyceride/decrease. • Decrease of serum high-density lipoprotein cholesterol/increase. • Increase of serum low-density lipoprotein cholesterol/inhibition. • Coronary artery risk index/reduction. • Atherosclerosis index/reduction. • Increase of the ratio of Firmicutes to Bacteroidetes/suppression.	[90]
Young animals			
Rats	25 or 250 mg/L in drinking water; from PND 1 to PND 60	• Body weight gain/attenuation. • Skeleton development/no effect on bone densitometry and biomechanical endurance.	[91]
Rats	250 mg/L in drinking water; from PND 1 to PND 21	• Body weight gain/attenuation. • Bone mineral density/no effect. • Morphological changes in jejunum/increase in both intestinal surface absorption area and mucosa thickness.	[46]
Rats	25 mg/L in drinking water; from PND 21 until 9th week of life	• Open field and locomotor activity tests/no effect. • Memory tests/no effect. • Depressive and anxiety tests/no effect. • Kynurenic acid content in blood and brain/no effect. • Kynurenine aminotransferases activity in brain tissue/no effect.	[92]

Because KYNA is water-soluble, it was administered in drinking water in most studies. This mode of administration is very convenient because it does not cause stress to the animal. In addition, water was available ad libitum, which allowed KYNA to be taken in the most natural way according to the daily pattern of drinking. The concentrations used ranged from 2.5 to 250 mg/L, approximating a dose of 0.25 to 25 mg/kg of KYNA per 1 kg body weight/day, respectively. Studies have been conducted on both young and adult animals. Generally, no toxic effects of KYNA administration have been reported. When administered to young animals, KYNA did not interfere with their overall growth and development. However, a moderate reduction in the rate of weight gain was observed. This effect was evident in young, but not adult, animals. On the other hand, the reduction of weight gain rate was present in adult rats kept on a high-fat diet (Table 2). These observations allowed for hypothesizing antiobesogenic properties of KYNA during early development [46]. Interestingly, KYNA has been found to stimulate intestinal mucosal growth in young rats and to cause, inter alia, an increase in the intestinal surface area. However, this affects neither the body composition nor bone mineralization and endurance capacity (Table 2). Importantly, the supplementation of KYNA in drinking water to developing rats for 2 months did not impair their brain functions measured in adulthood [92].

In healthy adult mice, the alimentary administration of KYNA did not affect blood hematological parameters. However, experiments performed in vitro on leukocytes and splenocytes obtained from drug supplemented animals revealed that KYNA exerted antioxidant and immunomodulatory effects [87,88]. In spontaneously hypertensive adult rats, the administration of KYNA in drinking water for 3 weeks did not affect the mean arterial pressure, but it moderately reduced heart rate [89] (Table 2).

Another method of the alimentary administration of the drug was utilized by Li et al. (2021) [90]. In this study, KYNA was applied intragastrically to adult mice kept on a high-fat diet, once a day for 8 weeks, in a dose of 5 mg/kg/day. It was found that such a regimen resulted in declined body weight gain and reduced daily energy intake. Moreover, the following serum metabolic parameters were improved: triglyceride, serum high-density lipoprotein cholesterol, and low-density lipoprotein levels. Finally, both the atherosclerosis index and the coronary artery risk index were significantly decreased [90]. Similar metabolic effects of KYNA injected intraperitoneally at a dose of 5 mg/kg/day, once a day for 1 to 4 weeks, to mice on a high-fat diet were described [93]. Very recently, it was reported that KYNA administered intraperitoneally three times decreased the colonization of the intestine by fungi and ameliorated intestinal injury, i.e., inhibited inflammation, promoted the expression of intestinal tight junction proteins, and protected from intestinal barrier damage caused by invasive *Candida albicans* infection in mice [94] (Table 2). Other data indicating multiple health-promoting effects of KYNA come from studies in which the drug was acutely injected intraperitoneally (Table S7). This route of administration is preferred by researchers because it allows for the accurate dosage and precise determination of the time of action of the substance. Historically, the earliest data relate to the antiulcer effects of KYNA. Glavin and Pinsky, in 1989, showed that KYNA significantly blocked restraint-cold stress ulcers, ethanol ulcers, and basal nonstimulated gastric acid secretion in normal rats. The authors premised both peripheral and cerebral effects of KYNA [95]. Protective effects of injected KYNA on the liver and the pancreas, and in disorders of the lower gastrointestinal tract, were later described (Table S7). More recently, numerous reports performed on animals on the beneficial effect of KYNA on the conditions commonly referred to as metabolic diseases in humans were published. Antiobesity, cholesterol-lowering, glucose tolerance improvement, and antiatherosclerotic effects were evidenced in appropriate animal models (Table S7). It is surprising that many of these effects observed after KYNA administration in animals can be therapeutic targets for metabolic syndromes in humans (Figure 4).

Similar disturbances were described as obese-related multimorbidity, when a low-caloric KYNA-enriched functional diet should be considered as supportive care. The effect of KYNA on bone metabolism is also of interest. A recent publication by Shi et al. (2022) revealed that KYNA administered in a relatively low dose of 5 mg/kg/day for 4 weeks alleviated the postmenopausal osteoporosis and highlighted the involvement of the GPR35 receptor, a molecular target of KYNA, in this action [97] (Table S7).

In addition, it has been shown that KYNA may have beneficial health effects in life-threatening conditions (Table S7), and this issue requires a separate commentary. Moroni et al. (2012) were the first to communicate that KYNA administered subcutaneously at doses of 500 mg/kg (single injection) or 200 mg/kg three times at 0, 3, and 6 h after LPS dramatically reduced LPS-induced death in mice [98]. The Hungarian group confirmed that KYNA protects against LPS-induced sepsis in subsequent publications, in which a much lower KYNA dose of 30 mg/kg, i.p., was used [99,100]. Most recently, Wang et al. (2022) demonstrated that intraperitoneally administered KYNA (5 mg/kg; three times at days 3, 6, and 9) reduced the mortality of mice infected with *Candida albicans* [94]. Hsieh et al. (2011) reported that KYNA administered intravenously at doses ranging from 30–100 mg/kg attenuated multiorgan dysfunction in rats exposed to heatstroke [101]. Kaszaki et al. (2008) found a profound anti-inflammatory action of KYNA administered in intravenous infusion in experimental colon obstruction in dogs [102]. Similarly, Marciniak, in 2013, demonstrated that the intravenous infusion of KYNA alleviated symptoms of experimental acute pancreatitis in rats [103]. These results deserve special attention because they indicate the feasibility of using KYNA administered as a bolus or an intravenous infusion in life-threatening conditions.

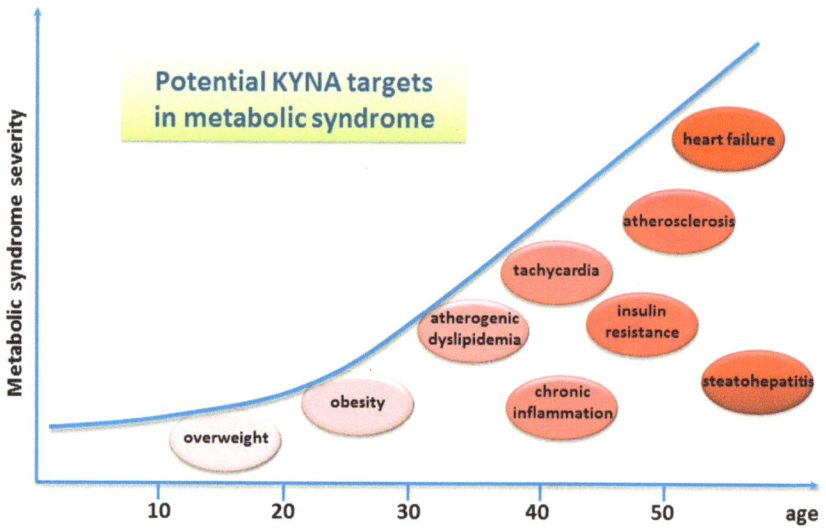

Figure 4. Graphic presentation of potential kynurenic acid (KYNA) targets in metabolic syndrome in humans. The effects of KYNA in specific pathological conditions drawn from animal studies are described in the text and are presented in Table S7. The graphic is based on [96]; however, only identified KYNA targets are presented.

The beneficial wound healing effects of KYNA (Table S7) after its external administration on the skin and cornea in rabbits are also worth mentioning [104,105]. It is worth noting that a clinical trial with the use of 0.5% KYNA dressing in people with skin scarring has already been successfully completed [106]. Furthermore, KYNA encapsulated in synthetic polymer microspheres implanted in a wound bed in rats was shown to reduce fibrotic tissue formation [107].

Detailed data on the health-promoting effects of KYNA administration in animals regardless of the route of administration are presented in Table S7 [26,87,90,93–95,97–106,108–123].

Since there are no substantial differences between the effects exerted by KYNA administered alimentary or infused by injection, it can be assumed that its supplementation by the oral route will produce similar effects as those described after infusion.

8.2. Clinical Trials

In the ClinicalTrials.gov database, only four registered studies were found in which KYNA was applied to humans. All studies were dedicated to examining the effect of the topical application of KYNA to skin (Table S8).

8.3. Patents

A survey of the PubChem database of patents in which the keyword KYNA appears revealed 23 patent applications dealing with the medical use of the drug (Table S9). Most of them relate to its oral or injectable administration and only a few assume the topical or local administration of KYNA. The most commonly claimed effect of KYNA is in digestive tract, liver, and pancreatic conditions. KYNA's effects have also been recommended in cardiovascular pathologies, lipid metabolism disorders, obesity, and kidney dysfunction. In addition, its use in fibrotic diseases, eye diseases, and mental stress is mentioned. In general, this is in line with the data obtained from scientific publications. Some novelty derived from the patent descriptions is KYNA's effect on skeletal muscles and its proposed use in sarcopenia or hangover control. In addition to the scientific content, it is worth noting that the number of patent applications on the medical use of KYNA has increased substantially since 2016.

9. Perspectives
9.1. Food as a Dietary Source of Kynurenic Acid

Although the presence of KYNA in food is a topic that has been addressed several times in various publications, the knowledge of its content in food products is still insufficient. It should be underlined that most of the studies come from Eurasia. There are almost no data from other continents and regions where diets are based on other products than in Europe. Thus, it is advisable to continue the search for rich sources of KYNA among various food products from all over the world.

Based on the current knowledge, it can be concluded that KYNA content in food and food products is generally low (Figure 3; Table S4) and, according to our calculation (Tables S10–S13), its daily intake is very small (Figure 5a) and quite marginal compared to its excretion (Table 1). The calculation of food-related KYNA intake was based on simulation of a dish of cruciferous, yellow, green, and other vegetables mixed equally, assuming that a single serving weighs 80 g according to Bensley et al. (2003) [124]. The KYNA ingested in red meat, poultry, eggs, and other extensively analyzed nutrients is omitted due to trace of their contents. Low intake was established as a consumption of three or fewer servings per week. High intake was established as consumption of more than 10 servings per week.

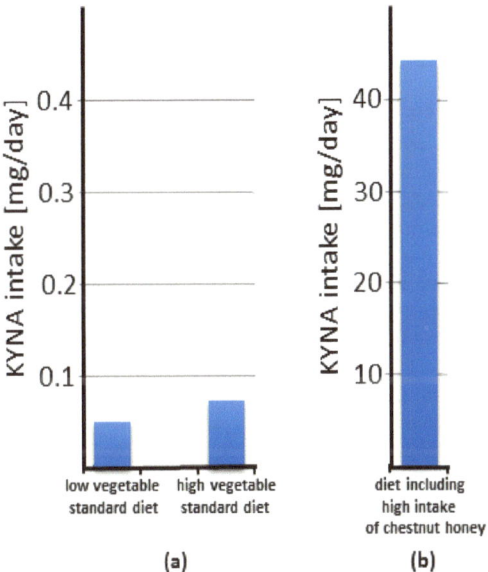

Figure 5. Estimation of the daily intake of kynurenic acid (KYNA) in standard diets and diets rich in chestnut honey. The columns reflect the value of the highest reported content of KYNA (see Table S4 for detail). Note that the scale on panel (**b**) is 100 times larger than on panel (**a**). The daily intake of KYNA in the diet was calculated as follows. The calculation of food-related KYNA intake was based on simulation of a dish of cruciferous, yellow, green and other vegetables mixed equally assuming that a single serving weighs 80 g according to Bensley et al. 2003 [124]. The KYNA ingested in red meat, poultry, eggs and other extensively analyzed nutrients is omitted due to trace of their contents. Low intake was established as consumption of three or fewer servings per week. High intake was established as consumption of more than 10 servings per week.

The calculated mean daily intake of KYNA as a food constituent was estimated to be approximately 0.065 mg in a diet that does not contain honey. The mean daily intake of KYNA derived from food is notably higher when chestnut honey is consumed in significant quantities and may account for 20.81 mg. However, it should be noted that chestnut honey is produced by bees that collect pollen in areas where chestnut trees grow. These regions are limited due to soil and climate requirements as well as cultivation culture [125]. Thus, it can be concluded that, for most of the human population, the daily amount of food-derived KYNA lies well below 0.1 mg. Taking into account that the daily requirement for KYNA in adult humans, calculated on the basis of its daily excretion, varies from 1.2 to 7 mg (Table 1), it can be concluded that, for most people, the food-derived KYNA does not exceed 10% of the daily requirement. In contrast, in people consuming chestnut honey in their diet, the supplied KYNA, approximating the value of 20 mg, almost triples the daily need. The latter estimation points to the safety of the alimentary administration of KYNA in amounts of up to 20 mg/day.

KYNA content in meat is very low, while in vegetables it is considerably higher but there are large differences between individual types of vegetables and their varieties. Moreover, it seems to depend on where and how the plants are grown. For these reasons, it is difficult to make rational dietary recommendations yet. In terms of KYNA content, chestnut honey is a particular exception among food products including other types of honey. On the other hand, almost nothing is known about the KYNA content in fruit. Interestingly, fermented food contains a higher level of KYNA in comparison to unprocessed food. This knowledge can be used to increase KYNA content in the human diet.

It is noteworthy that KYNA is present in breast milk from the beginning of newborn feeding and its content considerably rises over time [46]. The importance of this phenomenon is still far from being understood, but it should be noted that KYNA content in baby food formulas does not parallel its physiological changes.

9.2. Chestnut Honey as a Dietary Source of Kynurenic Acid

Summarizing the data collected so far, it is evident that KYNA possesses potential health-promoting relevance (Table S7). Its presence in food has been repeatedly confirmed, but its amount is relatively small. The exception is chestnut honey, in which the content of this substance can be even 1000 times higher than in other food products (Figure 3; Table S4). The uniqueness of chestnut honey is reflected by the fact that the consumption of only 10 g of honey provides such an amount of KYNA that corresponds to its average daily excretion. Greater consumption of chestnut honey in the amounts recommended for use for medical purposes [126] can result in the delivery of more than 3000 times KYNA per day than in a standard diet (Figure 5b). This creates a unique opportunity to verify whether the consumption of chestnut honey brings health benefits to humans. In fact, there are scientific reports on the effects of chestnut honey on diseases modeled in laboratory animals [127–131] (Table S14). Interestingly, similar to KYNA, chestnut honey administered by the alimentary route counteracts the effects of a high-fat diet in mice and also has an antiulcer effect in the alcohol model of the disease in rats [127,128]. Moreover, it was found to enhance the healing of CCl4-induced liver damage in rats [129]. When administered topically, it improves skin wound healing and the healing of corneal alkali burns [130,131]. Other effects described based on in vitro studies and biochemical analyses are summarized in Table S14 [132–141]. It should be noted that many of the reported effects of chestnut honey parallel those of KYNA. Therefore, it would be interesting to see if a health-promoting effect has been recognized in population-based studies. Unfortunately, we found no relevant studies in the available literature. This seems to be due to the fact that chestnut honey is not identified in publications on the dietary effects on human health. Furthermore, honey is rarely seen as a separate category in such studies. Therefore, we propose to reinvestigate previous data or to conduct such studies including chestnut honey consumption as a separate item in the menu, due to its exceptionally high KYNA content [13]. Such a study may be facilitated by the fact that chestnut honey is not widely consumed worldwide. It is primarily used in areas where chestnut trees grow. In many countries, its consumption is marginal or practically nonexistent. This allows for the matching of appropriate study groups with a high consumption of chestnut honey and a control group that does not consume chestnut honey. A brief analysis of the chestnut cultivation area indicates that it is typical of Mediterranean European countries, but also of some Asian countries. It also appears that many so-called Blue Zones, regions of the world thought to have a higher than usual number of people who live much longer than average, are located in areas where chestnut trees grow.

Chestnut honey is indeed a very rich source of KYNA, but it has some drawbacks and there are significant limitations to its consumption. First of all, honey contains about 50% monosaccharides and, for this reason, its high consumption is not popular nowadays. However, it should be realized that chestnut honey attenuates postprandial glycemic response and, therefore, is classified as a food with a low or medium glycemic index and glycemic load [142–144]. Second, due to the presence of bee- and pollen-derived proteins, honey can be allergenic. Young children should not eat honey. Third, the amount of honey produced by bees is limited and may not be enough to cover increased demands. Therefore, other sources of KYNA should be searched for, and at best its safety should be assessed and the use of KYNA as a supplement allowed.

9.3. Other Sources of Kynurenic Acid

Recent publications indicate that yeast may be an alternative source of KYNA [79,145,146]. The production of KYNA by yeast can be carried out on an industrial scale and does not require either suitable soil or climatic conditions, as do chestnut cultivation and honey production. This is a major advantage. However, the disadvantages are the relatively low efficiency of the production process and the limited amount of yeast that can be used for feeding. Therefore, further work is needed to improve the process of KYNA production by microorganisms. There is also a lack of data on the amount of KYNA production by the gut microbiome and how this process can be intensified.

10. Concluding Remarks

KYNA appears to be a very promising molecule with potential health-promoting importance and beneficial pharmacodynamics. The fact that it is found in very large amounts in chestnut honey, which is consumed only in limited areas, creates the opportunity to trace its effects on the human body without the need for long-term prospective studies. The rationale for such studies appears to be obvious. It is also imperative not to forget to be cautious, and to perform appropriate studies and closely follow information about its potential side effects before KYNA enters widely into food supplementation. Thus, it seems that the question should be when, not if, KYNA will be used as a dietary supplement.

Supplementary Materials: The following supporting information can be downloaded at: https://www.mdpi.com/article/10.3390/nu14194182/s1, Table S1. Content of kynurenic acid in human serum; Table S2. Content of kynurenic acid in human cerebrospinal fluid; Table S3. Excretion of kynurenic acid in human urine; Table S4. Content of kynurenic acid in food, beverages, herbs, and spices for cooking; Table S5. Content of kynurenic acid in medicinal herbs and supplements; Table S6. Content of kynurenic acid in human milk and baby food; Table S7. Health-related effects of kynurenic acid (KYNA) administration; Table S8. Clinical trials designed to investigate the kynurenic acid (KYNA) effect registered in ClinicalTrials.gov database; Table S9. Patents and patent applications claiming medical uses of kynurenic acid (KYNA); Table S10. Estimated daily intake of kynurenic acid as an ingredient of food; Table S11. Intake of kynurenic acid in vegetables; Table S12. Intake of kynurenic acid in meat, dairy, egg, and beverages; Table S13. Intake of kynurenic acid in single and daily dose of honey; Table S14. Effects of chestnut honey established in animals, in vitro and biochemical studies.

Author Contributions: Conceptualization, M.T.; methodology, M.T. and P.P.; formal analysis, M.T., P.P. and W.A.T.; writing—original draft preparation, J.P.-T., M.T., P.P. and W.A.T.; writing—review and editing, M.T.; visualization, M.T. and W.A.T.; supervision, J.P.-T. and M.T.; project administration, W.A.T.; funding acquisition, J.P.-T. and W.A.T. All authors have read and agreed to the published version of the manuscript.

Funding: The publication was supported by grants DS 394 and DS 448 from the Medical University of Lublin, Poland.

Institutional Review Board Statement: Not applicable.

Informed Consent Statement: Not applicable.

Data Availability Statement: Not applicable.

Conflicts of Interest: The authors declare no conflict of interest.

References

1. Turski, M.P.; Turska, M.; Paluszkiewicz, P.; Parada-Turska, J.; Oxenkrug, G.F. Kynurenic Acid in the Digestive System-New Facts, New Challenges. *Int. J. Tryptophan Res.* **2013**, *6*, 47–55. [CrossRef] [PubMed]
2. Kapolka, N.J.; Taghon, G.J.; Rowe, J.B.; Morgan, W.M.; Enten, J.F.; Lambert, N.A.; Isom, D.G. DCyFIR: A High-Throughput CRISPR Platform for Multiplexed G Protein-Coupled Receptor Profiling and Ligand Discovery. *Proc. Natl. Acad. Sci. USA* **2020**, *117*, 13117–13126. [CrossRef]
3. Collingridge, G.L.; Abraham, W.C. Glutamate Receptors and Synaptic Plasticity: The Impact of Evans and Watkins. *Neuropharmacology* **2022**, *206*, 108922. [CrossRef]
4. Stone, T.W. Does Kynurenic Acid Act on Nicotinic Receptors? An Assessment of the Evidence. *J. Neurochem.* **2020**, *152*, 627–649. [CrossRef]
5. Shore, D.M.; Reggio, P.H. The Therapeutic Potential of Orphan GPCRs, GPR35 and GPR55. *Front. Pharm.* **2015**, *6*, 69. [CrossRef] [PubMed]
6. Wang, J.; Simonavicius, N.; Wu, X.; Swaminath, G.; Reagan, J.; Tian, H.; Ling, L. Kynurenic Acid as a Ligand for Orphan G Protein-Coupled Receptor GPR35. *J. Biol. Chem.* **2006**, *281*, 22021–22028. [CrossRef] [PubMed]
7. O'Dowd, B.F.; Nguyen, T.; Marchese, A.; Cheng, R.; Lynch, K.R.; Heng, H.H.Q.; Kolakowski, L.F.; George, S.R. Discovery of Three Novel G-Protein-Coupled Receptor Genes. *Genomics* **1998**, *47*, 310–313. [CrossRef]
8. Okumura, S.; Baba, H.; Kumada, T.; Nanmoku, K.; Nakajima, H.; Nakane, Y.; Hioki, K.; Ikenaka, K. Cloning of a G-Protein-Coupled Receptor That Shows an Activity to Transform NIH3T3 Cells and Is Expressed in Gastric Cancer Cells. *Cancer Sci.* **2004**, *95*, 131–135. [CrossRef]
9. Kaya, B.; Melhem, H.; Niess, J.H. GPR35 in Intestinal Diseases: From Risk Gene to Function. *Front. Immunol.* **2021**, *12*, 717392. [CrossRef] [PubMed]
10. Quon, T.; Lin, L.-C.; Ganguly, A.; Tobin, A.B.; Milligan, G. Therapeutic Opportunities and Challenges in Targeting the Orphan G Protein-Coupled Receptor GPR35. *ACS Pharmacol. Transl. Sci.* **2020**, *3*, 801–812. [CrossRef] [PubMed]
11. Turska, M.; Rutyna, R.; Paluszkiewicz, M.; Terlecka, P.; Dobrowolski, A.; Pelak, J.; Turski, M.P.; Muszyńska, B.; Dabrowski, W.; Kocki, T.; et al. Presence of Kynurenic Acid in Alcoholic Beverages—Is This Good News, or Bad News? *Med Hypotheses* **2019**, *122*, 200–205. [CrossRef]
12. Kaihara, M.; Price, J.M.; Takahashi, H. The Conversion of Kynurenic Acid to Quinaldic Acid by Humans and Rats. *J Biol Chem* **1956**, *223*, 705–708.
13. Turski, M.P.; Chwil, S.; Turska, M.; Chwil, M.; Kocki, T.; Rajtar, G.; Parada-Turska, J. An Exceptionally High Content of Kynurenic Acid in Chestnut Honey and Flowers of Chestnut Tree. *J. Food Compos. Anal.* **2016**, *48*, 67–72. [CrossRef]
14. Turska, M.; Pelak, J.; Turski, M.P.; Kocki, T.; Dukowski, P.; Plech, T.; Turski, W. Fate and Distribution of Kynurenic Acid Administered as Beverage. *Pharm. Rep.* **2018**, *70*, 1089–1096. [CrossRef]
15. Li, P.; Zheng, J.; Bai, Y.; Wang, D.; Cui, Z.; Li, Y.; Zhang, J.; Wang, Y. Characterization of Kynurenine Pathway in Patients with Diarrhea-Predominant Irritable Bowel Syndrome. *Eur. J. Histochem.* **2020**, *64*. [CrossRef]
16. Iłzecka, J.; Kocki, T.; Stelmasiak, Z.; Turski, W.A. Endogenous Protectant Kynurenic Acid in Amyotrophic Lateral Sclerosis. *Acta Neurol. Scand.* **2003**, *107*, 412–418. [CrossRef] [PubMed]
17. Huang, J.; Tong, J.; Zhang, P.; Zhou, Y.; Cui, Y.; Tan, S.; Wang, Z.; Yang, F.; Kochunov, P.; Chiappelli, J.; et al. Effects of Neuroactive Metabolites of the Tryptophan Pathway on Working Memory and Cortical Thickness in Schizophrenia. *Transl. Psychiatry* **2021**, *11*, 198. [CrossRef]
18. Hartai, Z.; Klivenyi, P.; Janaky, T.; Penke, B.; Dux, L.; Vecsei, L. Kynurenine Metabolism in Plasma and in Red Blood Cells in Parkinson's Disease. *J. Neurol. Sci.* **2005**, *239*, 31–35. [CrossRef]
19. Zhang, Z.; Zhang, M.; Luo, Y.; Ni, X.; Lu, H.; Wen, Y.; Fan, N. Preliminary Comparative Analysis of Kynurenine Pathway Metabolites in Chronic Ketamine Users, Schizophrenic Patients, and Healthy Controls. *Hum. Psychopharmacol.* **2020**, *35*, e2738. [CrossRef] [PubMed]
20. Tömösi, F.; Kecskeméti, G.; Cseh, E.K.; Szabó, E.; Rajda, C.; Kormány, R.; Szabó, Z.; Vécsei, L.; Janáky, T. A Validated UHPLC-MS Method for Tryptophan Metabolites: Application in the Diagnosis of Multiple Sclerosis. *J. Pharm. Biomed. Anal.* **2020**, *185*, 113246. [CrossRef]
21. Kepplinger, B.; Baran, H.; Kainz, A.; Ferraz-Leite, H.; Newcombe, J.; Kalina, P. Age-Related Increase of Kynurenic Acid in Human Cerebrospinal Fluid—IgG and Beta2-Microglobulin Changes. *Neurosignals* **2005**, *14*, 126–135. [CrossRef] [PubMed]

22. Amirkhani, A.; Heldin, E.; Markides, K.E.; Bergquist, J. Quantitation of Tryptophan, Kynurenine and Kynurenic Acid in Human Plasma by Capillary Liquid Chromatography-Electrospray Ionization Tandem Mass Spectrometry. *J. Chromatogr. B Anal. Technol. Biomed. Life Sci.* **2002**, *780*, 381–387. [CrossRef]
23. Milart, P.; Urbańska, E.M.; Turski, W.A.; Paszkowski, T.; Sikorski, R. Intrapartum Levels of Endogenous Glutamate Antagonist-Kynurenic Acid in Amniotic Fluid, Umbilical and Maternal Blood. *Neurosci. Res. Comm.* **1999**, *24*, 173–178. [CrossRef]
24. Milart, P.; Sikorski, R. Kynurenic acid concentration in blood and urine during normal pregnancy. *Ginekol. Pol.* **1998**, *69*, 968–973. [PubMed]
25. Shestopalov, A.V.; Shatova, O.P.; Gaponov, A.M.; Moskaleva, N.E.; Appolonova, S.A.; Tutelyan, A.V.; Makarov, V.V.; Yudin, S.M.; Rumyantsev, S.A. The study of tryptophan metabolite concentrations in blood serum and fecal extracts from obese children. *Biomed. Khim.* **2020**, *66*, 494–501. [CrossRef] [PubMed]
26. Kuc, D.; Rahnama, M.; Tomaszewski, T.; Rzeski, W.; Wejksza, K.; Urbanik-Sypniewska, T.; Parada-Turska, J.; Wielosz, M.; Turski, W.A. Kynurenic Acid in Human Saliva–Does It Influence Oral Microflora? *Pharm. Rep.* **2006**, *58*, 393–398.
27. Paluszkiewicz, P.; Zgrajka, W.; Saran, T.; Schabowski, J.; Piedra, J.L.V.; Fedkiv, O.; Rengman, S.; Pierzynowski, S.G.; Turski, W.A. High Concentration of Kynurenic Acid in Bile and Pancreatic Juice. *Amino Acids* **2009**, *37*, 637–641. [CrossRef] [PubMed]
28. Walczak, K.; Dąbrowski, W.; Langner, E.; Zgrajka, W.; Piłat, J.; Kocki, T.; Rzeski, W.; Turski, W.A. Kynurenic Acid Synthesis and Kynurenine Aminotransferases Expression in Colon Derived Normal and Cancer Cells. *Scand. J. Gastroenterol.* **2011**, *46*, 903–912. [CrossRef] [PubMed]
29. Parada-Turska, J.; Zgrajka, W.; Majdan, M. Kynurenic Acid in Synovial Fluid and Serum of Patients with Rheumatoid Arthritis, Spondyloarthropathy, and Osteoarthritis. *J. Rheumatol.* **2013**, *40*, 903–909. [CrossRef] [PubMed]
30. Saran, T.; Turska, M.; Kocki, T.; Zawadka, M.; Zieliński, G.; Turski, W.A.; Gawda, P. Effect of 4-Week Physical Exercises on Tryptophan, Kynurenine and Kynurenic Acid Content in Human Sweat. *Sci. Rep.* **2021**, *11*, 11092. [CrossRef] [PubMed]
31. Alarcan, H.; Chaumond, R.; Emond, P.; Benz-De Bretagne, I.; Lefèvre, A.; Bakkouche, S.-E.; Veyrat-Durebex, C.; Vourc'h, P.; Andres, C.; Corcia, P.; et al. Some CSF Kynurenine Pathway Intermediates Associated with Disease Evolution in Amyotrophic Lateral Sclerosis. *Biomolecules* **2021**, *11*, 691. [CrossRef] [PubMed]
32. Rodrigues, F.B.; Byrne, L.M.; Lowe, A.J.; Tortelli, R.; Heins, M.; Flik, G.; Johnson, E.B.; De Vita, E.; Scahill, R.I.; Giorgini, F.; et al. Kynurenine Pathway Metabolites in Cerebrospinal Fluid and Blood as Potential Biomarkers in Huntington's Disease. *J. Neurochem.* **2021**, *158*, 539–553. [CrossRef] [PubMed]
33. Kepplinger, B.; Baran, H.; Kronsteiner, C.; Reuss, J. Increased Levels of Kynurenic Acid in the Cerebrospinal Fluid in Patients with Hydrocephalus. *Neurosignals* **2019**, *27*, 1–11. [CrossRef]
34. Nilsson, L.K.; Linderholm, K.R.; Engberg, G.; Paulson, L.; Blennow, K.; Lindström, L.H.; Nordin, C.; Karanti, A.; Persson, P.; Erhardt, S. Elevated Levels of Kynurenic Acid in the Cerebrospinal Fluid of Male Patients with Schizophrenia. *Schizophr. Res.* **2005**, *80*, 315–322. [CrossRef] [PubMed]
35. Erhardt, S.; Schwieler, L.; Engberg, G. Kynurenic Acid and Schizophrenia. *Adv. Exp. Med. Biol.* **2003**, *527*, 155–165. [CrossRef]
36. Rejdak, K.; Bartosik-Psujek, H.; Dobosz, B.; Kocki, T.; Grieb, P.; Giovannoni, G.; Turski, W.A.; Stelmasiak, Z. Decreased Level of Kynurenic Acid in Cerebrospinal Fluid of Relapsing-Onset Multiple Sclerosis Patients. *Neurosci. Lett.* **2002**, *331*, 63–65. [CrossRef]
37. Swartz, K.J.; Matson, W.R.; MacGarvey, U.; Ryan, E.A.; Beal, M.F. Measurement of Kynurenic Acid in Mammalian Brain Extracts and Cerebrospinal Fluid by High-Performance Liquid Chromatography with Fluorometric and Coulometric Electrode Array Detection. *Anal. Biochem.* **1990**, *185*, 363–376. [CrossRef]
38. Yamamoto, H.; Murakami, H.; Horiguchi, K.; Egawa, B. Studies on Cerebrospinal Fluid Kynurenic Acid Concentrations in Epileptic Children. *Brain Dev.* **1995**, *17*, 327–329. [CrossRef]
39. Turski, W.A.; Nakamura, M.; Todd, W.P.; Carpenter, B.K.; Whetsell, W.O.; Schwarcz, R. Identification and Quantification of Kynurenic Acid in Human Brain Tissue. *Brain Res.* **1988**, *454*, 164–169. [CrossRef]
40. Connick, J.H.; Carlà, V.; Moroni, F.; Stone, T.W. Increase in Kynurenic Acid in Huntington's Disease Motor Cortex. *J. Neurochem.* **1989**, *52*, 985–987. [CrossRef]
41. Moroni, F.; Russi, P.; Lombardi, G.; Beni, M.; Carlà, V. Presence of Kynurenic Acid in the Mammalian Brain. *J. Neurochem.* **1988**, *51*, 177–180. [CrossRef] [PubMed]
42. Baran, H.; Hainfellner, J.A.; Kepplinger, B.; Mazal, P.R.; Schmid, H.; Budka, H. Kynurenic Acid Metabolism in the Brain of HIV-1 Infected Patients. *J. Neural. Transm.* **2000**, *107*, 1127–1138. [CrossRef]
43. Baran, H.; Hainfellner, J.A.; Kepplinger, B. Kynurenic Acid Metabolism in Various Types of Brain Pathology in HIV-1 Infected Patients. *Int. J. Tryptophan Res.* **2012**, *5*, 49–64. [CrossRef]
44. Schwarcz, R.; Rassoulpour, A.; Wu, H.Q.; Medoff, D.; Tamminga, C.A.; Roberts, R.C. Increased Cortical Kynurenate Content in Schizophrenia. *Biol. Psychiatry* **2001**, *50*, 521–530. [CrossRef]
45. O'Rourke, L.; Clarke, G.; Nolan, A.; Watkins, C.; Dinan, T.G.; Stanton, C.; Ross, R.P.; Ryan, C.A. Tryptophan Metabolic Profile in Term and Preterm Breast Milk: Implications for Health. *J. Nutr. Sci.* **2018**, *7*, e13. [CrossRef]
46. Milart, P.; Paluszkiewicz, P.; Dobrowolski, P.; Tomaszewska, E.; Smolinska, K.; Debinska, I.; Gawel, K.; Walczak, K.; Bednarski, J.; Turska, M.; et al. Kynurenic Acid as the Neglected Ingredient of Commercial Baby Formulas. *Sci. Rep.* **2019**, *9*, 6108. [CrossRef]
47. Oluwagbemigun, K.; Anesi, A.; Clarke, G.; Schmid, M.; Mattivi, F.; Nöthlings, U. An Investigation into the Temporal Reproducibility of Tryptophan Metabolite Networks Among Healthy Adolescents. *Int. J. Tryptophan Res.* **2021**, *14*, 11786469211041376. [CrossRef]

48. Gomez-Gomez, A.; Marcos, J.; Aguilera, P.; To-Figueras, J.; Pozo, O.J. Comprehensive Analysis of the Tryptophan Metabolome in Urine of Patients with Acute Intermittent Porphyria. *J. Chromatogr. B Anal. Technol. Biomed. Life Sci.* **2017**, *1060*, 347–354. [CrossRef] [PubMed]
49. Furlanetto, S.; Tognini, C.; Carpenedo, R.; La Porta, E.; Pinzauti, S. Set-up and Validation of an Adsorptive Stripping Voltammetric Method for Kynurenic Acid Determination in Human Urine. *J. Pharm. Biomed. Anal.* **1998**, *18*, 67–73. [CrossRef]
50. Crow, B.; Bishop, M.; Paliakov, E.; Norton, D.; George, J.; Bralley, J.A. Analysis of Urinary Aromatic Acids by Liquid Chromatography Tandem Mass Spectrometry. *Biomed. Chromatogr.* **2008**, *22*, 1346–1353. [CrossRef] [PubMed]
51. Mawatari, K.; Iinuma, F.; Watanabe, M. Fluorometric Determination of Urinary Kynurenic Acid by Flow Injection Analysis Equipped with a "Bypass Line". *Anal. Biochem.* **1990**, *190*, 88–91. [CrossRef]
52. Yan, J.; Kuzhiumparambil, U.; Bandodkar, S.; Solowij, N.; Fu, S. Development and Validation of a Simple, Rapid and Sensitive LC-MS/MS Method for the Measurement of Urinary Neurotransmitters and Their Metabolites. *Anal. Bioanal. Chem.* **2017**, *409*, 7191–7199. [CrossRef]
53. Zhao, J.; Chen, H.; Ni, P.; Xu, B.; Luo, X.; Zhan, Y.; Gao, P.; Zhu, D. Simultaneous Determination of Urinary Tryptophan, Tryptophan-Related Metabolites and Creatinine by High Performance Liquid Chromatography with Ultraviolet and Fluorimetric Detection. *J. Chromatogr. B Anal. Technol. Biomed. Life Sci.* **2011**, *879*, 2720–2725. [CrossRef]
54. Leklem, J.E. Quantitative Aspects of Tryptophan Metabolism in Humans and Other Species: A Review. *Am. J. Clin. Nutr.* **1971**, *24*, 659–672. [CrossRef] [PubMed]
55. Shibata, K.; Hirose, J.; Fukuwatari, T. Method for Evaluation of the Requirements of B-Group Vitamins Using Tryptophan Metabolites in Human Urine. *Int. J. Tryptophan Res.* **2015**, *8*, 31–39. [CrossRef]
56. Hiratsuka, C.; Fukuwatari, T.; Shibata, K. Fate of Dietary Tryptophan in Young Japanese Women. *Int. J. Tryptophan Res.* **2012**, *5*, 33–47. [CrossRef]
57. Hiratsuka, C.; Fukuwatari, T.; Sano, M.; Saito, K.; Sasaki, S.; Shibata, K. Supplementing Healthy Women with up to 5.0 g/d of L-Tryptophan Has No Adverse Effects. *J. Nutr.* **2013**, *143*, 859–866. [CrossRef]
58. Nadour, Z.; Simian, C.; Laprévote, O.; Loriot, M.-A.; Larabi, I.A.; Pallet, N. Validation of a Liquid Chromatography Coupled to Tandem Mass Spectrometry Method for Simultaneous Quantification of Tryptophan and 10 Key Metabolites of the Kynurenine Pathway in Plasma and Urine: Application to a Cohort of Acute Kidney Injury Patients. *Clin. Chim. Acta* **2022**, *534*, 115–127. [CrossRef]
59. Uberos, J.; Romero, J.; Molina-Carballo, A.; Muñoz-Hoyos, A. Melatonin and Elimination of Kynurenines in Children with Down's Syndrome. *J. Pediatr. Endocrinol. Metab.* **2010**, *23*, 277–282. [CrossRef]
60. Molina-Carballo, A.; Cubero-Millán, I.; Fernández-López, L.; Checa-Ros, A.; Machado-Casas, I.; Jerez-Calero, A.; Blanca-Jover, E.; Cantarero-Malagón, A.-M.; Uberos, J.; Muñoz-Hoyos, A. Methylphenidate Ameliorates the Homeostatic Balance between Levels of Kynurenines in ADHD Children. *Psychiatry Res.* **2021**, *303*, 114060. [CrossRef]
61. Muñoz-Hoyos, A.; Molina-Carballo, A.; Macías, M.; Rodríguez-Cabezas, T.; Martín-Medina, E.; Narbona-López, E.; Valenzuela-Ruiz, A.; Acuña-Castroviejo, D. Comparison between Tryptophan Methoxyindole and Kynurenine Metabolic Pathways in Normal and Preterm Neonates and in Neonates with Acute Fetal Distress. *Eur. J. Endocrinol.* **1998**, *139*, 89–95. [CrossRef]
62. Muñóz-Hoyos, A.; Molina-Carballo, A.; Rodríguez-Cabezas, T.; Uberos-Fernández, J.; Ruiz-Cosano, C.; Acuña-Castroviejo, D. Relationships between Methoxyindole and Kynurenine Pathway Metabolites in Plasma and Urine in Children Suffering from Febrile and Epileptic Seizures. *Clin. Endocrinol.* **1997**, *47*, 667–677. [CrossRef]
63. Fukui, S.; Schwarcz, R.; Rapoport, S.I.; Takada, Y.; Smith, Q.R. Blood-Brain Barrier Transport of Kynurenines: Implications for Brain Synthesis and Metabolism. *J. Neurochem.* **1991**, *56*, 2007–2017. [CrossRef]
64. Füvesi, J.; Somlai, C.; Németh, H.; Varga, H.; Kis, Z.; Farkas, T.; Károly, N.; Dobszay, M.; Penke, Z.; Penke, B.; et al. Comparative Study on the Effects of Kynurenic Acid and Glucosamine-Kynurenic Acid. *Pharm. Biochem. Behav.* **2004**, *77*, 95–102. [CrossRef]
65. Varga, N.; Csapó, E.; Majláth, Z.; Ilisz, I.; Krizbai, I.A.; Wilhelm, I.; Knapp, L.; Toldi, J.; Vécsei, L.; Dékány, I. Targeting of the Kynurenic Acid across the Blood-Brain Barrier by Core-Shell Nanoparticles. *Eur. J. Pharm. Sci.* **2016**, *86*, 67–74. [CrossRef] [PubMed]
66. Goeden, N.; Notarangelo, F.M.; Pocivavsek, A.; Beggiato, S.; Bonnin, A.; Schwarcz, R. Prenatal Dynamics of Kynurenine Pathway Metabolism in Mice: Focus on Kynurenic Acid. *Dev. Neurosci.* **2017**, *39*, 519–528. [CrossRef] [PubMed]
67. Brown, R.R.; Price, J.M. Quantitative Studies on Metabolites of Tryptophan in the Urine of the Dog, Cat, Rat, and Man. *J. Biol. Chem.* **1956**, *219*, 985–997. [CrossRef]
68. Turski, W.A.; Schwarcz, R. On the Disposition of Intrahippocampally Injected Kynurenic Acid in the Rat. *Exp. Brain Res.* **1988**, *71*, 563–567. [CrossRef]
69. Dong, F.; Hao, F.; Murray, I.A.; Smith, P.B.; Koo, I.; Tindall, A.M.; Kris-Etherton, P.M.; Gowda, K.; Amin, S.G.; Patterson, A.D.; et al. Intestinal Microbiota-Derived Tryptophan Metabolites Are Predictive of Ah Receptor Activity. *Gut Microbes* **2020**, *12*, 1–24. [CrossRef] [PubMed]
70. Human Feces. Available online: https://en.wikipedia.org/wiki/Human_feces (accessed on 13 September 2022).
71. Uttekar, P. How Much Does an Average Person Sweat in a Day? 2021. Available online: https://www.medicinenet.com/how_much_does_an_average_person_sweat_in_a_day/article.htm (accessed on 5 September 2022).
72. Perspiration. Available online: https://en.wikipedia.org/wiki/Perspiration (accessed on 13 September 2022).

73. Turski, M.P.; Turska, M.; Zgrajka, W.; Kuc, D.; Turski, W.A. Presence of Kynurenic Acid in Food and Honeybee Products. *Amino Acids* **2009**, *36*, 75–80. [CrossRef] [PubMed]
74. Beretta, G.; Artali, R.; Caneva, E.; Orlandini, S.; Centini, M.; Facino, R.M. Quinoline Alkaloids in Honey: Further Analytical (HPLC-DAD-ESI-MS, Multidimensional Diffusion-Ordered NMR Spectroscopy), Theoretical and Chemometric Studies. *J. Pharm. Biomed. Anal.* **2009**, *50*, 432–439. [CrossRef]
75. Muszynska, B.; Sutkowska-Ziaja, K.; Ekiert, H. Indole Compounds in Some Culinary-Medicinal Higher Basidiomycetes from Poland. *Int. J. Med. Mushrooms* **2011**, *13*, 449–454. [CrossRef]
76. Turski, M.P.; Kamiński, P.; Zgrajka, W.; Turska, M.; Turski, W.A. Potato- an Important Source of Nutritional Kynurenic Acid. *Plant Foods Hum. Nutr.* **2012**, *67*, 17–23. [CrossRef]
77. Turski, M.P.; Turska, M.; Kocki, T.; Turski, W.A.; Paluszkiewicz, P. Kynurenic Acid Content in Selected Culinary Herbs and Spices. *J. Chem.* **2015**, *2015*, 1–6. [CrossRef]
78. Yılmaz, C.; Gökmen, V. Determination of Tryptophan Derivatives in Kynurenine Pathway in Fermented Foods Using Liquid Chromatography Tandem Mass Spectrometry. *Food Chem.* **2018**, *243*, 420–427. [CrossRef]
79. Yılmaz, C.; Gökmen, V. Formation of Amino Acid Derivatives in White and Red Wines during Fermentation: Effects of Non-Saccharomyces Yeasts and Oenococcus Oeni. *Food Chem.* **2021**, *343*, 128415. [CrossRef]
80. Kim, J.; Kim, D.; Lee, S. Quantitative Analysis of Kynurenic Acid in Chestnut Honey from Different Regions and Method Validation. *Korean J. Pharmacogn.* **2022**, *53*, 111–118. [CrossRef]
81. Kita, A.; Kołodziejczyk, M.; Michalska-Ciechanowska, A.; Brzezowska, J.; Wicha-Komsta, K.; Turski, W. The Effect of Thermal Treatment on Selected Properties and Content of Biologically Active Compounds in Potato Crisps. *Appl. Sci.* **2022**, *12*, 555. [CrossRef]
82. Turski, M.P.; Turska, M.; Zgrajka, W.; Bartnik, M.; Kocki, T.; Turski, W.A. Distribution, Synthesis, and Absorption of Kynurenic Acid in Plants. *Planta Med* **2011**, *77*, 858–864. [CrossRef]
83. Zgrajka, W.; Turska, M.; Rajtar, G.; Majdan, M.; Parada-Turska, J. Kynurenic Acid Content in Anti-Rheumatic Herbs. *Ann Agric Environ. Med.* **2013**, *20*, 800–802.
84. Turski, M.P.; Zgrajka, W.; Siwicki, A.K.; Paluszkiewicz, P. Presence and Content of Kynurenic Acid in Animal Feed. *J. Anim. Physiol. Anim. Nutr.* **2015**, *99*, 73–78. [CrossRef]
85. Sathyasaikumar, K.V.; Notarangelo, F.M.; Kelly, D.L.; Rowland, L.M.; Hare, S.M.; Chen, S.; Mo, C.; Buchanan, R.W.; Schwarcz, R. Tryptophan Challenge in Healthy Controls and People with Schizophrenia: Acute Effects on Plasma Levels of Kynurenine, Kynurenic Acid and 5-Hydroxyindoleacetic Acid. *Pharmaceuticals* **2022**, *15*, 1003. [CrossRef]
86. Turski, W.A.; Małaczewska, J.; Marciniak, S.; Bednarski, J.; Turski, M.P.; Jabłoński, M.; Siwicki, A.K. On the Toxicity of Kynurenic Acid in Vivo and in Vitro. *Pharm. Rep.* **2014**, *66*, 1127–1133. [CrossRef] [PubMed]
87. Małaczewska, J.; Siwicki, A.K.; Wójcik, R.M.; Kaczorek, E.; Turski, W.A. Effect of Oral Administration of Kynurenic Acid on the Activity of the Peripheral Blood Leukocytes in Mice. *Cent. Eur. J. Immunol.* **2014**, *39*, 6–13. [CrossRef] [PubMed]
88. Małaczewska, J.; Siwicki, A.K.; Wójcik, R.M.; Turski, W.A.; Kaczorek, E. The Effect of Kynurenic Acid on the Synthesis of Selected Cytokines by Murine Splenocytes—In Vitro and Ex Vivo Studies. *Cent. Eur. J. Immunol.* **2016**, *41*, 39–46. [CrossRef] [PubMed]
89. Bądzyńska, B.; Zakrocka, I.; Turski, W.A.; Olszyński, K.H.; Sadowski, J.; Kompanowska-Jezierska, E. Kynurenic Acid Selectively Reduces Heart Rate in Spontaneously Hypertensive Rats. *Naunyn. Schmiedebergs Arch. Pharm.* **2020**, *393*, 673–679. [CrossRef]
90. Li, J.; Zhang, Y.; Yang, S.; Lu, Z.; Li, G.; Wu, S.; Wu, D.-R.; Liu, J.; Zhou, B.; Wang, H.-M.D.; et al. The Beneficial Effects of Edible Kynurenic Acid from Marine Horseshoe Crab (Tachypleus Tridentatus) on Obesity, Hyperlipidemia, and Gut Microbiota in High-Fat Diet-Fed Mice. *Oxid. Med. Cell. Longev.* **2021**, *2021*, 8874503. [CrossRef]
91. Tomaszewska, E.; Muszyński, S.; Kuc, D.; Dobrowolski, P.; Lamorski, K.; Smolińska, K.; Donaldson, J.; Świetlicka, I.; Mielnik-Błaszczak, M.; Paluszkiewicz, P.; et al. Chronic Dietary Supplementation with Kynurenic Acid, a Neuroactive Metabolite of Tryptophan, Decreased Body Weight without Negative Influence on Densitometry and Mandibular Bone Biomechanical Endurance in Young Rats. *PLoS ONE* **2019**, *14*, e0226205. [CrossRef]
92. Kozlowska, M. Biochemical, Genetic and Behavioural Aspects of Dietary Supplementation with Kynurenic Acid in Rats. Doctoral Dissertation. Medical University of Lublin, Lublin, Poland, 2018.
93. Agudelo, L.Z.; Ferreira, D.M.S.; Cervenka, I.; Bryzgalova, G.; Dadvar, S.; Jannig, P.R.; Pettersson-Klein, A.T.; Lakshmikanth, T.; Sustarsic, E.G.; Porsmyr-Palmertz, M.; et al. Kynurenic Acid and Gpr35 Regulate Adipose Tissue Energy Homeostasis and Inflammation. *Cell Metab.* **2018**, *27*, 378–392.e5. [CrossRef]
94. Wang, Z.; Yin, L.; Qi, Y.; Zhang, J.; Zhu, H.; Tang, J. Intestinal Flora-Derived Kynurenic Acid Protects Against Intestinal Damage Caused by Candida Albicans Infection via Activation of Aryl Hydrocarbon Receptor. *Front. Microbiol.* **2022**, *13*, 934786. [CrossRef]
95. Glavin, G.B.; Pinsky, C. Kynurenic Acid Attenuates Experimental Ulcer Formation and Basal Gastric Acid Secretion in Rats. *Res. Commun. Chem. Pathol. Pharm.* **1989**, *64*, 111–119.
96. Dobrowolski, P.; Prejbisz, A.; Kuryłowicz, A.; Baska, A.; Burchard, P.; Chlebus, K.; Dzida, G.; Jankowski, P.; Jaroszewicz, J.; Jaworski, P.; et al. Zespół metaboliczny—Nowa definicja i postępowanie w praktyce. *Lek. POZ* **2022**, *8*, 147–170.
97. Shi, T.; Shi, Y.; Gao, H.; Ma, Y.; Wang, Q.; Shen, S.; Shao, X.; Gong, W.; Chen, X.; Qin, J.; et al. Exercised Accelerated the Production of Muscle-Derived Kynurenic Acid in Skeletal Muscle and Alleviated the Postmenopausal Osteoporosis through the Gpr35/NFκB P65 Pathway. *J. Orthop. Transl.* **2022**, *35*, 1–12. [CrossRef] [PubMed]

98. Moroni, F.; Cozzi, A.; Sili, M.; Mannaioni, G. Kynurenic Acid: A Metabolite with Multiple Actions and Multiple Targets in Brain and Periphery. *J. Neural Transm.* **2012**, *119*, 133–139. [CrossRef] [PubMed]
99. Juhász, L.; Rutai, A.; Fejes, R.; Tallósy, S.P.; Poles, M.Z.; Szabó, A.; Szatmári, I.; Fülöp, F.; Vécsei, L.; Boros, M.; et al. Divergent Effects of the N-Methyl-D-Aspartate Receptor Antagonist Kynurenic Acid and the Synthetic Analog SZR-72 on Microcirculatory and Mitochondrial Dysfunction in Experimental Sepsis. *Front. Med.* **2020**, *7*, 566582. [CrossRef]
100. Poles, M.Z.; Nászai, A.; Gulácsi, L.; Czakó, B.L.; Gál, K.G.; Glenz, R.J.; Dookhun, D.; Rutai, A.; Tallósy, S.P.; Szabó, A.; et al. Kynurenic Acid and Its Synthetic Derivatives Protect Against Sepsis-Associated Neutrophil Activation and Brain Mitochondrial Dysfunction in Rats. *Front. Immunol.* **2021**, *12*, 717157. [CrossRef]
101. Hsieh, Y.; Chen, R.; Yeh, Y.; Lin, M.; Hsieh, J.; Chen, S. Kynurenic Acid Attenuates Multiorgan Dysfunction in Rats after Heatstroke. *Acta Pharm. Sin.* **2011**, *32*, 167–174. [CrossRef]
102. Kaszaki, J.; Palásthy, Z.; Erczes, D.; Rácz, A.; Torday, C.; Varga, G.; Vécsei, L.; Boros, M. Kynurenic Acid Inhibits Intestinal Hypermotility and Xanthine Oxidase Activity during Experimental Colon Obstruction in Dogs. *Neurogastroenterol. Motil.* **2008**, *20*, 53–62. [CrossRef]
103. Marciniak, A. Rola Kwasu Kynureninowego w Utrzymaniu Integralności Układu Zewnątrzwydzielniczego Trzustki w Doświadczalnym Ceruleinowym Ostrym Zapaleniu Trzustki. Habilitation Dissertation. Medical University of Lublin, Lublin, Poland, 2013.
104. Poormasjedi-Meibod, M.-S.; Hartwell, R.; Kilani, R.T.; Ghahary, A. Anti-Scarring Properties of Different Tryptophan Derivatives. *PLoS ONE* **2014**, *9*, e91785. [CrossRef]
105. Matysik-Woźniak, A.; Turski, W.A.; Turska, M.; Paduch, R.; Łańcut, M.; Piwowarczyk, P.; Czuczwar, M.; Rejdak, R. Kynurenic Acid Accelerates Healing of Corneal Epithelium In Vitro and In Vivo. *Pharmaceuticals* **2021**, *14*, 753. [CrossRef]
106. Nestor, M.S.; Berman, B.; Fischer, D.L.; Han, H.; Gade, A.; Arnold, D.; Lawson, A. A Randomized, Double-Blind, Active- and Placebo-Controlled Trial Evaluating a Novel Topical Treatment for Keloid Scars. *J. Drugs Derm.* **2021**, *20*, 964–968. [CrossRef] [PubMed]
107. Nabai, L.; Ghahary, A.; Jackson, J. Localized Controlled Release of Kynurenic Acid Encapsulated in Synthetic Polymer Reduces Implant—Induced Dermal Fibrosis. *Pharmaceutics* **2022**, *14*, 1546. [CrossRef] [PubMed]
108. Wejksza, K.; Rzeski, W.; Turski, W.A. Kynurenic Acid Protects against the Homocysteine-Induced Impairment of Endothelial Cells. *Pharm. Rep.* **2009**, *61*, 751–756. [CrossRef]
109. Zhao, C.; Wu, K.; Bao, L.; Chen, L.; Feng, L.; Liu, Z.; Wang, Y.; Fu, Y.; Zhang, N.; Hu, X. Kynurenic Acid Protects against Mastitis in Mice by Ameliorating Inflammatory Responses and Enhancing Blood-Milk Barrier Integrity. *Mol. Immunol.* **2021**, *137*, 134–144. [CrossRef]
110. Csáti, A.; Edvinsson, L.; Vécsei, L.; Toldi, J.; Fülöp, F.; Tajti, J.; Warfvinge, K. Kynurenic Acid Modulates Experimentally Induced Inflammation in the Trigeminal Ganglion. *J. Headache Pain* **2015**, *16*, 99. [CrossRef]
111. Varga, G.; Erces, D.; Fazekas, B.; Fülöp, M.; Kovács, T.; Kaszaki, J.; Fülöp, F.; Vécsei, L.; Boros, M. N-Methyl-D-Aspartate Receptor Antagonism Decreases Motility and Inflammatory Activation in the Early Phase of Acute Experimental Colitis in the Rat. *Neurogastroenterol. Motil.* **2010**, *22*, 217–225.e68. [CrossRef]
112. Benbow, T.; Teja, F.; Sheikhi, A.; Exposto, F.G.; Svensson, P.; Cairns, B.E. Peripheral N-Methyl-D-Aspartate Receptor Activation Contributes to Monosodium Glutamate-Induced Headache but Not Nausea Behaviours in Rats. *Sci. Rep.* **2022**, *12*, 13894. [CrossRef]
113. Körtési, T.; Tuka, B.; Tajti, J.; Bagoly, T.; Fülöp, F.; Helyes, Z.; Vécsei, L. Kynurenic Acid Inhibits the Electrical Stimulation Induced Elevated Pituitary Adenylate Cyclase-Activating Polypeptide Expression in the TNC. *Front. Neurol.* **2017**, *8*, 745. [CrossRef]
114. Oláh, G.; Herédi, J.; Menyhárt, A.; Czinege, Z.; Nagy, D.; Fuzik, J.; Kocsis, K.; Knapp, L.; Krucsó, E.; Gellért, L.; et al. Unexpected Effects of Peripherally Administered Kynurenic Acid on Cortical Spreading Depression and Related Blood-Brain Barrier Permeability. *Drug Des. Dev.* **2013**, *7*, 981–987. [CrossRef]
115. Knyihar-Csillik, E.; Mihaly, A.; Krisztin-Peva, B.; Robotka, H.; Szatmari, I.; Fulop, F.; Toldi, J.; Csillik, B.; Vecsei, L. The Kynurenate Analog SZR-72 Prevents the Nitroglycerol-Induced Increase of c-Fos Immunoreactivity in the Rat Caudal Trigeminal Nucleus: Comparative Studies of the Effects of SZR-72 and Kynurenic Acid. *Neurosci. Res.* **2008**, *61*, 429–432. [CrossRef]
116. Ramírez Ortega, D.; Ugalde Muñiz, P.E.; Blanco Ayala, T.; Vázquez Cervantes, G.I.; Lugo Huitrón, R.; Pineda, B.; González Esquivel, D.F.; Pérez de la Cruz, G.; Pedraza Chaverrí, J.; Sánchez Chapul, L.; et al. On the Antioxidant Properties of L-Kynurenine: An Efficient ROS Scavenger and Enhancer of Rat Brain Antioxidant Defense. *Antioxidants* **2021**, *11*, 31. [CrossRef] [PubMed]
117. Glavin, G.B.; Bose, R.; Pinsky, C. Kynurenic Acid Protects against Gastroduodenal Ulceration in Mice Injected with Extracts from Poisonous Atlantic Shellfish. *Prog. Neuropsychopharmacol. Biol. Psychiatry* **1989**, *13*, 569–572. [CrossRef]
118. Mei, J.; Zhou, Y.; Yang, X.; Zhang, F.; Liu, X.; Yu, B. Active Components in Ephedra Sinica Stapf Disrupt the Interaction between ACE2 and SARS-CoV-2 RBD: Potent COVID-19 Therapeutic Agents. *J. Ethnopharmacol.* **2021**, *278*, 114303. [CrossRef] [PubMed]
119. Lima, V.S.S.; Mariano, D.O.C.; Vigerelli, H.; Janussi, S.C.; Baptista, T.V.L.; Claudino, M.A.; Pimenta, D.C.; Sciani, J.M. Effects of Kynurenic Acid on the Rat Aorta Ischemia-Reperfusion Model: Pharmacological Characterization and Proteomic Profiling. *Molecules* **2021**, *26*, 2845. [CrossRef]
120. Wyant, G.A.; Yu, W.; Doulamis, I.P.; Nomoto, R.S.; Saeed, M.Y.; Duignan, T.; McCully, J.D.; Kaelin, W.G. Mitochondrial Remodeling and Ischemic Protection by G Protein-Coupled Receptor 35 Agonists. *Science* **2022**, *377*, 621–629. [CrossRef] [PubMed]
121. Marciniak, S.; Wnorowski, A.; Smolińska, K.; Walczyna, B.; Turski, W.; Kocki, T.; Paluszkiewicz, P.; Parada-Turska, J. Kynurenic Acid Protects against Thioacetamide-Induced Liver Injury in Rats. *Anal. Cell. Pathol.* **2018**, *2018*, 1270483. [CrossRef] [PubMed]

122. Pyun, D.H.; Kim, T.J.; Kim, M.J.; Hong, S.A.; Abd El-Aty, A.M.; Jeong, J.H.; Jung, T.W. Endogenous Metabolite, Kynurenic Acid, Attenuates Nonalcoholic Fatty Liver Disease via AMPK/Autophagy- and AMPK/ORP150-Mediated Signaling. *J. Cell Physiol.* **2021**, *236*, 4902–4912. [CrossRef]
123. Dolecka, J.; Urbanik-Sypniewska, T.; Skrzydło-Radomańska, B.; Parada-Turska, J. Effect of Kynurenic Acid on the Viability of Probiotics in Vitro. *Pharm. Rep.* **2011**, *63*, 548–551. [CrossRef]
124. Bensley, L.; Van Eenwyk, J.; Bruemmer, B.A. Measuring Fruit and Vegetable Consumption: Providing Serving Size Information Doubles Estimated Percent Eating Five per Day. *J. Am. Diet. Assoc.* **2003**, *103*, 1530–1532. [CrossRef]
125. Mellano, M.G.; Beccaro, G.L.; Donno, D.; Marinoni, D.T.; Boccacci, P.; Canterino, S.; Cerutti, A.K.; Bounous, G. Castanea Spp. Biodiversity Conservation: Collection and Characterization of the Genetic Diversity of an Endangered Species. *Genet Resour Crop. Evol.* **2012**, *59*, 1727–1741. [CrossRef]
126. Honey. Available online: https://www.rxlist.com/honey/supplements.htm (accessed on 13 September 2022).
127. Terzo, S.; Calvi, P.; Nuzzo, D.; Picone, P.; Galizzi, G.; Caruana, L.; Di Carlo, M.; Lentini, L.; Puleio, R.; Mulè, F.; et al. Preventive Impact of Long-Term Ingestion of Chestnut Honey on Glucose Disorders and Neurodegeneration in Obese Mice. *Nutrients* **2022**, *14*, 756. [CrossRef] [PubMed]
128. Sahin, H.; Kaltalioglu, K.; Erisgin, Z.; Coskun-Cevher, S.; Kolayli, S. Protective Effects of Aqueous Extracts of Some Honeys against HCl/Ethanol-Induced Gastric Ulceration in Rats. *J. Food Biochem.* **2019**, *43*, e13054. [CrossRef] [PubMed]
129. Saral, Ö.; Yildiz, O.; Aliyazicioğlu, R.; Yuluğ, E.; Canpolat, S.; Öztürk, F.; Kolayli, S. Apitherapy Products Enhance the Recovery of CCL4-Induced Hepatic Damages in Rats. *Turk. J. Med. Sci.* **2016**, *46*, 194–202. [CrossRef] [PubMed]
130. Nisbet, H.O.; Nisbet, C.; Yarim, M.; Guler, A.; Ozak, A. Effects of Three Types of Honey on Cutaneous Wound Healing. *Wounds* **2010**, *22*, 275–283. [PubMed]
131. Atalay, K.; Cabuk, K.S.; Kirgiz, A.; Caglar, A.K. Treatment of Corneal Alkali Burn with Chestnut Honey, Royal Jelly, and Chestnut Honey-Royal Jelly Mixture. *Beyoglu. Eye J.* **2019**, *4*, 196–201. [CrossRef]
132. Seyhan, M.F.; Yılmaz, E.; Timirci-Kahraman, Ö.; Saygılı, N.; Kısakesen, H.İ.; Eronat, A.P.; Ceviz, A.B.; Bilgiç Gazioğlu, S.; Yılmaz-Aydoğan, H.; Öztürk, O. Anatolian Honey Is Not Only Sweet but Can Also Protect from Breast Cancer: Elixir for Women from Artemis to Present. *IUBMB Life* **2017**, *69*, 677–688. [CrossRef] [PubMed]
133. Yildiz, O.; Karahalil, F.; Can, Z.; Sahin, H.; Kolayli, S. Total Monoamine Oxidase (MAO) Inhibition by Chestnut Honey, Pollen and Propolis. *J. Enzym. Inhib. Med. Chem* **2014**, *29*, 690–694. [CrossRef] [PubMed]
134. Sahin, H. Honey as an Apitherapic Product: Its Inhibitory Effect on Urease and Xanthine Oxidase. *J. Enzym. Inhib. Med. Chem.* **2016**, *31*, 490–494. [CrossRef] [PubMed]
135. Combarros-Fuertes, P.; M Estevinho, L.; Teixeira-Santos, R.; G Rodrigues, A.; Pina-Vaz, C.; Fresno, J.M.; Tornadijo, M.E. Antibacterial Action Mechanisms of Honey: Physiological Effects of Avocado, Chestnut, and Polyfloral Honey upon Staphylococcus Aureus and Escherichia Coli. *Molecules* **2020**, *25*, 1252. [CrossRef]
136. Ronsisvalle, S.; Lissandrello, E.; Fuochi, V.; Petronio Petronio, G.; Straquadanio, C.; Crascì, L.; Panico, A.; Milito, M.; Cova, A.M.; Tempera, G.; et al. Antioxidant and Antimicrobial Properties of Casteanea Sativa Miller Chestnut Honey Produced on Mount Etna (Sicily). *Nat. Prod. Res.* **2019**, *33*, 843–850. [CrossRef] [PubMed]
137. Pereira, C.; Barreira, J.C.M.; Calhelha, R.C.; Lopes, M.; Queiroz, M.J.R.P.; Vilas-Boas, M.; Barros, L.; Ferreira, I.C.F.R. Is Honey Able to Potentiate the Antioxidant and Cytotoxic Properties of Medicinal Plants Consumed as Infusions for Hepatoprotective Effects? *Food Funct.* **2015**, *6*, 1435–1442. [CrossRef]
138. Kolayli, S.; Can, Z.; Yildiz, O.; Sahin, H.; Karaoglu, S.A. A Comparative Study of the Antihyaluronidase, Antiurease, Antioxidant, Antimicrobial and Physicochemical Properties of Different Unifloral Degrees of Chestnut (Castanea Sativa Mill.) Honeys. *J. Enzym. Inhib. Med. Chem.* **2016**, *31*, 96–104. [CrossRef]
139. Can, Z.; Yildiz, O.; Sahin, H.; Akyuz Turumtay, E.; Silici, S.; Kolayli, S. An Investigation of Turkish Honeys: Their Physico-Chemical Properties, Antioxidant Capacities and Phenolic Profiles. *Food Chem.* **2015**, *180*, 133–141. [CrossRef]
140. Truzzi, C.; Illuminati, S.; Annibaldia, A.; Finale, C.; Rossetti, M.; Scarponi, G. Physicochemical Properties of Honey from Marche, Central Italy: Classification of Unifloral and Multifloral Honeys by Multivariate Analysis. *Nat. Prod. Commun.* **2014**, *9*, 1595–1602. [CrossRef]
141. Escuredo, O.; Míguez, M.; Fernández-González, M.; Carmen Seijo, M. Nutritional Value and Antioxidant Activity of Honeys Produced in a European Atlantic Area. *Food Chem.* **2013**, *138*, 851–856. [CrossRef]
142. Atayoğlu, A.T.; Soylu, M.; Silici, S.; İnanç, N. Glycemic Index Values of Monofloral Turkish Honeys and the Effect Oftheir Consumption on Glucose Metabolism. *Turk. J. Med. Sci.* **2016**, *46*, 483–488. [CrossRef]
143. Gourdomichali, T.; Papakonstantinou, E. Short-Term Effects of Six Greek Honey Varieties on Glycemic Response: A Randomized Clinical Trial in Healthy Subjects. *Eur. J. Clin. Nutr.* **2018**, *72*, 1709–1716. [CrossRef] [PubMed]
144. Deibert, P.; König, D.; Kloock, B.; Groenefeld, M.; Berg, A. Glycaemic and Insulinaemic Properties of Some German Honey Varieties. *Eur. J. Clin. Nutr.* **2010**, *64*, 762–764. [CrossRef] [PubMed]
145. Wróbel-Kwiatkowska, M.; Turski, W.; Kocki, T.; Rakicka-Pustułka, M.; Rymowicz, W. An Efficient Method for Production of Kynurenic Acid by Yarrowia Lipolytica. *Yeast* **2020**, *37*, 541–547. [CrossRef]
146. Rakicka-Pustułka, M.; Ziuzia, P.; Pierwoła, J.; Szymański, K.; Wróbel-Kwiatkowska, M.; Lazar, Z. The Microbial Production of Kynurenic Acid Using Yarrowia Lipolytica Yeast Growing on Crude Glycerol and Soybean Molasses. *Front. Bioeng. Biotechnol.* **2022**, *10*, 936137. [CrossRef]

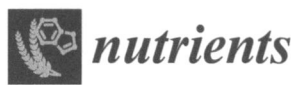

Review

Extracts Rich in Nutrients as Novel Food Ingredients to Be Used in Food Supplements: A Proposal Classification

Ricardo López-Rodríguez, Laura Domínguez, Virginia Fernández-Ruiz and Montaña Cámara *

Nutrition and Food Science Department, Pharmacy Faculty, Complutense University of Madrid (UCM), Plaza Ramón y Cajal, s/n, E-28040 Madrid, Spain
* Correspondence: mcamara@ucm.es; Tel.: +34-923941802; Fax: +34-913941799

Abstract: Consumers' commitment to healthy lifestyles and a varied diet has experienced rapid growth in recent decades, causing an increase in the demand of better food quality and variety. The food industry has opted for innovation and the search for new sources of food, and these trends led to the need to develop a European regulatory framework. Novel foods are under Regulation (EU) 2015/2283 (formerly Regulation (EC) No 258/97), and this concept includes all food not used in an important measure for human consumption in the EU before 15 May 1997, and which is included in any of the food categories established. Currently, there are 26 extracts authorized as novel foods or ingredients, being one of the most numerous groups. These extracts are concentrated sources of nutrients, and 23 of them can be used in food supplements. Given their heterogeneous composition and the perceptive risk assessments performed, sometimes, the authorizations are limited to certain population groups. The present work is a comprehensive review of the extracts rich in nutrients authorized as novel ingredients to be used in food supplements within the EU. A classification is proposed according to their source of origin, resulting in four main groups: extracts of plant, animal, algae, and fungal origins. A description of each extract as well as the evaluation of the potential use restriction and health benefits are also addressed.

Keywords: novel foods; novel ingredients; extracts; food supplements; risk assessment

Citation: López-Rodríguez, R.; Domínguez, L.; Fernández-Ruiz, V.; Cámara, M. Extracts Rich in Nutrients as Novel Food Ingredients to Be Used in Food Supplements: A Proposal Classification. *Nutrients* 2022, *14*, 3194. https://doi.org/10.3390/nu14153194

Academic Editor: Anna Gramza-Michałowska

Received: 1 July 2022
Accepted: 30 July 2022
Published: 4 August 2022

Publisher's Note: MDPI stays neutral with regard to jurisdictional claims in published maps and institutional affiliations.

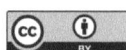

Copyright: © 2022 by the authors. Licensee MDPI, Basel, Switzerland. This article is an open access article distributed under the terms and conditions of the Creative Commons Attribution (CC BY) license (https://creativecommons.org/licenses/by/4.0/).

1. Introduction

Consumers' commitment to increasingly healthy lifestyles and a varied diet has experienced rapid growth in recent decades, which has led to an increase in demand in terms of the quality and variety of food and food supplements they consume. The population is increasingly aware that health encompasses something more than the mere fact of not suffering from a disease, which is why they seek to improve their well-being through an optimized diet. Thus, consumers need to acquire products such as food supplements that complement their diet in order to improve or maintain health [1,2].

The definition of food supplements, established in Directive 2002/46/EC of the European Parliament and of the Council of 10 June 2002 on the approximation of the laws of the Member States relating to food supplements, postulates them as food products whose purpose is to supplement the normal diet and consisting of concentrated sources of nutrients or other substances that have a nutritional or physiological effect, in simple or combined form, marketed in dosage form such as capsules, pastilles, tablets, pills, and other similar forms, sachets of powders, liquid ampoules, dropper bottles, and other similar forms of liquids and powders that are taken in small unit quantities [3].

Food supplements are products in the frontier of food-pharma and have a specific regulatory framework in which the legislative provisions related to extracts authorized as novel foods must be considered [1]. In this context, the food industry has opted for innovation through the application of new technological processes and the search for new sources of food and food supplements that allow it to meet these demands and thus maintain its competitiveness in a globalized market [4,5]. However, the consumers' perception of its safety and the cost benefits associated with its consumption will be crucial in the final introduction of a novel food product on the market.

When innovations are applied to traditional foods or products, their acceptance by consumers will largely depend on the type of food and applied innovation, being well accepted those that provide relevant benefits without substantially modifying the food in question [6]. The lack of positive consumer perception regarding the potential benefits of these products can lead most consumers to question the need and usefulness of this novel product, and may even have the opposite effect, increasing the perception of risk [7]. That is why it is common to carry out consumer studies (during the stages of identifying a new product, its development, or the tests before its commercialization) as a step prior to launching a new product on the market [8].

These innovation trends in the market caused the need to develop an adequate regulatory framework in the European Union, thus giving rise to the so-called novel foods. The concept of novel food, initially established by Regulation (EC) No. 258/97, concerning novel foods and novel food ingredients, and currently in force according to Regulation (EU) 2015/2283, includes any food that has not been used in an important measure for human consumption in the European Union before 15 May 1997, and that is included in any of the food categories established in the aforementioned Regulation [9].

The authorization procedure for extracts as novel foods has followed different paths depending on whether the authorization took place [9]. Until 1 January 2018 (date of entry into force of the current Regulation (EU) 2015/2283), the applicant must present a request to the Member State in which the novel food was placed on the market for the first time. The Member State in question issued an initial assessment report with the conclusions about the safety of the novel food. If no substantiated objection was raised, the novel food could be placed on the market. If additional evaluations were required, the novel food had to be the subject of a further assessment by the European Food Safety Authority (EFSA) [10]. After completing the evaluation requested, the EFSA sent it to the European Commission who, in turn, prepared a draft Decision. This draft was sent to the Standing Committee on the Food Chain and Animal Health (SCFCAH), where the Decision was definitively adopted by authorizing or denying the placing on the market of the novel food in question.

Parallel to the general authorization procedure for novel foods, Article 5 of Regulation (EC) No. 258/97 established a simplified procedure called notification, applicable to those foods and food ingredients that were substantially equivalent to existing foods or food ingredients regarding their composition, nutritional value, metabolism, intended use, and content of undesirable substances, in accordance with the scientific data available, recognized by general form and/or opinions issued by one of the competent bodies. In this procedure, the applicant had to notify the placing of the product on the market to the European Commission. This notification had to be accompanied by a favorable scientific opinion issued by a competent body of one of the Member States.

After the entry into the force of the current Regulation (EU) 2015/2283, all valid applications for the evaluation of novel foods are sent by the European Commission to the EFSA, which has a maximum period of 9 months to proceed with its evaluation and issue an opinion on the safety of the novel food. Once its evaluation is complete, the EFSA publishes its opinion and transmits it to the Commission, the Member States, and the applicant. Within 7 months from the date of publication of the EFSA's opinion, the Commission will submit to the Standing Committee on Plants, Animals, Food and Feed (SCPAFF) a draft implementing act, in accordance with the procedure laid down in Regulation (EU) No. 182/2011, which authorizes the marketing of the novel food in the European Union and updates the so-called Union list of novel foods established in Regulation (EU) 2017/2470 [11,12]. Novel foods are under the food legislation approved in the European Union so that they must meet the labeling provisions established by Regulation (EU) No. 1169/2011 [9]. Additional labeling requirements regarding a particular characteristic or property of the novel food in question (nutritional composition and value, intended use, restriction of use in specific population groups, etc.) are included in Commission Implementing Regulation (EU) 2017/2470, which establishes the Union list of novel foods in accordance with Regulation (EU) 2015/2283 of the European Parliament and of the Council on novel foods. The objective of the present work is to study the authorized extracts as novel foods or food ingredients for its use in food supplements in the European Union since 1997. In order to group the different types of extracts authorized, a classification of these extracts is proposed by the authors of the present work. A description of each extract as well as the evaluation of the potential use restriction and health benefits are also addressed in this study.

2. Materials and Methods

A search for scientific opinions, regulations, and bibliographies has been carried out using official databases such as Web of Science and Science Direct. A literature review of the current and available scientific evidence about the potential health benefits attributed to these extracts rich in nutrients was performed in scientific databases and resources such as Pubmed and Google Scholar, using the name of each extract plus "health benefits" as selected keywords. Scientific studies published in the English language and during the last 11-year period (2011–2022) were considered in the present review.

The authorization procedure for extracts as novel foods for its use in food supplements has taken place through different pathways, established both in Regulation (EC) No. 258/97 and in Regulation (EU) 2015/2283. The analysis of the different authorization decisions and regulations, and the reports of initial and complementary evaluations of the different extracts, allows us to know their main characteristics as sources of nutrients and the main aspects related to their safety evaluations, as well as establishes a classification of the same.

This study focused only on those novel foods of which the word 'extract' is included in the title of the EU decision as a classification and selection purpose. The authors are aware that other novel foods already approved include an extraction process; however, those are not approved as extracts, and are thus not included in this proposed classification.

3. Results and Discussion

To date, a total of 26 extracts has been approved as novel foods and novel food ingredients in the European Union. The great majority of these extracts (23/26) has been authorized to be used in food supplements (FS). Out of these 23 extracts, 20 were authorized under the former Regulation (EC) No. 258/97 on novel foods. The authorization of red cranberry powder extract and three-root extract (*Cynanchum wilfordii* Hemsley, *Phlomis umbrosa* Turcz., and *Angelica gigas* Nakai) was requested through the former Regulation; however, their evaluation had not been completed when the current Regulation (EU) 2015/2283 entered into force on 1 January 2018, therefore the authorization process of these two extracts took place under the current Regulation, after a new assessment of their safety by the EFSA. Finally, the remaining extract (extract of *Panax notoginseng* and *Astragalus membranaceus*) was evaluated and authorized following the current procedure established by Regulation (EU) 2015/2283 [9].

The great majority of the extracts (15/23) were placed on the market through the notification procedure (substantial equivalence), while another five extracts were authorized through decisions. The three remaining extracts have been authorized through implementing regulations, in accordance with the procedure established in Regulation (EU) 2015/2283 [9].

In order to group the different types of extracts authorized for use in food supplements, a classification of these extracts is proposed by the authors of the present work according to the extract origin, distinguishing for these four main groups: extracts of plant origin (18/23), algae extracts (2/23), extracts of animal origin (1/23), and extracts of fungal origin (2/23) (Figure 1). Extracts of plant origin can be further classified into four subgroups: seed extracts; extracts of leaves, fruits, and roots; plant cell culture extracts; and other extracts of plant origin. In each group, the date of the authorization of each extract has been considered as a criterion for ordering them.

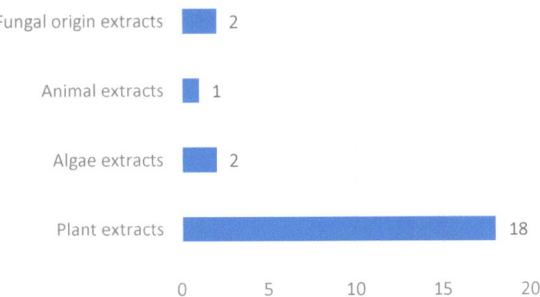

Figure 1. Distribution of 23 extracts authorized to be used in food supplements according with Novel Food Regulation.

In the case of extracts authorized as novel foods for its use in food supplements, the group of extracts of plant origin is the largest and, therefore, the most likely to be studied in the scientific literature. Another factor to take into account is that many food supplements have a complex composition, resulting from the mixture of several substances, therefore it may not be easy to identify the origin of an adverse effect. The review of the scientific literature has made it possible to identify some examples of possible adverse effects associated with this type of substances.

3.1. Extracts of Plant Origin

The use of substances of plant origin is common in the elaboration of food supplements, and particularly those based on botanical products and plant extracts have also experienced rapid growth [13]. This fast rise has led to numerous scientific studies' investigation of the potential beneficial or adverse effects associated with its consumption [14,15].

A total of 18 extracts are included in this group, being the largest group of extracts authorized to date to be used in food supplements. Within this category, the subgroups of extracts of seeds and the extracts of leaves, fruits, and roots would be the most numerous, including six and seven extracts, respectively, followed by the subgroup of plant cell culture extracts with four extracts (Figure 2).

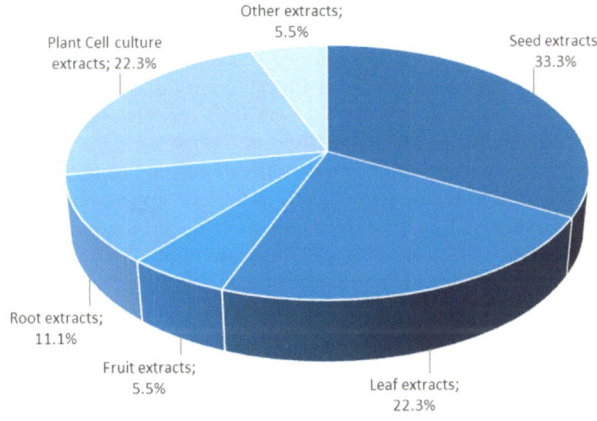

Figure 2. Distribution of extracts of plant origin considered in this study.

3.1.1. Seed Extracts

This group includes six extracts: sunflower oil extract, extract of defatted cocoa powder, low fat cocoa extract, fermented soybean extract, fermented black bean extract, and spermidine-rich wheat germ extract (*Triticum aestivum*) (Table 1).

Table 1. Seed extracts authorized as novel foods for its use in food supplements.

Extract	Maximum Levels in Food Supplements	Initial Evaluation	Authorization
Sunflower oil extract	1.1 g/day	France	Substantial equivalence [16,17]
Extract of defatted cocoa powder	1.0 g/day	Ireland	Substantial equivalence [17,18]
Low fat cocoa extract	1.2 g/day	Ireland	Substantial equivalence [17,19]
Fermented soybean extract	100 mg/day	Belgium	Decision (EU) 2017/115 [20]
Fermented black bean extract	4.5 g/day	United Kingdom	Decision (EU) 2011/497/EU [20]
Spermidine-rich wheat germ extract	6 mg/day spermidine	Austria	Substantial equivalence [17,21]

The first extract marketed within this group was the sunflower oil extract, placed on the market for the first time in 2009 through the notification procedure, when substantial equivalence was established for its use in food supplements with the corn germ oil extract with a high content of unsaponifiable material, which had previously been authorized as a novel food by Decision 2006/723/EC. Substantial equivalence was established on a weighted basis of 1 g of sunflower oil extract with 2 g of corn oil extract [16]. This sunflower oil extract is characterized by its high content of oleic and linoleic acids (20 and 70%, respectively) in addition to phytosterols (5.5%) and tocopherols (1.1%) [12]. According to the results of the European Project "Using rapeseed and sunflower meal as novel ingredients" (November 2017–December 2021), side products obtained from sunflower oil can be used as potential novel ingredients in the food industry. For instance, de-oiled sunflower kernels can be considered as a promising new protein source with some food applications, such as a meat analogue [22].

With regard to cocoa extracts, both were marketed for the first time through the notification procedure, having established substantial equivalences with a defatted cocoa powder, in the case of extract of defatted cocoa powder (for its use in food supplements and other foods) [18], and with a natural cocoa powder in the case of low fat cocoa extract for its use in food supplements [19]. Defatted extract and low fat cocoa extract are rich in polyphenols (minimum 55% gallic acid equivalent) and flavonols (minimum 300 mg/g), respectively. These high contents gave rise to additional specific labeling requirements in order to inform consumers that they should not consume neither more than 600 mg of polyphenols per day, which is equivalent to 1.1 g of the extract of defatted cocoa powder, nor more than 600 mg of cocoa flavanols per day, in the case of low fat cocoa extract [12]. Oddoye et al. (2013) reported that some by-products of cocoa beans such as cocoa pulp juice, also known as "sweatings", are used as ingredients in several food products. Cocoa pulp juice stands out for its natural content in sugars (glucose, fructose, and sucrose) and minerals (calcium, magnesium, and potassium, among others) [23]. This by-product can be added to refreshing drinks, either alone or in combination with other fruit juices. It can be used for making jam as well. Other food applications, such as the production of alcoholic beverages (gin, brandy, wine) and vinegar, can be obtained with the fermentation of the sugars naturally present in cocoa pulp juice [23].

On the other hand, two of the other extracts included in this group have their source in soybeans. The fermented black bean extract, authorized by Decision 2011/497/EU for its use in food supplements [20], is rich in protein (≥55%) and contains an alpha-glucosidase inhibitor. This extract was subject to a complementary assessment by the EFSA (2011) as the initial evaluation report received several comments and objections related, among others, to the toxicological information provided. Even though the toxicological and clinical studies provided limited evidence on the safety of the extract in question, the EFSA considered that it did not pose a concern. The target population of food supplements containing this extract were adults who wanted to inhibit the digestion of carbohydrates in order to control their weight [24]. In this sense, it should be highlighted that the authorization of a novel food is based on its safety, so that any health claims must be authorized in accordance with the procedure established for this purpose in Regulation (EC) No. 1924/2006 on nutrition and health claims on foods [25]. Regarding the potential health benefits, Kim et al. (2011) carried out in vitro, in vivo, and ex vivo clinical trials with black soybean extract to investigate its effect on platelet activation, an important risk factor in cardiovascular diseases [26]. The results suggested that black soybean extract could be able to attenuate thrombosis through the inhibition of collagen-induced platelet activation, opening the doors for this extract's use as a novel food supplement in the management of cardiovascular disorders and for the improvement of blood circulation [26].

Regarding the fermented soybean extract, it contains the enzyme nattokinase (20,000–28,000 UF/g) extracted from natto, which results from the fermentation of non-genetically modified soybeans (*Glycine max* L.) to which a selected strain of *Bacillus subtilis* var. Natto is added. This parenterally administered enzyme has fibrinolytic activity in vitro and thrombolytic activity in vivo in animals, as revealed by EFSA (2016a) in its complementary evaluation [27]. Due to this activity, it was established as a specific requirement for additional labeling that food supplements containing this extract contain a warning stating that people taking medicines must consume the product exclusively under medical supervision [28]. In addition to this specific requirement, the two soy extracts must be labeled in accordance with Annex II of Regulation (EU) No. 1169/2011, given that the risk of allergic reaction to these soy extracts is similar to that of other soy products [9]. Park et al. (2013) performed an in vitro study with soybean extract and demonstrated a potential modulation of retinoic acid-related gene expression of skin and photo-protective effects in human keratinocytes [29]. These preliminary results could be a good starting point to further investigate the use of soybean extract in food supplements intended to protect skin from the damage caused by UVB irradiation [29].

The spermidine-rich wheat germ extract is the last extract of this group authorized (December 2017) by means of substantial equivalence with the wheat germ of *Triticum aestivum* (common wheat) for its use in food supplements [21]. This extract is characterized by its contents of spermidine (0.8–2.4 mg/g) and spermine (0.4–1.2 mg/g). Scientific studies carried out on supplementation with spermidine, an autophagy-inducing agent, have shown a protective effect against neurodegeneration and cognitive impairment in animal models [30]. Nutritional and functional composition of wheat germ, an important by-product of the flour milling industry, is characterized by its content of protein (26–35%), sugars (17%), lipids (10–15%), minerals (4%), fiber (1.5–4.5%), as well as significant amounts of certain bioactive compounds such as tocopherols (300–740 mg/kg dry matter), phytosterols (24–50 mg/kg), and carotenoids (4–38 mg/kg) [31]. According to several in vitro and in vivo clinical trials, the fermented wheat germ extract, a food supplement commercialized under the name of Avemar®, has shown potential health benefits in rheumatoid arthritis, cardiac remodeling, and metabolic symptoms [32,33].

The fermented soybean extract, resulting from the fermentation of non-genetically modified soybean (*Glycine max* L.), can be considered as an example of seed extract for which potential adverse effects have been identified in the scientific literature. Di Lorenzo et al. (2014) identified 95 scientific publications regarding adverse effects associated with *Glycine max* (L.), mainly related to its allergenic potential or its isoflavone content (used to reduce menopausal symptoms) [34–36].

3.1.2. Extracts of Leaves, Fruits, and Roots

This group includes four leaf extracts: alfalfa leaf extract (*Medicago sativa*), Aloe macroclada Baker leaf extract, aqueous extracts of dried leaves of *Ilex guayusa* and *Epigallocatechin gallate* as purified extract of green tea leaves (*Camellia sinensis*); one fruit extract: powdered cranberry extract; and two root extracts: three-root extract (*Cynanchum wilfordii* Hemsley,

Phlomis umbrosa Turcz., and *Angelica gigas* Nakai), and *Panax notoginseng* and *Astragalus membranaceus* extract (Table 2).

Table 2. Leaf, fruit, and root extracts authorized as novel foods for its use in food supplements.

	Extract	Maximum Levels in Food Supplements	Initial Evaluation	Authorization
Leaf extracts	Lucerne leaf extract from *Medicago sativa* (Alfalfa leaf extract)	10 g/day	France	Decision 2009/826/EC [37]
	Epigallocatechin gallate as purified extract from green tea leaves (*Camellia sinensis*)	150 mg in one portion	Ireland	Substantial equivalence [17,38]
	Aloe macroclada Baker leaf extract	In line with normal use in food supplements of the similar gel derived from *Aloe vera* (L.) Burm.	Ireland	Substantial equivalence [17,39]
	Aqueous extracts of dried leaves of *Ilex guayusa*	In line with normal use in herbal infusions and food supplements of a similar aqueous extract of dried leaves of *Ilex paraguariensis*.	Ireland	Substantial equivalence [17,40]
Fruit extracts	Cranberry extract powder	350 mg/day.	France	Regulation (EU) 2018/1631 [41]
Root extracts	Extract of three herbal roots (*Cynanchum wilfordii* Hemsley, *Phlomis umbrosa* Turcz. and *Angelica gigas* Nakai)	175 mg/day (for adult population).	Ireland	Regulation (EU) 2018/469 [42]
	Extract from *Panax notoginseng* and *Astragalus membranaceus*	35 mg/day (for adult population).	EFSA	Regulation (EU) 2020/1821 [43]

Extracts of Leaves

Alfalfa leaf extract is the only one of this group authorized by Commission Decision. It is an extract rich in proteins (45–60%) whose use is only authorized in food supplements [37]. During its initial assessment carried out by the French competent authorities, various safety issues were highlighted, leading the initial assessment report to conclude that a further evaluation was necessary. It is an extract that has used since 1992 in third-world countries outside the European Union to combat malnutrition without adverse effects having been detected. The complementary evaluation carried out by the EFSA (2009) focused on the presence of phytoestrogens (Coumestrol and isoflavones) and L-canavanine, ruling out the presence of adverse effects based on studies in humans and animals [44]. In this sense, maximum contents were set for these substances in the specifications. Another key aspect to assess was the allergenic potential, concluding that the existence of a cross-reaction in subjects allergic to peanuts could not be ruled out. The final authorization decision (Decision 2009/826/EC) did not establish any specific provision regarding this issue [37]; however, Regulation (EU) No. 1169/2011, on food information provided to the consumer, is applicable and establishes as mandatory the mentioning of any ingredient or technological aid that appears in its annex II or derives from a substance or product that appears in that annex that causes allergies or intolerances and is used in the manufacture or processing of a food and is still present in the finished product, even if in a modified form [9]. The nutritional and functional composition of alfalfa leaf has been widely studied in the scientific literature. Alfalfa leaf contains interesting amounts of fiber, vitamins, minerals, chlorophylls, carotenoids, and phytoestrogens. Moreover, it has been reported that alfalfa leaf can be considered a good source of phenolic compounds (quercetin, naringenin, kaempferol, medicarpin, luteolin, myricetin, apigenin, etc.) and bioactive compounds with an important antioxidant activity and potential antimicrobial, anti-inflammatory, and immunomodulatory properties. On the other hand, and in accordance with some preclinical studies, alfalfa leaf extract enriched with vitamin C could strengthen and enhance the immune system. It has also been suggested that the use of this extract as a food supplement could be beneficial in some disorders of the digestive tract as well as in malnutrition and ischemic disease. However, further studies are needed to confirm these potential health effects in human organisms [45].

Regarding the other three extracts, it should be noted that they were placed on the market for the first time through the notification procedure for their use in food supplements. *Epigallocatechin gallate* extract, as a purified extract ($\geq$90%) of green tea (*Camellia sinensis*) leaves, was commercialized upon the establishment of substantial equivalence to other green tea extracts with a history of safe use prior to 1997 [38]. *Epigallocatechin gallate* is the main component of the polyphenolic fraction of green tea, responsible for most of the therapeutic effects attributed to its consumption, highlighting its antioxidant and anti-adipogenic potential [46,47]. A systematic review carried out by Momose et al. (2016) resulted in 17 human trials showing a potential capacity of *Epigallocatechin gallate* extract in decreasing LDL levels after 4–14 weeks of supplementation [48]. Recently, Chatree et al. (2020) performed an in vitro study with human adipocytes and revealed that the administration of *Epigallocatechin gallate* extract reduced triglycerides concentrations as well as systolic and diastolic blood pressure after 8 weeks of supplementation [49].

In the case of the *Aloe macroclada* Baker leaf extract, substantial equivalence was established with an *Aloe vera* L. leaf extract with a history of safe use in food supplements prior to 1997 [39]. It stands out for its content in dietary fibers (28.6%), polysaccharides (9.5%), and glucose (8.9%) [12]. According to the scientific literature, Aloe gel obtained from the leaf has potentially showed antiviral and immunological properties as well as hypoglycemic activity in human clinical trials. For that reason, Aloe gel has been used in some food supplements for the management of different diseases or disorders such as acquired immune deficiency syndrome and diabetes [50].

The systematic review carried out by Di Lorenzo et al. (2014), regarding the possible adverse effects of *Camellia sinensis* (L.) Kuntze [34], identified 34 publications, 29 of which were considered as sufficiently documented to assess their causality. Among the side effects described, acute hepatotoxicity is underlined, including cases with clinical effects described as a slight increase in serum aminotransferases levels or even hepatitis [34].

These potential adverse effects were associated with different degrees of causality, with food supplements based on green tea extracts, including hydroalcoholic extracts, and with aqueous extracts of green tea consumed either as a tea or in capsules, being the gallic esters of catechins, and in particular of Epigallocatechin-3-gallate, the compounds most frequently identified as responsible in cases of hepatotoxicity [40]. However, it is necessary to highlight that most of the cases described were classified as "certain/probable" or "possible" when considering the potential contribution of other factors such as age, concomitant pathological conditions, the presence of other ingredients, or even adulteration or contamination [34].

Aqueous extracts of dried leaves of *Ilex guayusa* were considered to be substantially equivalent to aqueous extracts of *Ilex paraguariensis* for its use in food supplements and infusions. This extract stands out for its caffeine content (19.8–57.7 mg/100 g)—one of the main study parameters when establishing equivalence, as differences related to caffeine content were found between both extracts. Natural variability based on the location, the type of crop, the collection, and the extraction process could be the reason for such differences [51]. Among the main potential beneficial effects of guayusa, it is important to highlight its stimulant and antioxidant properties. A systematic review performed by Radice et al. (2016) with an extract of dried leaves of *Ilex guayusa* [52] reported a reduction in hyperglycemia in animal models. Further scientific studies are needed to elucidate the potential use of this extract in nutraceutical formulations.

Extracts of Fruits

To date, this subgroup is made up of a single authorized extract: cranberry extract powder, characterized by its high content of phenols (>46.2%, expressed as gallic acid equivalents) and proanthocyanidins (55.0–60.0% or 15.0–18.0%, depending on the analytical method used). The initial application included its use in various types of beverages and by several population groups, including children. In this sense, during their initial evaluation, emphasis was placed on the possible risks existing for children aged 1–3 years old due to the potential excessive consumption of polyphenols through the novel food and other sources present in the diet of these children [41]. This issue, along with other objections, led to a further evaluation by the EFSA (2017) and the modification of the application excluding infants, young children, and adolescents from its use, focusing the requested uses only on adults. The EFSA concluded that the use of this extract in the proposed conditions was safe considering the estimation of the intake together with the results of clinical studies in humans without adverse effects [53].

However, the European Commission continued to show concern about the risk that infants, young children, and adolescents could consume these drinks with the extract in question. For this reason, the alternative of authorizing cranberry extract for its use in food supplements intended for the adult population was proposed. This authorization is currently in force according to Regulation (EU) 2018/1631 [41].

It is well known that cranberry extracts are commonly used in food supplements to alleviate some symptoms of acute and uncomplicated urinary tract infections. A systematic review carried out by Gbinigie et al. (2020) [54], found some human studies in which cranberry extract capsules were associated with a within-group improvement in urinary symptoms.

A comprehensive review carried out by Kowalska and Olejnik (2016), [55], comprising 7 human studies and 10 animal studies suggested that cranberry extract could be used as an effective complement in individuals with metabolic complications as it could be able to ameliorate insulin resistance, improve plasma lipid profile, and reduce diet-induced weight gain and visceral obesity as well as different markers of oxidative stress. Peixoto et al. (2018) demonstrated that cranberry extract [56], could enhance the metabolic profile and decrease the oxidative damage and steatosis in rats with a high-fat diet. These studies suggest that the administration of cranberry extracts through food supplements could be helpful in managing obesity-related disorders along with the pharmacological treatment.

Extracts of Roots

This group is made up of two extracts: the extract formed by three herbal roots (*Cynanchum wilfordii* Hemsley, *Phlomis umbrosa* Turcz., and *Angelica gigas* Nakai), and the extract from *Panax notoginseng* and *Astragalus membranaceus*.

The extract of three herbal roots (*Cynanchum wilfordii* Hemsley, *Phlomis umbrosa* Turcz., and *Angelica gigas* Nakai) is characterized by its content of some compounds such as phenols (13.0–40.0 mg/g), coumarins (13.0–40.0 mg/g), and iridoids (13.0–40.0 mg/g). The proportion of this mixture of roots is the following: 32.5% (p/p) of *Cynanchum wilfordii*, 32.5% (p/p) of *Phlomis umbrosa*, and 35.0% (p/p) of *Angelica gigas* [12]. The initial application, which established its use in food supplements aimed at postmenopausal women, was the subject of a complementary evaluation by the EFSA (2016) wherein the safety of this extract was not established for the requested maximum intake level (514 mg/day), as this exceeds the level of intake considered safe. However, the EFSA concluded that the extract was safe for adults if it was added to food supplements at a maximum daily dose (175 mg/day), which was significantly lower than that initially requested, and which corresponded to the safe intake level. Likewise, it was considered that the risk of allergic reaction to *Angelica gigas* Nakai did not differ from celery, since both plants belong to the same botanical family (*Apiaceae*) [57]. After providing additional information by the applicant, the EFSA carried out a new evaluation, where it reaffirmed the conclusions of its first report [58].

The final authorization of this extract for its use in food supplements intended for the adult population [42], established as a specific labeling requirement that food supplements containing the extract of the mixture of the three herbal roots will include, next to the list of ingredients, the indication that it should not be consumed by people allergic to celery, in accordance with the provisions of Regulation (EU) No. 1169/2011 [9].

An in vivo study performed by Oh et al. (2018) [59], suggested a potential improvement of stress-induced depression in mice after supplementation with the extract of three herbal roots (*Cynanchum wilfordii* Hemsley, *Phlomis umbrosa* Turcz., and *Angelica gigas* Nakai). These authors indicated that those potential health effects could be attributed to the antagonistic activity on the 5-HT6 receptor. Due to its possible antidepressant effects, this extract is starting to attract the attention of both food and pharmaceutical industries; however, human studies are needed to confirm these preliminary findings.

The extract from *Panax notoginseng* and *Astragalus membranaceus* is the last authorized extract (in 2020) as a novel food [60]. It is a mixture of two extracts: an ethanol extract from the roots of *Astragalus membranaceus* (Fisch.), Bunge, and a hot water extract from the roots of *Panax notoginseng* (Burkill) F.H. Chen, fundamentally characterized by a content of carbohydrates ($\geq$90%), proteins ($\leq$4.5%), and saponins (1.5–5%) [43].

This extract is authorized by Regulation (EU) 2020/1821 for its use in food supplements (maximum content 35 mg/day), as defined in Directive 2002/46/EC, for the general adult population, except food supplements for pregnant women, after having been the subject of a risk assessment by the EFSA (2020), in which, among other issues, the extensive history of the use of the two plants used was revealed, especially in traditional Chinese medicine. Regarding its toxicity, a safe intake of 0.5 mg/kg body weight/day (corresponding to a maximum daily intake of 35 mg) was established based on a no adverse effect level (NOAEL) of 100 mg/day/kg body weight/day, derived from a subchronic toxicity study, and applying a safety factor of 200. Furthermore, the presented studies ruled out any concern regarding genotoxicity. Another aspect evaluated by the EFSA was its potential allergenicity, given the presence of proteins ($\leq$4.5%) in its composition. Considering the extensive history of the use of the two plants used in the production of the extract, it was concluded that the risk of possible allergic reactions, although unknown, was expected to be low in the case of the general population [60].

As a specific additional labeling requirement, Regulation (EU) 2020/1821 establishes that the labeling of food supplements containing *Panax notoginseng* and *Astragalus membranaceus* extract will include a statement highlighting that these food supplements should not be consumed by individuals under the age of 18 years old or pregnant women [43].

According to Zhou et al. (2012) [61], *Panax notoginseng* and *Astragalus membranaceus* are considered Chinese medicinal plants. *Panax notoginseng* contains ginsenosides, bioactive compounds with potential health effects such as immunological and anti-fatigue functions. *Astragalus membranaceus* is known as a tonic to strengthen the immune system and, in combination with ginseng, it is used in Chinese medicine to manage certain ailments.

3.1.3. Plant Cell Culture Extracts

A total of four extracts are included in this group: *Ajuga reptans* extract, *Echinacea angustifolia* extract, dried extract of *Lippia citriodora*, and *Echinacea purpurea* extract. All of them were placed on the market for the first time through the notification procedure for their use in food supplements, with the *Echinacea purpurea* extract being the last one commercialized (2017) (Table 3).

Table 3. Cell culture extracts authorized as novel foods for their use in food supplements.

Extract	Maximum Levels in Food Supplements	Initial Evaluation	Authorization
Ajuga reptans extract from cell cultures	In line with normal use in food supplements of a similar extract of the flowering aerial parts of *Ajuga reptans*	Italy	Substantial equivalence [17,62]
Echinacea angustifolia extract from cell cultures	In line with normal use in food supplements of a similar extract from the root of *Echinacea angustifolia*	Italy	Substantial equivalence [17,63]
Dried extract of *Lippia citriodora* from cell cultures	In line with normal use in food supplements of a similar extract from the leaves of *Lippia citriodora*	Italy	Substantial equivalence [17,64]
Echinacea purpurea extract from cell cultures	In line with normal use in food supplements of a similar extract from florets within the flower head of *Echinacea purpurea*	Italy	Substantial equivalence [17,65]

Regarding the substantial equivalences established with foods with histories of safe uses, the *Ajuga reptans* extract was substantially equivalent to the extracts of the flowering aerial parts of *Ajuga reptans* obtained through traditional cultivation [62]; *Echinacea angustifolia* extract to the root extract of *Echinacea angustifolia* obtained in ethanol-water titrated to 4% echinacoside [63]; *Lippia citriodora* extract to a similar extract of leaves of *Lippia citriodora* obtained by traditional cultures [64]; and *Echinacea purpurea* extract to a similar extract of the flower of the chapter of *Echinacea purpurea* [65].

Unlike other authorized extracts, no specifications about their composition or the content of undesirable substances have been established in the Union List [12] for the four abovementioned cell culture extracts. Only specifications about the description of these cell culture extracts have been set. No specific maximum amounts have been established for its use in food supplements; however, reference is made to quantities consistent with a normal use of the extracts with which the substantial equivalences were established.

Di Lorenzo et al. (2014) identified 20 publications related to possible adverse effects of *Echinacea purpurea* (L.); however, these side effects are mainly associated with aqueous and hydroalcoholic extracts of roots and herbs, while the one authorized as a novel food is a dry extract and was authorized in 2017 [34].

Reported effects include allergenicity, mainly due to IgE-mediated hypersensitivity as a consequence of the immunostimulatory properties of *Echinacea purpurea* [34,66,67] and acute hepatotoxicity [68,69].

Esposito et al. (2020) performed a study on *Ajuga reptans* extract. The results showed that this extract could decrease the reactive oxygen species levels in cancer cell lines, opening the doors for its use as an active ingredient for nutraceutical or pharmaceutical purposes [70]. Toso and Melandri (2011) investigated the possible benefits attributed to *Echinacea angustifolia* extract from cell cultures in intensive human sport. A significant reduction in lipoperoxides levels (oxidative stress marker) in 20 humans under high physical training was demonstrated after a daily supplementation during 4 weeks with an *Echinacea angustifolia* plant cell culture extract that contained of 2.5 mg echinacoside [71]. In an in vitro study, Ghasempour et al. (2016) suggested the antifungal activity of an ethanolic extract of *Lippia citriodora*, which could be a good starting point to further investigate in vivo its efficacy and properties [72]. Motamedi et al. (2018) confirmed that *Echinacea purpurea* extract has beneficial effects on sperm characteristics in mice. According to the results of this in vivo study, the extract in question significantly increased the sperm count as well as its motility and mobility [73]. In addition, Banica et al. (2020) indicated that food supplements and extracts of *Echinacea purpurea* have antiviral, antibacterial, or antioxidant activities [74]. Among the main active substances present in *Echinacea purpurea*, polyphenols mainly derived from caffeic acid should be highlighted.

3.1.4. Other Extracts of Plant Origin

A taxifolin-rich extract from the wood of Dahurian Larch (*Larix gmelinii* (Rupr.) Rupr), which had no history of safe use in the European Union, is included in this group. This extract stands out for its high content of the flavonoid taxifolin ($\geq$90.0% of dry weight), an antioxidant used in a wide range of food products, including food supplements [75,76].

In 2010, the initial application of this extract included several uses (alcoholic beverages, chocolate products, yoghurts, and food supplements) which were initially evaluated by the competent authorities of the United Kingdom [75]. Subsequently, the abovementioned uses were subject to a positive complementary evaluation by the EFSA, basing the risk characterization on the calculation of the margin of exposure (MOE) of the combined intake [77]. However, its use was only authorized in food supplements intended for the general population, excluding infants, young children, children, and adolescents under 14 years of age [78]. Then, the Commission requested a new evaluation from the EFSA about the rest of the uses and levels of use whose authorization had not finally been granted. After informing the applicant, the applicant requested a further extension of the use and conditions of use in dairy products intended for the general population, as well as a change in the chemical name of taxifolin. Finally, after the evaluation carried out by the EFSA, based on the estimation of the exposure for the new uses and calculation of the MOE, Regulation (EU) 2018/461 authorized the rest of the uses initially requested and the extension to the dairy products [79,80].

Wang et al. (2011) suggested that extract rich in taxifolin and other flavonoids from the wood sawdust of *Larix gmelinii* showed a remarkable antioxidant activity measured by the DPPH and BHT assays [81]. These antioxidant properties are important since scientific evidence has demonstrated that oxidative stress caused by reactive oxygen species (ROS) is considered one important risk factor for the appearance of different chronic diseases and disorders. However, more studies are crucial to clarify the potential health effects of this extract as well as its use in the food and pharmaceutical industries.

3.2. Algae Extracts

This group comprises two fucoidan extracts from the algae *Fucus vesiculosus* and *Undaria pinnatifida*, both placed on the market for the first time in 2017 by the notification procedure for their use in foods and food supplements after a joint evaluation of their safety [82] (Table 4).

Table 4. Algae extracts authorized as novel foods for its use in food supplements.

Extract	Maximum Levels in Food Supplements	Initial Evaluation	Authorization
Fucoidan extract from the seaweed *Fucus vesiculosus*	250 mg/day	Belgium	Substantial equivalence [17,82]
Fucoidan extract from the seaweed *Undaria pinnatifida*	250 mg/day	Belgium	Substantial equivalence [17,82]

Both fucoidan extracts from the algae *Fucus vesiculosus* and *Undaria pinnatifida* are allowed to be commercialized in two types of extracts depending on the concentration of fucoidan. Thus, in the case of *Undaria pinnatifida*, the concentration of this compound varies between 75–95% in one of the extracts and 50–55% in the other, while, in the case of *Fucus vesiculosus*, the concentrations of fucoidan vary between 75–95% and 60–65% [12].

Fucoidan is a sulfated polysaccharide characterized by its high content of L-fucose and sulfate, as well as other minor components such as xylose, galactose, mannose, and glucuronic acid. As examples of its biological activity, some authors include the antioxidant, anti-inflammatory, antiviral, or antitumor activities as well as its effect on osteoblastic differentiation [83].

Bae et al. (2020) [84], evaluated the potential effect of fucoidan extracted from *Fucus vesiculosus* on ovarian cancer. The preliminary results revealed that this extract was able to inhibit in vitro the development of human ovarian cancer through different mechanisms, suggesting the potential use of this fucoidan extract in the pharmaceutical industry [84]. According to the review published by Zhao et al. (2018) [85], fucoidan extracted from *Undaria pinnatifida* could be considered an interesting source for nutraceuticals and functional foods given its antioxidant and antiviral properties.

3.3. Extracts of Animal Origin

A protein extract from pig kidneys is included in this group. This extract of animal origin was placed on the EU market for the first time in 2012 through the notification procedure for its use in food supplements and foods for special medical uses [17,86].

It is an extract with a natural content of the enzyme diamine oxidase (DAO) that was initially formulated as enteric-coated capsules to target the active sites of digestion and with its use limited to three capsules daily (0.9 mg/day DAO). This authorized use was extended by Regulation (EU) 2020/973 [87], without an evaluation by the EFSA, to include enteric-coated tablets, so that the maximum quantity currently authorized in food supplements is "3 capsules or 3 tablets/day; equivalent to 12.6 mg of pig kidney extract per day. Diamine oxidase (DAO) content: 0.9 mg/day (3 capsules or 3 tablets with a DAO content of 0.3 mg/capsule or 0.3 mg/tablet)" [12].

To the authors knowledge, there is no scientific evidence about the potential health effects of pig kidney extract. The literature review in different scientific databases carried out by the authors of the present work did not find any study assessing these effects.

3.4. Extracts of Fungal Origin

To date, only two extracts have been authorized within this group: mushroom chitosan extract (*Agaricus bisporus*; *Aspergillus niger*) and shiitake mushroom mycelium extract (*Lentinula edodes*) (Table 5).

Table 5. Extracts of fungal origin authorized as novel foods for its use in food supplements.

Extract	Maximum Levels in Food Supplements	Initial Evaluation	Authorization
Chitosan extract from fungi (*Agaricus bisporus*; *Aspergillus niger*)	In line with normal use in food supplements of chitosan from crustaceans	Belgium	Substantial equivalence [17,88]
Mycelial extract from Shiitake mushroom (*Lentinula edodes*)	2.5 mL/day	United Kingdom	Decision 2011/73/EU [89]

On one hand, the chitosan extract from fungi (*Agaricus bisporus*; *Aspergillus niger*) stands out for having been the first extract authorized as a novel food in 2008 for its use in food supplements, and which was placed on the EU market for the first time through the notification procedure as substantial equivalence with a crustacean chitosan extract has been established [88]. This extract is characterized by its chitosan content ($\geq 85\%$) which, in turn, mainly contains poly D-glucosamine. A maximum amount of use in food supplements has not been established, but it will be in line with the normal use in these food supplements of chitosan from crustaceans with which substantial equivalence was established [12].

Among the uses of chitosan, the formulation of food supplements and its use in the treatment of hypercholesterolemia or the prevention of cardiovascular risks should be highlighted [90,91].

On the other hand, the mycelial extract from Shiitake mushroom (*Lentinula edodes*) is a sterile aqueous extract obtained from the mycelium of *Lentinula edodes* cultivated in submerged fermentation. This extract was authorized by Decision 2011/73/EU [89] for its use as a novel food ingredient in various foods and in food supplements, standing out for its lentinan content (0.8–1.2 mg/mL), a modifier of the biological response with immunostimulatory properties [92]. The competent authorities of the United Kingdom evaluated the safety of this β-glucan and its estimation of exposure [93], which were in turn one of the aspects that the EFSA underlined in its complementary evaluation along with its potential allergenicity. Its risk was not considered higher than that derived from the consumption of the *Lentinula edodes* mushroom and other sources of β-glucan [94].

Shiitake mushroom has traditionally and commonly been used as a food ingredient in the Asian culture, specifically in China and Japan, whereas its use in American and European cuisines is currently increasing. Scientific evidence about the potential medicinal value of shiitake mushrooms (*Lentinula edodes*) is scarce. It has been suggested that shiitake mushrooms have immune-modulating, antitumor, and antiviral properties; however, further randomized, double-blind, and controlled clinical trials need to be performed to clarify these benefits [95]. Regarding the mushroom chitosan extract (*Agaricus bisporus*; *Aspergillus niger*), no specific scientific studies were found in the literature review performed.

4. Conclusions

After an intensive study of the extracts rich in nutrients and bioactive compounds authorized as novel food ingredients to be used in food supplements within the European Union, the results indicate that the extracts are one of the largest groups within the novel foods or novel food ingredients authorized, with currently 26 extracts authorized. These extracts are characterized as concentrated sources of nutrients. Out of the 26 authorized extracts, 23 of them include food supplements among their authorized uses. Given its heterogeneous composition, and considering the perceptive risk assessments carried out, the authorizations are limited, in some cases, to the use of the extract in food supplements to certain population groups. A classification of these extracts according to their source of origin was proposed by authors in the present work, and this results in four main groups: (a) extracts of plant origin (classified into four subgroups: seed extracts; extracts of leaves, fruits, and roots; plant cell culture extracts; and other extracts of plant origin), (b) algae extracts, (c) extracts of animal origin, and (d) extracts of fungal origin. This proposed classification could be considered a useful approach to obtain an organized description of each extract and a useful tool in the evaluation of their potential use restriction.

The use of plant-based substances is common in the production of food supplements, which have also experienced a rapid growth, particularly those based on botanical products and plant extracts. This fast rise has meant that the potential beneficial or adverse effects associated with its consumption have become subject of study in numerous scientific studies.

In the case of extracts authorized as novel foods for its use in food supplements, the group of extracts of plant origin is the largest and, therefore, the most likely group to be studied in the scientific literature, although a greater part of them have been authorized in the last 4 years. Another factor to consider is that many food supplements have a complex composition, resulting from the mixture of several substances, therefore it may not be easy to identify the origin of an adverse effect. The review of the scientific literature performed in the present work has made it possible to identify some examples of adverse effects associated with this type of substances.

The potential health effects attributed to the extracts rich in nutrients have been identified in the scientific literature. Among the most interesting benefits suggested, the possible use of some of these extracts in cardiovascular diseases (fermented black bean extract, Alfalfa leaf extract), rheumatoid arthritis (fermented wheat germ extract), metabolism disorders (fermented wheat germ extract, cranberry extract), disorders of the digestive tract (Alfalfa leaf extract), urinary tract infections (cranberry extract), ovarian cancer (fucoidan extracted from *Fucus vesiculosus*), stress-induced depression (extract of three herbal roots: *Cynanchum wilfordii* Hemsley, *Phlomis umbrosa* Turcz., and *Angelica gigas* Nakai), hyperpigmentation (Aloe leaf extract), skin protection (soybean extract), hyperglycemia (extract of dried leaves of *Ilex guayusa*), maintenance of normal blood pressure and cholesterol levels (*Epigallocatechin gallate* extract), strengthening of the immune system (Alfalfa leaf extract, extracts from *Panax notoginseng* and *Astragalus membranaceus*), improvement of physical performance (*Echinacea angustifolia* extract) and sperm characteristics (*Echinacea purpurea* extract), antifungal activity (ethanolic extract of *Lippia citriodora*), and antiviral properties (fucoidan extracted from *Undaria pinnatifida*) could be highlighted. Regarding the pig kidney extract and mushroom chitosan extract (*Agaricus bisporus*; *Aspergillus niger*), no scientific evidence about their possible health effects was found in the literature review carried out by the authors of the present work.

In conclusion, these extracts could be used as novel ingredients in functional products such as functional foods, food supplements, and even nutraceuticals to complement the daily diet and contribute to the maintenance of an adequate health status. However, further studies in humans are necessary to clearly demonstrate and confirm these preliminary results, as most of the studies found in the scientific literature were carried out in vitro.

Author Contributions: Conceptualization, R.L.-R., V.F.-R. and M.C.; Funding acquisition, M.C.; Investigation, R.L.-R., V.F.-R. and M.C.; Methodology, R.L.-R., V.F.-R. and M.C.; Supervision, V.F.-R. and M.C.; Validation, V.F.-R. and M.C.; Writing—original draft, R.L.-R., L.D., V.F.-R. and M.C. Writing—review & editing, R.L.-R., L.D., V.F.-R. and M.C. All authors have read and agreed to the published version of the manuscript.

Funding: This research was funded by UCM ALIMNOVA Research Group ref: 951505 and Project OTRI Art. 83 ref: 317-2020, UCM-Fundación Sabor y Salud. Laura Domínguez is grateful to her PhD grant (UCM-Santander; Ref: CT42/18-CT43/18).

Institutional Review Board Statement: Not applicable.

Informed Consent Statement: Not applicable.

Conflicts of Interest: The authors declare no conflict of interest.

References

1. Domínguez Díaz, L.; Fernández-Ruiz, V.; Cámara, M. The frontier between nutrition and pharma: The international regulatory framework of functional foods, food supplements and nutraceuticals. *Crit. Rev. Food Sci. Nutr.* **2019**, *60*, 1738–1746. [CrossRef]
2. Domínguez, L.; Fernández-Ruiz, V.; Morales, P.; Sánchez-Mata, M.-C.; Cámara, M. Assessment of Health Claims Related to Folic Acid in Food Supplements for Pregnant Women According to the European Regulation. *Nutrients* **2021**, *13*, 937. [CrossRef]
3. European Parliament and Council of the European Union. Directive 2002/46/EC of the European Parliament and of the Council of 10 June 2002 on the approximation of the laws of the Member States relating to food supplements. *Off. J. Eur. Union* **2002**, *L183*, 51. Available online: http://eur-lex.europa.eu/legal-content/EN/ALL/?uri=CELEX:32002L0046 (accessed on 30 May 2022).
4. Barrena, R.; Sánchez, M. Neophobia, personal consumer values and novel food acceptance. *Food Qual. Prefer* **2013**, *27*, 72–84. [CrossRef]
5. De Roos, B.; Bronze Aura, A.M.; Cassidy, A.; Garcia Conesa, M.T.; Gibney, E.R.; Greyling, A.; Kaput, J.; Kerem, Z.; Knežević, N.; Kroon, P.; et al. Targeting the delivery of dietary plant bioactives to those who would benefit most: From science to practical applications. *Eur. J. Nutr.* **2019**, *58*, 65–73. [CrossRef]
6. Knežević, M.; Grbavac, S.; Palfi, M.; Sabolović, M.B.; Brnčić, S.R. Novel food legislation and consumer acceptance. *Emir. J. Food Agric.* **2021**, *33*, 93–100. [CrossRef]
7. Rollin, F.; Kennedy, J.; Wills, J. Consumers and new food technologies. *Trends Food Sci. Technol.* **2011**, *22*, 99–111. [CrossRef]
8. Van Kleef, E.; Hans, C.M.; van Trijp, P.L. Consumer research in the early stages of new product development: A critical review of methods and techniques. *Food Qual. Prefer.* **2005**, *16*, 181–201. [CrossRef]
9. European Parliament; Council of the European Union. Regulation (EU) 2015/2283 of the European Parliament and of the Council of 25 November 2015 on novel foods, amending Regulation (EU) No 1169/2011 of the European Parliament and of the Council and repealing Regulation (EC) No 258/97 of the European Parliament and of the Council and Commission Regulation (EC) No 1852/2001. *Off. J. Eur. Union* **2015**, *L327/1*, 1–22. Available online: https://eur-lex.europa.eu/legal-content/en/ALL/?uri=CELEX:32015R2283 (accessed on 29 May 2022).
10. European Parliament; Council of the European Union. Regulation (EC) No 178/2002 of the European Parliament and of the Council of 28 January 2002 laying down the general principles and requirements of food law, establishing the European Food Safety Authority and laying down procedures in matters of food safety. *Off. J. Eur. Union* **2002**, *L31/1*, 1–24. Available online: https://eur-lex.europa.eu/legal-content/EN/ALL/?uri=celex%3A32002R0178 (accessed on 30 May 2022).

11. European Parliament; Council of the European Union. Regulation (EU) No 182/2011 of the European Parliament and of the Council of 16 February 2011 laying down the rules and general principles concerning mechanisms for control by Member States of the Commission's exercise of implementing powers. *Off. J. Eur. Union* **2011**, *L55/13*, 13–18. Available online: https://eur-lex.europa.eu/legal-content/EN/ALL/?uri=celex%3A32011R0182 (accessed on 28 May 2022).
12. European Commission; Directorate-General for Health and Food Safety. Commission Implementing Regulation (EU) 2017/2470 of 20 December 2017 establishing the Union list of novel foods in accordance with Regulation (EU) 2015/2283 of the European Parliament and of the Council on novel foods. *Off. J. Eur. Union* **2017**, *L351/72*, 72–102. Available online: https://eur-lex.europa.eu/legal-content/EN/ALL/?uri=CELEX:32017R2470 (accessed on 30 May 2022).
13. Fibigr, J.; Šatínský, D.; Solich, P. Current trends in the analysis and quality control of food supplements based on plant extracts. *Anal. Chim. Acta* **2018**, *1036*, 1–15. [CrossRef]
14. Faisal, R.; Shinwari, L.; Aziz, I.; Khalil, A.T. Therapeutic and adverse effects of commonly used medicinal plants: Standardization and quality assurance: Adverse effects of commonly used herbs. *Proc. Pak. Acad. Sci. B Life Environ. Sci.* **2019**, *56*, 1–9.
15. Veiga, M.; Costa, E.M.; Silva, S.; Pintado, M. Impact of plant extracts upon human health: A review. *Crit. Rev. Food Sci. Nutr.* **2020**, *60*, 873–886. [CrossRef]
16. AFSSA (Agence Française de Sécurité Sanitaire des Aliments). Avis de l'Agence Française de Sécurité Sanitaire des Aliments Relative à L'évaluation de L'équivalence Substantielle D'un Extrait D'huile de Tournesol avec un Extrait D'huile de Germe de maïs. Available online: https://www.anses.fr/fr/content/avis-de-l%E2%80%99agence-fran%C3%A7aise-de-s%C3%A9curit%C3%A9-sanitaire-des-aliments-relatif-%C3%A0-l%C3%A9valuation-de-5 (accessed on 22 June 2022).
17. European Commission. Notifications of Novel Foods under the Former Novel Food Regulation. Available online: https://ec.europa.eu/food/safety/novel_food/authorisations/list_authorisations_en (accessed on 20 June 2022).
18. FSAI (Food Safety Authority or Ireland). Substantial Equivalence Opinion. Extract of Defatted Cocoa Poder. Available online: https://www.fsai.ie/uploadedFiles/Science_and_Health/Novel_Foods/Notifications/2011%20Omnicoa%2055.pdf (accessed on 22 June 2022).
19. FSAI (Food Safety Authority or Ireland). Substantial Equivalence Opinion. Cocoa Extract. Available online: https://www.fsai.ie/uploadedFiles/Science_and_Health/Novel_Foods/Notifications/2015%20Cocoa%20extract.pdf (accessed on 19 June 2022).
20. European Commission. Decision 2011/497/EU authorising the placing on the market of fermented black bean extract as a novel food ingredient under Regulation (EC) No 258/97 of the European Parliament and of the Council. *Off. J. Eur. Union* **2011**, *L205/33*. Available online: https://eur-lex.europa.eu/legal-content/EN/TXT/HTML/?uri=CELEX:32011D0497&from=ES (accessed on 12 June 2022).
21. AGES (Austrian Agency for Health and Food Safety). Opinion on the Substantial Equivalence of Spermidine-Rich Wheat Germ Extract (*Triticum aestevium*) 2017. Notifications Pursuant to Article 5 of Regulation (EC) no 258/97 of the European Parliament and of the Council. Available online: https://food.ec.europa.eu/system/files/2018-06/novel-food_notifications_en.pdf (accessed on 25 July 2022).
22. Wageningen University & Research. Using Rapeseed and Sunflower Meal as Novel Ingredients. Available online: https://www.wur.nl/en/project/Using-rapeseed-and-sunflower-meal-as-novel-ingredients.htm (accessed on 17 June 2022).
23. Oddoye, E.O.; Agyente-Badu, C.K.; Gyedu-Akoto, E. Cocoa and its by-products: Identification and utilization. In *Chocolate in Health and Nutrition*; Humana Press: Totowa, NJ, USA, 2013; pp. 23–27.
24. EFSA (European Food Safety Authority). Panel on Dietetic Products, Nutrition and Allergies (NDA). Scientific Opinion on the safety of "fermented black bean extract" (Touchi) as a Novel Food ingredient. *EFSA J.* **2011**, *9*, 2136.
25. European Parliament and Council of the European Union. Regulation (EC) No 1924/2006 of the European Parliament and of the Council of 20 December 2006 on nutrition and health claims made on food. *Off. J. Eur. Union* **2006**, *L404*, 9. Available online: http://eurlex.europa.eu/legal-content/EN/ALL/?uri=CELEX%3A02006R1924-20121129 (accessed on 22 June 2022).
26. Kim, K.; Lim, K.M.; Kim, C.W.; Shin, H.J.; Seo, D.B.; Lee, S.J.; Chung, J.H. Black soybean extract can attenuate thrombosis through inhibition of collagen-induced platelet activation. *J. Nutr. Biochem.* **2011**, *22*, 964–970. [CrossRef]
27. EFSA (European Food Safety Authority). Panel on Dietetic Products, Nutrition and Allergies. Scientific opinion on the safety of fermented soybean extract NSK-SD®as a novel food pursuant to Regulation (EC) No 258/97. *EFSA J.* **2016**, *14*, 4541.
28. European Commission. Commission implementing Decision (EU) 2017/115 of 20 January 2017 authorising the placing on the market of fermented soybean extract as a novel food ingredient under Regulation (EC) No 258/97 of the European Parliament and of the Council. *Off. J. Eur. Union* **2017**, *L18/50*. Available online: https://eur-lex.europa.eu/legal-content/EN/TXT/HTML/?uri=CELEX:32017D0115&from=ES (accessed on 21 June 2022).
29. Park, N.H.; Park, J.S.; Kang, Y.G.; Bae, J.H.; Lee, H.K.; Yeom, M.H.; Na, Y.J. Soybean extract showed modulation of retinoic acid-related gene expression of skin and photo-protective effects in keratinocytes. *Int. J. Cosmet. Sci.* **2013**, *35*, 136–142. [CrossRef]
30. Schwarz, C.; Stekovic, S.; Wirth, M.; Benson, G.; Royer, P.; Sigrist, S.J.; Pieber, T.; Dammbrueck, C.; Magnes, C.; Eisenberg, T.; et al. Safety and tolerability of spermidine supplementation in mice and older adults with subjective cognitive decline. *Clin. Neurophysiol.* **2018**, *129*, e91. [CrossRef]
31. Brandolini, A.; Hidalgo, A. Wheat germ: Not only a by-product. *Int. J. Food Sci. Nutr.* **2012**, *63*, 71–74. [CrossRef]
32. Bálint, G.; Apathy, A.; Gaál, M.; Telekes, A.; Resetar, A.; Blazso, G.; Hidvégi, M. Effect of Avemar®-a fermented wheat germ extract-on rheumatoid arthritis. Preliminary data. *Clin. Exp. Rheumatol.* **2006**, *24*, 325.

33. Iyer, A.; Brown, L. Fermented wheat germ extract (Avemar) in the treatment of cardiac remodeling and metabolic symptoms in rats. *Evid. Based Complementary Altern.* **2011**, *47*. [CrossRef]
34. Di Lorenzo, C.; Ceschi, A.; Kupferschmidt, H.; Lüde, S.; De Souza Nascimento, E.; Dos Santos, A.; Colombo, F.; Frigerio, G.; Norby, K.; Plumb, J.; et al. Adverse effects of plant food supplements and botanical preparations: A systematic review with critical evaluation of causality. *Br. J. Clin. Pharmacol.* **2014**, *79*, 578–592. [CrossRef]
35. Kwack, S.J.; Kim, K.B.; Kim, H.S.; Yoon, K.S.; Lee, B.M. Risk assessment of soybean-based phytoestrogens. *J. Toxicol. Environ. Health A* **2009**, *72*, 1254–1261. [CrossRef]
36. Ricketts, M.L.; Moore, D.D.; Banz, W.J.; Mezei, O.; Shay, N.F. Molecular mechanisms of action of the soy isoflavones includes activation of promiscuous nuclear receptors. A review. *J. Nutr. Biochem.* **2005**, *16*, 321–330. [CrossRef]
37. European Commission. Commission Decision 2009/826/EC, of 13 October 2009, authorising the placing on the market of a leaf extract from Lucerne (Medicago sativa) as novel food or novel food ingredient under Regulation (EC) No 258/97 of the European Parliament and of the Council. *Off. J. Eur. Union* **2009**, *L294/12*. Available online: https://eur-lex.europa.eu/legal-content/EN/TXT/HTML/?uri=CELEX:32009D0826&from=ES (accessed on 21 June 2022).
38. FSAI (Food Safety Authority or Ireland). Substantial Equivalence Opinion. Purified Green Tea Extract. Available online: https://www.fsai.ie/uploadedFiles/Science_and_Health/Novel_Foods/Notifications/2009%20Teavigo.pdf (accessed on 24 June 2022).
39. FSAI (Food Safety Authority or Ireland). Substantial Equivalence Opinion. Aloe Macroclada Baker—Gel Extract. Available online: https://www.fsai.ie/uploadedFiles/Science_and_Health/Novel_Foods/Notifications/2016%20Stemtech%20Aloe%20gel%20extract.pdf (accessed on 25 June 2022).
40. FSAI (Food Safety Authority or Ireland). Substantial Equivalence Opinion. Ilex Guayusa. Available online: https://www.fsai.ie/uploadedFiles/Science_and_Health/Novel_Foods/Notifications/2017%20SE%20opinion%20Ilex%20Guayusa.pdf (accessed on 21 June 2022).
41. European Commission; Directorate-General for Health and Food Safety. Commission Implementing Regulation (EU) 2018/1631 of 30 October 2018 authorising the placing on the market of cranberry extract powder as a novel food under Regulation (EU) 2015/2283 of the European Parliament and of the Council and amending Commission Implementing Regulation (EU) 2017/2470. *Off. J. Eur. Union* **2018**, *L272/17*. Available online: https://eur-lex.europa.eu/legal-content/EN/TXT/HTML/?uri=CELEX:32018R1631&from=en (accessed on 23 June 2022).
42. European Commission; Directorate-General for Health and Food Safety. Commission Implementing Regulation (EU) 2018/469 of 21 March 2018 authorising the placing on the market of an extract of three herbal roots (Cynanchum wilfordii Hemsley, Phlomis umbrosa Turcz. and Angelica gigas Nakai) as a novel food under Regulation (EU) 2015/2283 of the European Parliament and of the Council, and amending Commission Implementing Regulation (EU) 2017/2470. *Off. J. Eur. Union* **2018**, *L79/11*. Available online: https://eur-lex.europa.eu/legal-content/EN/TXT/HTML/?uri=CELEX:32018R0469&from=EN (accessed on 22 June 2022).
43. European Commission; Directorate-General for Health and Food Safety. Commission Implementing Regulation (EU) 2020/1821 of 2 December 2020 authorising the placing on the market of an extract from Panax notoginseng and Astragalus membranaceus as a novel food under Regulation (EU) 2015/2283 of the European Parliament and of the Council and amending Commission Implementing Regulation (EU) 2017/2470. *Off. J. Eur. Union* **2020**, *L406/34*. Available online: https://eur-lex.europa.eu/legal-content/EN/TXT/HTML/?uri=CELEX:32020R1821&from=EN (accessed on 19 June 2022).
44. EFSA (European Food Safety Authority). Opinion on the safety of 'Alfalfa protein concentrate' as food. Scientific Opinion of the Panel on Dietetic Products, Nutrition and Allergies. *EFSA J.* **2009**, *997*, 997.
45. Soto-Zarazúa, M.G.; Bah, M.; Costa, A.S.G.; Rodrigues, F.; Pimentel, F.B.; Rojas-Molina, I.; Oliveira, M.B.P.P. Nutraceutical potential of new alfalfa (Medicago sativa) ingredients for beverage preparations. *J. Med. Food* **2017**, *20*, 1039–1046. [CrossRef]
46. Bartosikova, L.; Necas, J. Epigallocatechin gallate: A review. *Vet. Med.* **2018**, *63*, 443–467. [CrossRef]
47. Javaid, M.S.; Latief, N.; Ijaz BAshfaq, U.A. Epigallocatechin Gallate as an anti-obesity therapeutic compound: An in silico approach for structure-based drug designing. *Nat. Prod. Res.* **2018**, *32*, 2121–2125. [CrossRef]
48. Momose, Y.; Maeda-Yamamoto, M.; Nabetani, H. Systematic review of green tea epigallocatechin gallate in reducing low-density lipoprotein cholesterol levels of humans. *Int. J. Food Sci. Nutr.* **2016**, *67*, 606–613. [CrossRef]
49. Chatree, S.; Sitticharoon, C.; Maikaew, P.; Pongwattanapakin, K.; Keadkraichaiwat, I.; Churintaraphan, M.; Tapechum, S. Epigallocatechin gallate decreases plasma triglyceride, blood pressure, and serum kisspeptin in obese human subjects. *Exp. Biol. Med.* **2021**, *246*, 163–176. [CrossRef]
50. Rodríguez Rodríguez, E.; Darias Martín, J.; Díaz Romero, C. Aloe vera as a Functional Ingredient in Foods. *Crit. Rev. Food Sci. Nutr.* **2010**, *50*, 305–326. [CrossRef]
51. Wise, G.; Negrin, A. A critical review of the composition and history of safe use of guayusa: A stimulant and antioxidant novel food. *Crit. Rev. Food Sci. Nutr.* **2020**, *60*, 2393–2404. [CrossRef]
52. Radice, M.; Cossio, N.; Scalvenzi, L. *Ilex Guayusa*: A Systematic Review of its traditional uses, chemical constituents, biological activities and biotrade opportunities. In Proceedings of the MOL2NET 2016, International Conference on Multidisciplinary Sciences, Puyo, Ecuador-Porto, Portugal, 15–20 October 2016. Available online: https://sciforum.net/paper/view/3868 (accessed on 1 July 2022).
53. EFSA (European Food Safety Authority). EFSA Panel on Dietetic Products, Nutrition and Allergies. Scientific Opinion on the safety of cranberry extract powder as a novel food ingredient pursuant to Regulation (EC) No. 258/97. *EFSA J.* **2017**, *15*, 4777.

54. Gbinigie, O.A.; Spencer, E.A.; Heneghan, C.J.; Lee, J.J.; Butler, C.C. Cranberry extract for symptoms of acute, uncomplicated urinary tract infection: A systematic review. *Antibiotics* **2020**, *10*, 12. [CrossRef]
55. Kowalska, K.; Olejnik, A. Beneficial effects of cranberry in the prevention of obesity and related complications: Metabolic syndrome and diabetes–A review. *J. Funct. Foods* **2016**, *20*, 171–181. [CrossRef]
56. Peixoto, T.C.; Moura, E.G.; de Oliveira, E.; Soares, P.N.; Guarda, D.S.; Bernardino, D.N.; Lisboa, P.C. Cranberry (*Vaccinium macrocarpon*) extract treatment improves triglyceridemia, liver cholesterol, liver steatosis, oxidative damage and corticosteronemia in rats rendered obese by high fat diet. *Eur. J. Nutr.* **2018**, *57*, 1829–1844. [CrossRef]
57. EFSA (European Food Safety Authority). Panel on Dietetic Products, Nutrition and Allergies. Safety of EstroG-100TM as a novel food pursuant to Regulation (EC) No 258/97. *EFSA J.* **2016**, *14*, 4589.
58. EFSA (European Food Safety Authority). EFSA Panel on Dietetic Products, Nutrition and Allergies. Statement on the safety of EstroG-100TM as a novel food pursuant to Regulation (EC) No 258/97. *EFSA J.* **2017**, *15*, 4778.
59. Oh, K.N.; Oh, D.R.; Jung, M.A.; Kim, Y.; Choi, E.J.; Hong, J.; Choi, C.Y. Antidepressant effects of *Cynanchum wilfordii* Hemsley, *Phlomis umbrosa* Turcz, and *Angelica gigas* Nakai via inhibition of 5-HT6 receptor-mediated cyclic AMP activity. *J. Physiol. Pathol. Korean Med.* **2018**, *32*, 247–254. [CrossRef]
60. EFSA (European Food Safety Authority). Safety of a botanical extract derived from Panax notoginseng and Astragalus membranaceus (AstraGinTM) as a novel food pursuant to Regulation (EU) 2015/2283. *EFSA J.* **2020**, *18*, 6099.
61. Zhou, J.; Kulkarni, M.G.; Huang, L.Q.; Guo, L.P.; Van Staden, J. Effects of temperature, light, nutrients and smoke-water on seed germination and seedling growth of *Astragalus membranaceus*, *Panax notoginseng* and *Magnolia officinalis*—Highly traded Chinese medicinal plants. *S. Afr. J. Bot.* **2012**, *79*, 62–70. [CrossRef]
62. DSPVNSA. Ministero della Salute-Dipartimento per la Sanità Pubblica Veterinaria, la Nutrizione e la Sicurezza degli Alimenti. Substantial Equivalence for *Ajuga reptans* Extracts from Plant Tissue Cultures, 2008. Notifications Pursuant to Article 5 of Regulation (EC) no 258/97 of the European Parliament and of the Council. Available online: https://food.ec.europa.eu/system/files/2018-06/novel-food_notifications_en.pdf (accessed on 25 July 2022).
63. DSPVNSA. Ministero della Salute-Dipartimento per la Sanità Pubblica Veterinaria, la Nutrizione e la Sicurezza degli Alimenti. Substantial Equivalence for *Echinacea angustifolia* Extract from Plant Tissue Cultures, 2009. Notifications Pursuant to Article 5 of Regulation (EC) no 258/97 of the European Parliament and of the Council. Available online: https://food.ec.europa.eu/system/files/2018-06/novel-food_notifications_en.pdf (accessed on 25 July 2022).
64. DSPVNSA. Ministero della Salute-Dipartimento per la Sanità Pubblica Veterinaria, la Nutrizione e la Sicurezza degli Alimenti. Richiesta di, Sostanziale Equivalenza, ai Sensi dell'ari. 5 del Regolamento (CE) 258/97, di Estratto di Aloysia Citriodora Palau [sin. *Lippia citriodora* (Palau) Kunth] da Colture di Tessuto Vegetale Rispetto ad Estratto Commerciale di Foglie da Coltura Tradizionale (ditta Solimè)n ai Sensi dell'articolo 5 del Regolamento (CE) 258/97 sui Nuovi Alimenti (Novel Food) Presentata dalla ditta IRB, 2015. Notifications Pursuant to Article 5 of Regulation (EC) no 258/97 of the European Parliament and of the Council. Available online: https://food.ec.europa.eu/system/files/2018-06/novel-food_notifications_en.pdf (accessed on 25 July 2022).
65. DSPVNSA. Ministero della Salute-Dipartimento per la Sanità Pubblica Veterinaria, la Nutrizione e la Sicurezza degli Alimenti. Substantial Equivalence for *Echinacea purpurea* Extract from Cell Cultures HTN®Vb, 2017. Notifications Pursuant to Article 5 of Regulation (EC) no 258/97 of the European Parliament and of the Council. Available online: https://food.ec.europa.eu/system/files/2018-06/novel-food_notifications_en.pdf (accessed on 25 July 2022).
66. Barrett, B. *Echinacea*: A safety review. *HerbalGram* **2003**, *57*, 36–39.
67. Mullins, R.J.; Heddle, R. Adverse reactions associated with echinacea: The Australian experience. *Ann. Allergy Asthma Immunol.* **2002**, *88*, 42–51. [CrossRef]
68. Kocaman, O.; Hulagu, S.; Senturk, O. Echinacea-induced severe acute hepatitis with features of cholestatic autoimmune hepatitis. *Eur. J. Intern. Med.* **2008**, *19*, 148–152. [CrossRef]
69. Jacobsson, I.; Jönsson, A.K.; Gerdén, B.; Hägg, S. Spontaneously reported adverse reactions in association with complementary and alternative medicine substances in Sweden. *Pharmacoepidemiol. Drug Saf.* **2009**, *18*, 1039–1047. [CrossRef]
70. Esposito, T.; Sansone, F.; Auriemma, G.; Franceschelli, S.; Pecoraro, M.; Picerno, P.; Mencherini, T. Study on *ajuga reptans* extract: A natural antioxidant in microencapsulated powder form as an active ingredient for nutraceutical or pharmaceutical purposes. *Pharmaceutics* **2020**, *12*, 671. [CrossRef] [PubMed]
71. Dal Toso, R.; Melandri, F. *Echinacea angustifolia* cell culture extract. *Nutrafoods* **2011**, *10*, 19–24. [CrossRef]
72. Ghasempour, M.; Omran, S.M.; Moghadamnia, A.A.; Shafiee, F. Effect of aqueous and ethanolic extracts of *Lippia citriodora* on candida albicans. *Electron. Physician* **2016**, *8*, 2752. [CrossRef]
73. Motamedi, S.; Asghari, A.; Jahandideh, A.; Abedi, G.; Mortazavi, P. Effects of *Echinacea purpurea* extract on sperm characteristics and hematology following testicular ischemia-reperfusion injury in rat. *Crescent J. Med. Biol. Sci.* **2018**, *5*, 119–122.
74. Banica, F.; Bungau, S.; Tit, D.M.; Behl, T.; Otrisal, P.; Nechifor, A.C.; Nemeth, S. Determination of the total polyphenols content and antioxidant activity of Echinacea purpurea extracts using newly manufactured glassy carbon electrodes modified with carbon nanotubes. *Processes* **2020**, *8*, 833. [CrossRef]
75. FSA (Food Standards Agency. Initial opinion). Opinion on a Taxifolin-Rich Extract from Dahurian Larch. Available online: https://webarchive.nationalarchives.gov.uk/ukgwa/20200406003919/https://acnfp.food.gov.uk/assess/fullapplics/taxifolin (accessed on 25 June 2022).

76. Moura, F.C.S.; Machado, C.L.D.; Paula, F.R. Taxifolin stability: In silico prediction and in vitro degradation with HPLC-UV/UPLC-ESI-MS monitoring. *J. Pharm. Anal.* **2020**, *11*, 232–240. [CrossRef]
77. EFSA (European Food Safety Authority). EFSA Panel on Dietetic Products, Nutrition and Allergies. Scientific Opinion on taxifolin-rich extract from Dahurian Larch (*Larix gmelinii*). *EFSA J.* **2017**, *15*, 4682.
78. European Commission; Directorate-General for Health and Food Safety. Commission implementing Decision (EU) 2017/2079, of 10 November 2017, authorising the placing on the market of taxifolin-rich extract as a novel food ingredient under Regulation (EC) No 258/97 of the European Parliament and of the Council. *Off. J. Eur. Union* **2017**, *L295/81*. Available online: https://eur-lex.europa.eu/legal-content/EN/TXT/HTML/?uri=CELEX:32017D2079&from=ES (accessed on 23 June 2022).
79. EFSA (European Food Safety Authority). EFSA Panel on Dietetic Products, Nutrition and Allergies. Statement on the safety of taxifolin-rich extract from Dahurian Larch (*Larix gmelinii*). *EFSA J.* **2017**, *15*, 5059.
80. European Commission; Directorate-General for Health and Food Safety. Commission Implementing Regulation (EU) 2018/461 of 20 March 2018 authorising an extension of use of taxifolin-rich extract as a novel food under Regulation (EU) 2015/2283 of the European Parliament and of the Council, and amending Commission Implementing Regulation (EU) 2017/2470. *Off. J. Eur. Union* **2018**, *L78/7*, 7–10. Available online: https://eur-lex.europa.eu/legal-content/EN/ALL/?uri=CELEX%3A32018R0461 (accessed on 24 June 2022).
81. Wang, Y.; Zu, Y.; Long, J.; Fu, Y.; Li, S.; Zhang, D.; Efferth, T. Enzymatic water extraction of taxifolin from wood sawdust of Larix gmelinii (Rupr.) Rupr. and evaluation of its antioxidant activity. *Food Chem.* **2011**, *126*, 1178–1185. [CrossRef]
82. CSS (Conseil Supérieur de la Santé). Opinion on the Substancail Equivalence of Focodian Extracted from *Undaria pinnatifida* and Fucoidan Extracted from *Fucus vesiculosus*, 2017. Notifications Pursuant to Article 5 of Regulation (EC) no 258/97 of the European Parliament and of the Council. Available online: https://food.ec.europa.eu/system/files/2018-06/novel-food_notifications_en.pdf (accessed on 25 July 2022).
83. Cho, Y.S.; Jung, W.-K.; Kim, J.-A.; Choi, I.-W.; Kim, S.-K. Beneficial effects of fucoidan on osteoblastic MG-63 cell differentiation. *Food Chem.* **2009**, *116*, 990–994. [CrossRef]
84. Bae, H.; Lee, J.Y.; Yang, C.; Song, G.; Lim, W. Fucoidan derived from *Fucus vesiculosus* inhibits the development of human ovarian cancer via the disturbance of calcium homeostasis, endoplasmic reticulum stress, and angiogenesis. *Mar. Drugs* **2020**, *18*, 45. [CrossRef]
85. Zhao, Y.; Zheng, Y.; Wang, J.; Ma, S.; Yu, Y.; White, W.L.; Lu, J. Fucoidan extracted from *Undaria pinnatifida*: Source for nutraceuticals/functional foods. *Mar. Drugs* **2018**, *16*, 321. [CrossRef]
86. AGES (Austrian Agency for Health and Food Safety). Gutachten—Stellungnahme zum Antrag auf Notifikation von DAOSIN®nach Art. 5 der Novel Food VO (EG) 258/97, 2012. Notifications Pursuant to Article 5 of Regulation (EC) no 258/97 of the European Parliament and of the Council. Available online: https://food.ec.europa.eu/system/files/2018-06/novel-food_notifications_en.pdf (accessed on 25 July 2022).
87. European Commission; Directorate-General for Health and Food Safety. Commission Implementing Regulation (EU) 2020/973 of 6 July 2020 authorising a change of the conditions of use of the novel food 'protein extract from pig kidneys' and amending Implementing Regulation (EU) 2017/2470. *Off. J. Eur. Union* **2020**, *L215/7*. Available online: https://eur-lex.europa.eu/legal-content/EN/TXT/HTML/?uri=CELEX:32020R0973&from=ES (accessed on 25 June 2022).
88. CSS (Conseil Supérieur de la Santé). Avis du Conseil Supérieur de la Santé N° 8319 Chitosane (KIOnutrime-Cs™) Équivlence Substantielle, 2008. Notifications Pursuant to Article 5 of Regulation (EC) no 258/97 of the European Parliament and of the Council. Available online: https://food.ec.europa.eu/system/files/2018-06/novel-food_notifications_en.pdf (accessed on 25 July 2022).
89. European Commission. Commission Decision of 2 February 2011 authorising the placing on the market of a mycelial extract from Lentinula edodes (Shiitake mushroom) as a novel food ingredient under Regulation (EC) No 258/97 of the European Parliament and of the Council. *Off. J. Eur. Union* **2011**, *L29/30*, 30–31. Available online: https://eur-lex.europa.eu/legal-content/EN/ALL/?uri=CELEX%3A32011D0073 (accessed on 26 June 2022).
90. Apetroaei, M.R.; Rau, I.; Paduretu, C.C.; Lilios, G.; Schroder, V. Pharmaceutical Applications of Chitosan Extracted from Local Marine Sources. *Rev. Chim.* **2019**, *70*, 2618–2621. [CrossRef]
91. Vargas, M.; González-Martínez, C. Recent patents on food applications of chitosan. *Recent Pat. Food Nutr. Agric.* **2010**, *2*, 121–128. [CrossRef] [PubMed]
92. McCormack, E.; Skavland, J.; Mujic, M.; Bruserud, O.; Gjertsen, B.T. Lentinan: Hematopoietic, Immunological, and Efficacy Studies in a Syngeneic Model of Acute Myeloid Leukemia. *Nutr. Cancer* **2010**, *62*, 574–583. [CrossRef] [PubMed]
93. FSA (Food Standards Agency). Initial Opinion. Opinion on a Beta-Glucan Rich Extract from *lentinus edodes*. Available online: https://webarchive.nationalarchives.gov.uk/ukgwa/20200405232715/https://acnfp.food.gov.uk/assess/fullapplics/lentinanglycanova (accessed on 17 June 2022).
94. EFSA (European Food Safety Authority). Panel on Dietetic Products, Nutrition and Allergies (NDA). Scientific Opinion on the safety of "*Lentinus edodes* extract" as a Novel Food ingredient. *EFSA J.* **2010**, *8*, 1685. [CrossRef]
95. Hobbs, C. Medicinal value of *Lentinus edodes* (Berk.) Sing. (Agaricomycetideae). A literature review. *Int. J. Med. Mushrooms* **2000**, *2*, v2.i4.90. [CrossRef]

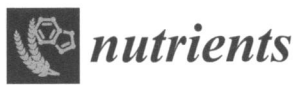

Article

Resveratrol Food Supplement Products and the Challenges of Accurate Label Information to Ensure Food Safety for Consumers

Maja Bensa [1,2,3], Irena Vovk [1,*] and Vesna Glavnik [1]

[1] Laboratory for Food Chemistry, National Institute of Chemistry, Hajdrihova 19, SI-1000 Ljubljana, Slovenia
[2] Faculty of Agriculture and Life Sciences, University of Maribor, Pivola 10, SI-2311 Hoče, Slovenia
[3] Faculty of Health Sciences, University of Ljubljana, Zdravstvena pot 5, SI-1000 Ljubljana, Slovenia
* Correspondence: irena.vovk@ki.si; Tel.: +386-1476-0341

Abstract: The food supplement market is growing as many consumers wish to complement their nutrient intake. Despite all the regulations in place to ensure food supplements safety, there are still many cases of irregularities reported especially connected to internet sales. Twenty resveratrol food supplement products sold on the Slovenian market were evaluated on their compliance of declared vs. determined resveratrol content, as well as the compliance of labels with the European Union (EU) and Slovenian regulatory requirements. Both the ingredient contents and food information are important parts of food safety. Analyses of 20 food supplements performed using high-performance thin-layer chromatography (HPTLC) coupled with densitometry showed that 95% of products had contents different from what was declared and 55% of products contained higher contents than declared. In 25% of the products the determined content per unit exceeded the maximum level (150 mg/day) specified in EU novel food conditions for food supplement with *trans*-resveratrol. Evaluation of the 20 food supplement labels included mandatory and voluntary food information, food supplement information, novel food information, health claims and nutrition claims. Most labels contained the necessary information, but multiple errors were observed ranging from typos to misleading practices. From a food safety perspective there is still a lot of improvement needed in the field of food supplements.

Keywords: *trans*-resveratrol; dietary supplements; food safety; regulation; labels; health claims; nutrition claims; novel foods; high-performance thin-layer chromatography; HPTLC

Citation: Bensa, M.; Vovk, I.; Glavnik, V. Resveratrol Food Supplement Products and the Challenges of Accurate Label Information to Ensure Food Safety for Consumers. *Nutrients* 2023, 15, 474. https://doi.org/10.3390/nu15020474

Academic Editors: Laura Domínguez Díaz, Montaña Cámara, Virginia Fernández-Ruiz and Mari Maeda-Yamamoto

Received: 15 December 2022
Revised: 10 January 2023
Accepted: 12 January 2023
Published: 16 January 2023

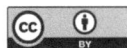

Copyright: © 2023 by the authors. Licensee MDPI, Basel, Switzerland. This article is an open access article distributed under the terms and conditions of the Creative Commons Attribution (CC BY) license (https://creativecommons.org/licenses/by/4.0/).

1. Introduction

1.1. Food Supplements: Safety and Labels

Food supplements are concentrated sources of nutrients (e.g., vitamins, minerals and other bioactive compounds) taken in dose forms to supplement the normal diet [1]. A healthy, varied diet and a healthy lifestyle are important to maintain good health, but consumers also look at food supplements as additional support for maintaining good health. The market of food supplements is growing on a global scale. The safety of food supplements is of great importance for the health and well-being of consumers. Food supplements are considered as food, and are also regulated as food, even though some forms of food supplements (e.g., capsules, tablets, etc.) can visually resemble medication.

Despite the many regulations in place, there are still many cases of irregularities and food fraud when it comes to food supplements. The 2021 Annual Report of the Alert and Cooperation Network [2] includes information about food noncompliances with EU legislation. The Alert and Cooperation Network (ACN) consists of three networks: the Rapid Alert System for Food and Feed network (RASFF), the Administrative Assistance and Cooperation network (AAC) and the Agri-Food Fraud Network (FFN). The ACN report states that the second highest number (approximately 10%) of noncompliance reports made for food categories in 2021 was for the category of food supplements, dietetic foods and fortified foods [2]. Only the fruit and vegetables category had more reports—about 14% [2]. With regard to food supplements the report also mentions the problematic use of nonauthorized health claims [2]. With regard to food fraud the most concerning practices are: (1) the differences between the declared or marketed contents of substances (e.g., vitamin D) and the actual content in food supplements, (2) the presence of nonauthorized substances that can be harmful to health as well as (3) incomplete or missing information concerning the list of ingredients or responsible food business operators [2]. An increase in the use of food supplements, especially due to internet sales, occurred during the COVID-19 pandemic. Food supplements purchased online often pose a health risk due to many illegal products and food fraud. Half of the RASFF notifications regarding products bought via the internet concerned the food supplement, dietetic foods and fortified foods [2]. While searching for fraudulent practices will probably remain a big challenge for the food sector and regulatory authorities, a lot has already been done in the European Union (EU) to unify the requirements and standards for food products.

EU regulation of food supplements covers several important aspects: food supplements [1], food labeling [3], novel foods [4], as well as health and nutrition claims [5]. Labels are intended to provide the consumer with correct and clear information to help the consumer make informed purchase choices. Labels are not allowed to be misleading or confusing for the consumer. Labels of food supplements include: mandatory information, voluntary information, health and nutrition claims, as well as information required for food supplements and novel foods (if applicable).

1.2. Mandatory and Voluntary Food Information

Regulation (EU) No 1169/2011 lists the requirements for food information, both mandatory and voluntary. Food information should be accurate and understandable for consumers. Food labels should not be misleading and should not connect the food's properties with preventing or treating disease. Regulation (EU) No 1169/2011 lists 12 categories of mandatory information for food products: (1) name of the food, (2) list of ingredients, (3) allergens, (4) quantities of certain ingredients or categories of ingredients, (5) net quantity of the food, (6) date of minimum durability, (7) any special storage conditions and/or conditions of use, (8) name and address of the food business operator, (9) country of origin or place of provenance, (10) instructions for use, (11) nutrition declaration, as well as (12) alcoholic strength by volume for alcoholic beverages [3]. For each of the 12 items there are additional rules, details and conditions for providing the information. The degree to which each of the 12 items is mandatory depends on the food product.

The list of ingredients must include the word "ingredients" in the title. Allergenic ingredients need to be included in the list and written in a different font (e.g., bold). Any nano materials also need to be labeled. Certain information, such as country of origin, is mandatory if without this information the consumer could be misled. Instructions for use are mandatory if the product cannot be used without them. Special storage conditions are also required depending on the product. The nutrition declaration is not used for food supplements [1] except when health or nutrition claims are included on the label [5]. Regulation (EU) No 1169/2011 [3] specifies the daily reference intakes for vitamins and minerals as well as reference intakes for energy and other selected nutrients. Voluntary food label information is also regulated [3] and can include information about the following: unintentional presence of allergens, suitability for vegetarians or vegans, reference intakes for specific population groups as well as absence or reduced presence of gluten. Regulation (EU) No 1169/2011 [3] is clear that voluntary information must be based on scientific evidence, understandable to the consumers and must not overtake the space for mandatory food information. Quite common are claims connected to the absence or reduced presence of gluten or lactose, which is also regulated in other regulations (e.g., Regulation (EU) No 828/2014 [6]).

1.3. Health and Nutrition Claims

Food supplement and other food product labels often include health and nutrition claims. The rules about nutrition and health claims are provided in the Regulation (EC) No 1924/2006 [5]. Claims on labels must be comprehensive and scientifically proven. Misleading claims are not allowed. Only authorized claims can be used. Authorized and nonauthorized health claims are available in the EU register of Nutrition and Health Claims [7], which also includes authorized nutrition claims.

Nutrition claims describe properties related to the energy and nutrients or other substances (1) provided, (2) provided in an increased or decreased amount or (3) not provided).

Health claims describe the connection between food and health. Regulation (EC) 1924/2006 also sets the conditions for using nutrition and health claims [5]. The substance for which the claim is made needs to be in a form that can be used by the body and must be present in a sufficient quantity for producing the claimed nutritional or physiological effect. The labels can include health and nutrition claims if the effects they describe are understood by the average consumer [5]. For health claims to be permitted, the labeling needs to include the following four statements: (1) warning for products that are likely to present health risks if consumed to excess, (2) persons who should avoid using the food, (3) the quantity of the food and pattern of consumption required to obtain the claimed beneficial effects, and (4) the importance of a varied and balanced diet, and a healthy lifestyle.

1.4. Food Supplements and Novel Foods

To protect consumers from possible misinformation and health risks only food supplements fulfilling the requirements of the Directive 2002/46/EC [1] can be sold in the EU market. The Directive 2002/46/EC [1] lists the vitamins and minerals that can be included among food supplement ingredients together with the permitted sources of vitamins and minerals. The Directive [1] also prescribes units of vitamins and minerals that are to be used on food supplement labels. All food supplements need to be declared as "food supplement" on the label [1]. Advertising of food supplement products is not allowed to claim disease prevention or healing properties. Food supplement labels need to include: (1) the names of the categories of nutrients; (2) the portion of product recommended for daily consumption; (3) a warning not to exceed the stated recommended daily dose; (4) a warning that food supplements should not be used as a substitute for a varied diet; (5) a warning to store the products out of the reach of young children; (6) the amount of minerals or vitamins in specified units and as a percentage of the reference values; and (7) the amount of nutrients or substances with nutritional or physiological effect present in the product and per daily dose.

Sometimes, due to the nature of the food supplement products or their ingredients food supplements are regulated as novel foods. Examples of novel food are resveratrol food supplements with resveratrol from Japanese knotweed extract or microbial source. Novel foods are foods that were not used as human food on a larger scale in the EU before 1997 [8]. The novel foods listed in the Commission Implementing Regulation (EU) 2017/2470 can be sold in the EU. The authorized novel food is *trans*-resveratrol in the food category of food supplements with maximum levels of 150 mg/day. Labels of resveratrol food supplements must include "*trans*-resveratrol" and a statement for patients using medicines to only consume the product under medical supervision.

Despite the regulations in place, many reports of food fraud and misleading practices concerning food supplements have been reported through Rapid Alert System for Food and Feed RASFF [2]. The reports reveal products that were not compliant and harmful to health as well as a lack of control of internet sales. These problems underscore the importance of developing analytical methods that enable fast and effective analysis of food supplements, ensuring consumer's safety.

Different phenolic compounds are frequently found among the ingredients of food supplements. Resveratrol is a good example as it is included in many food supplement products. Resveratrol is a stilbene with two isomeric forms (*cis* and *trans*). It is also present in different foods (such as grapes, peanuts, pistachio, strawberries, currants and blackberries). Resveratrol has been linked to protection of the heart and blood vessels as well as the following bioactivities: anticarcinogenic; antioxidative; anti-inflammatory; antitumor and antiviral activity [9]. Studies also showed the inhibitory activity of resveratrol against influenza virus replication and the potential of resveratrol in combination with pterostilbene as antiviral compounds to inhibit severe acute respiratory syndrome coronavirus 2 (SARS-CoV-2) infection [10]. Thus, it is not surprising that resveratrol is present in many food supplements. Resveratrol can either be extracted from plants (e.g., Japanese knotweed and grapes) or their products (e.g., wine) or obtained with biochemical and genetic engineering [11].

The aim of this study was to examine resveratrol food supplements purchased on the Slovenian market in the spring 2022 from two points of view: first, the compliance of declared resveratrol contents with the contents determined using high performance thin-layer chromatography (HPTLC), and second, the overall labeling compliance with EU regulatory requirements for mandatory and voluntary food information [3], nutrition and health claims on food [5], food supplements [1] and novel foods [4].

2. Materials and Methods

2.1. Chemicals

All chemicals were at least of analytical grade. Ethyl acetate, *n*-hexane, formic acid (98–100%), acetic acid (glacial, 100%) sulfuric acid (95–97%) and *p*-methoxybenzaldehyde (anisaldehyde) were from Merck (Darmstadt, Germany). Methanol (HPLC grade) was from J.T. Baker (Deventer, the Netherlands). Standard *trans*-resveratrol (99%) was purchased from Sigma-Aldrich (St. Louis, MO, USA).

2.2. Food Supplements with Resveratrol

In the spring of 2022, 20 resveratrol food supplement products were purchased in pharmacies and specialized stores in Slovenia. The food supplements were manufactured by 15 producers from 10 countries (4 samples from 1 producer, 2 samples from another 2 producers and only 1 sample from each of the remaining 12 producers) (Figure 1). Food supplements were in three forms (Figure 2): powder packet (sample 14), tablets (samples 1, 5, 6, 11) and capsules (the remaining 15 samples: 2, 3, 4, 7, 8, 9, 10, 12, 13, 15, 16, 17, 18, 19, 20). In addition to resveratrol, the food supplements analyzed in this study contained several other ingredients, such as plant parts (leaves, sprouts, rhizomes or roots, and fruits), plant extracts, carotenoids, amino acids, vitamins, minerals, etc.

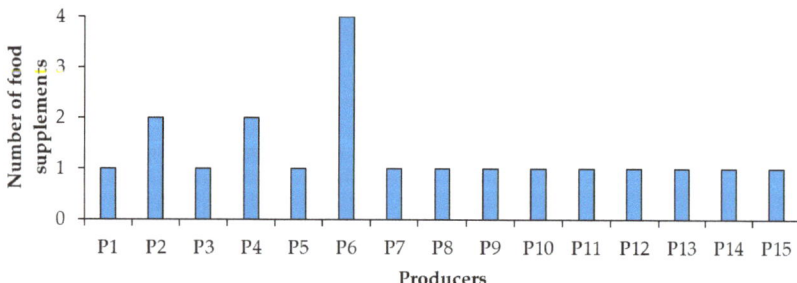

Figure 1. Number of food supplement products and producers.

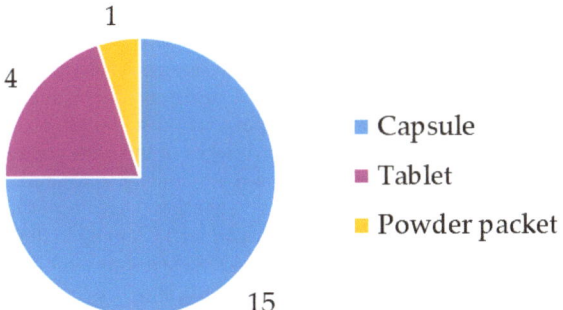

Figure 2. Forms of food supplement products.

2.3. Preparation of Standard Solutions

A standard stock solution of *trans*-resveratrol (1 mg/mL) was prepared in methanol. Working standard solutions of *trans*-resveratrol (0.1 mg/mL, 0.02 mg/mL, 0.01 mg/mL) were prepared by diluting a standard stock solution with methanol. All standard solutions were stored in amber glass storage vials at −80 °C.

2.4. Preparation of Sample Test Solutions (STSs) of Food Supplements

Sample test solutions (STSs) of food supplements were prepared using five units of each food supplement, where one unit was represented by one tablet or one capsule or one powder packet. The tablets were ground into powder in a grinder (mortar and pestle). The capsules were opened and the contents (powder or paste) were emptied. Each powdered or paste sample was homogenized by mixing. Afterwards each homogenized sample was applied for the extraction performed in three replicates. Homogenized powders or pastes of food supplement material were dispersed in methanol. The suspensions obtained were vortexed (5 s at 2800 rpm; IKA Vortex 1, IKA, Staufen, Germany) followed by ultrasound assisted extraction (15 min at 50 Hz; ultrasonic bath Sonis 3 GT, Iskra Pio d.o.o., Šentjernej, Slovenia). The supernatants obtained after 5 min centrifugation at 4200 rpm (Centric 322 A, Tehtnica, Železniki, Slovenia) were filtered through a 0.45 µm polyvinylidene fluoride (PVDF) membrane filter (Millipore, Billerica, MA, USA) into amber glass storage vials, which were stored at −20 °C. These undiluted STSs were then analyzed by HPTLC. Based on the differences in the declared contents of resveratrol in the food supplement samples STSs (triplicates) were prepared with the following concentrations: 0.2 mg/mL (samples: 1, 2, 4, 7, 8, 10, 12, 15, 19, 20), 1 mg/mL (samples: 3, 13, 17, 18) and 10 mg/mL (samples: 5, 6, 9, 11, 14, 16).

2.5. HPTLC Analyses

HPTLC analyses were performed on 20 cm × 10 cm glass backed HPTLC silica gel plates (Merck, Art. No. 1.05641). Standard solutions and STSs of food supplements were applied on the plates by means of an automatic TLC Sampler 4 (Camag, Muttenz, Switzerland). Applications were performed as 8 mm bands, 8 mm from the bottom of the plate and 15 mm from the left edge. For quantitative analysis the solution of *trans*-resveratrol standard (1, 2, 4, 8, 10 and 15 µL; 0.02 mg/mL) and three replicates of STSs of two food supplements were applied on each plate. Each of the three replicates of STSs was applied on the plate twice using data-pair technique (one application on the left and the other on the right half of the plate). Application volumes of STSs were as follows: 1 µL (samples 2, 4, 7, 8, 10, 11, 15, 17, 20), 2 µL (samples 1, 3, 9, 12, 13, 18, 19), 3 µL (sample 16), 5 µL (sample 6), 7 µL (sample 5) and 10 µL (sample 14). The plates were developed up to 9 cm in a saturated (15 min) twin-trough chamber (Camag) for 20 cm × 10 cm plates using 10 mL of the developing solvent *n*-hexane–ethyl acetate–formic acid (20:19:1, *v/v*) [12,13]. Development time was 25 min. After development and drying in a stream of warm air for 1 min, post-chromatographic derivatization was performed by dipping the plate for 2 s into anisaldehyde detection reagent by means of a Chromatogram immersion device III (Camag). Anisaldehyde detection reagent was prepared by mixing glacial acetic acid (20 mL) and methanol (170 mL). During cooling with cold water, 16 mL of sulfuric acid was added in a dropwise manner and subsequently anisaldehyde (1 mL) was added to the mixture [14] (pp. 195–196). Images of the plates were documented with a DigiStore 2 documentation system (Camag) at white light, 254 nm, 366 nm after development and after post-chromatographic derivatization. Densitometric scanning was performed by a slit-scanning densitometer TLC Scanner 3 (Camag) in the absorption/reflectance mode at 303 nm (before derivatization) or 500 nm (10 min after derivatization). The dimensions of the slit were: length 6 mm, width 0.3 mm; and the scanning speed 20 mm/s. All instruments were controlled by the winCATS software (Camag; Version 1.4.9.2001).

2.6. Validation of HPTLC Method

The HPTLC method for quantification of resveratrol (*cis*- and *trans*-resveratrol in one chromatographic zone) in food supplements was validated. Validation parameters included: system precision, limit of detection (LOD), limit of quantification (LOQ), linearity, accuracy (intraday precision and recovery) and were performed by the same person and laboratory equipment. Experimentally determined LOD was 10 ng, while LOQ was 20 ng. System precision was tested with nine applications of *trans*-resveratrol standard at 20 ng (LOQ) and at 80 ng (near the amount of resveratrol in applied test solutions of food supplements). Relative standard deviation (RSD) of resveratrol amount at 20 ng was 6.9%, while RSD at 80 ng was 4.4%, which met the established criteria (RSD < 10% at LOQ and RSD < 5% at the amount of resveratrol in the applied food supplement test solution). The regression coefficient for three polynomial calibration curves (20 ng, 40 ng, 80 ng, 160 ng, 200 ng and 300 ng) of resveratrol standard was 0.999, which satisfied the established criterion. Samples 12 (conc. 0.2 mg/mL), 18 (conc. 1 mg/mL) and 5 (conc. 10 mg/mL) were selected for testing the accuracy of the method. Six food supplement test solutions in each concentration were prepared simultaneously for intraday precision of the method. Three food supplement test solutions with addition of *trans*-resveratrol standard for each concentration were simultaneously prepared. Analysis for each concentration was performed on one HPTLC plate. Each solution with the addition of resveratrol standard was applied twice with six food supplement test solutions for intraday precision and resveratrol standard solution for calibration curve. RSD ($n = 6$) for intraday precision of food supplements test solutions prepared in 0.2 mg/mL was 5.49%, for food supplement test solutions prepared in 1 mg/mL was 4.58% and for food supplement test solutions prepared in 5 mg/mL was 4.60%. The obtained results met the established criteria (RSD < 10%). Recovery for sample 5 was 99.7%, for sample 18 97.1%, and for sample 12 102.3%. All values for recovery of all samples met the established criteria, which was 75–120%.

2.7. Label Regulatory Compliance

The EU regulatory compliance of the 20 food supplement products was checked for the following aspects: food labeling [3], health and nutrition claims [5], food supplements [1] and novel foods [4]. A checklist (Table 1) was created to see if all required information was provided on the labels and if the stated information was compliant with the requirements (units, fonts, necessary warnings and statements, etc.). Special attention was paid to any possible misleading practices that could have a negative effect on consumers.

Table 1. Regulatory compliance checklist for food supplement labels for the regulation topics of food labeling, health and nutrition claims, food supplements and novel foods.

Regulation Topic	Information
	Regulatory Compliance Checklist for Food Supplement Labels
Mandatory food information	Name of the food
	List of ingredients
	Allergens
	Quantity of certain ingredients or categories of ingredients
	Net quantity of the food
	Date of minimum durability
	Any special storage conditions and/or conditions of use
	Name or business name and address of the food business operator
	Country of origin or place of provenance
	Instructions for use
	Nutrition declaration *
Voluntary food information	Absence or reduced presence of gluten in food
	Reference intakes for specific population groups
	Suitability of a food for vegetarians or vegans
	Unintentional presence of allergens
Nutrition and health claims	Nutrition claims
	Health claims
	Warning for products that are likely to present a health risk if consumed to excess
	Persons who should avoid using the food
	Quantity of the food and pattern of consumption required to obtain the claimed beneficial effect
	Importance of a varied and balanced diet and a healthy lifestyle
	Nutrition declaration
Food supplements	"Food supplement"
	Names of the categories of nutrients
	Portion of product recommended for daily consumption
	Do not exceed the stated recommended daily dose
	Food supplements should not be used as a substitute for a varied diet
	Store out of the reach of young children
	Amount of the minerals/vitamins (in specified units and as a percentage of the reference values)
	Amount of nutrients/substances with nutritional/physiological effect present in the product & per daily dose
Novel foods	"*trans*-resveratrol"
	People using medicines should only consume the product under medical supervision

* Mandatory only for food supplements with nutrition and/or health claims.

3. Results and Discussion

3.1. HPTLC Quantification of Resveratrol and Assessment of Compliance of Declared and Determined Resveratrol Contents

An overview of the 20 food supplement products included in this study showed that only seven of them (samples 1, 2, 7, 8, 11, 17, 18) were labeled to contain *trans*-resveratrol. For the remaining 13 samples it is, therefore, unclear if they contain a mixture of both isomers (*cis*- and *trans*-resveratrol, although only *trans*-resveratrol is approved as a novel food) or if the manufacturers chose to not write "*trans*-" and for a reason unknown declared what should be the *trans*-resveratrol content as resveratrol content. Therefore, it was decided to analyze the content of total resveratrol (both *cis*- and *trans*-resveratrol) within the scope of this study. HPTLC quantification of resveratrol was performed for 20 food supplement products claiming to contain resveratrol. Based on the results of the HPTLC analyses (Table 2) compliance of the declared resveratrol content with the average (n = 3) determined resveratrol content in food supplements was evaluated. For some samples the contents of resveratrol were higher than 70 mg/unit (Figure 3) and for others they were lower than 50 mg/unit (Figure 4). Various deviations of the average (n = 3) determined resveratrol contents from the declared contents (Figures 3 and 4) were observed. The declared resveratrol contents ranged from 1 mg to 233 mg per unit (capsule, tablet, powder packet), while the average resveratrol contents determined ranged from 2 to 269 mg per unit (Figures 3 and 4). In five food supplements (samples 1, 2, 4, 12, 19), representing 25% of the analyzed food supplements, the declared content was higher than 150 mg/unit, which the Commission Implementing Regulation (EU) 2017/2470 [4] sets as the maximum level (150 mg/day) for *trans*-resveratrol in food supplements. In eight food supplements (samples 1, 2, 4, 7, 8, 10, 19, 20), representing 40% of the analyzed food supplements, the average (n = 3) determined resveratrol contents were higher than 150 mg/unit (Table 2 and Figure 3). Of the 20 food supplements analyzed only one food supplement (sample 15) was found to have the same determined and declared resveratrol contents (Figure 3 and Table 2). In other words, in 95% of the analyzed food supplements the determined resveratrol content was either higher or lower than declared (Figures 3 and 4). In twelve food supplements (samples 1, 2, 3, 4, 7, 8, 9, 10, 13, 18, 19, 20), representing 60% of the analyzed food supplements, the determined resveratrol contents were higher than declared (Figures 3 and 4). In seven food supplements (samples 5, 6, 11, 12, 14, 16, 17), representing 35% of the analyzed food supplements, the determined resveratrol contents were lower than declared (Figures 3 and 4).

Table 2. Average resveratrol content (mg/unit ± SD) determined in 20 food supplements.

Sample	Average Determined Resveratrol Content (mg/unit ± SD) [1]	RSD (%) [1]
1	205.92 ± 6.36	3.09
2	203.10 ± 1.56	0.77
3	31.35 ± 0.52	1.67
4	215.00 ± 0.89	0.41
5	1.52 ± 0.03	2.23
6	1.54 ± 0.05	3.15
7	189.85 ± 4.63	2.44
8	164.28 ± 1.92	1.17
9	2.34 ± 0.01	0.34
10	176.29 ± 4.37	2.48
11	6.78 ± 0.09	1.28
12	124.27 ± 3.28	2.64
13	42.21 ± 1.22	2.88
14	1.94 ± 0.13	6.49
15	125.41 ± 0.63	0.50
16	3.33 ± 0.07	2.01
17	73.76 ± 2.84	3.85
18	28.92 ± 0.37	1.28
19	269.14 ± 4.70	1.75
20	182.80 ± 3.48	1.90

[1] n = 3.

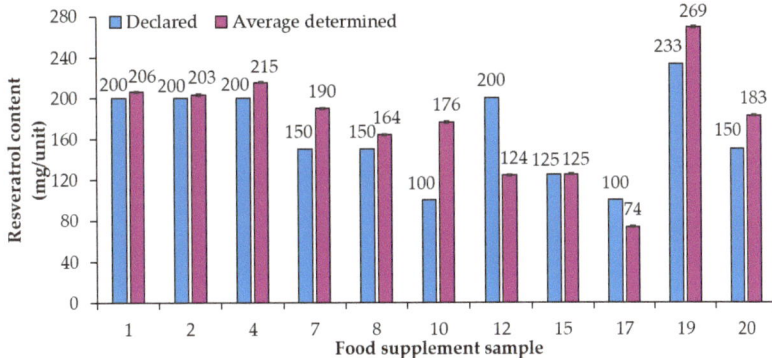

Figure 3. Comparison of declared contents vs. the average (*n* = 3) determined resveratrol contents in food supplements with contents of resveratrol higher than 70 mg/unit.

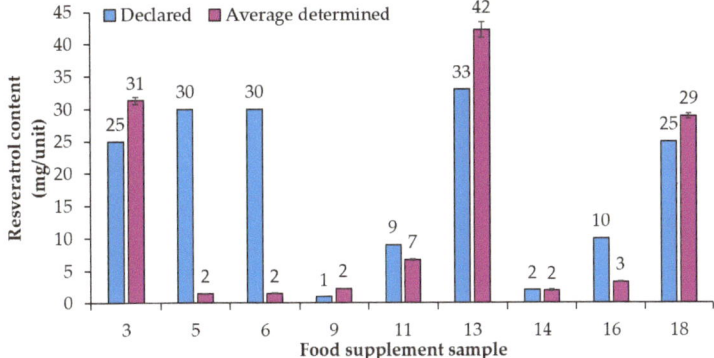

Figure 4. Comparison of declared contents vs. the average (*n* = 3) determined resveratrol contents in food supplements with contents of resveratrol lower than 50 mg/unit.

Using the declared resveratrol contents and the contents of resveratrol determined by quantitative analyses, the percent of declared resveratrol contents in food supplements (Figure 5) and the deviation of determined content from declared content (Figure 6) were calculated. Only in sample 15 was the percent of declared resveratrol content 100% (Figure 5). In the remaining 95% of resveratrol food supplements the determined contents of resveratrol were different from the declared contents and consequently percent of the declared resveratrol content were higher or lower than 100% with differences ranging from 5% to 234% (Figure 5). In five food supplements (samples 1, 2, 4, 8, 14), representing 25% of the food supplements analyzed, the deviation of determined content from declared content (Figure 6) was 10% or less than 10% (percent of declared resveratrol contents ranged between 97% and 110%, Figure 5). In 14 food supplements (samples 3, 5, 6, 7, 9, 10, 11, 12, 13, 16, 17, 18, 19, 20), representing 70% of the food supplements analyzed, the deviation of determined content from declared content (Figure 6) was higher than 10% (more than 10% higher or 10% lower than declared). In eight of those 14 food supplements (samples 3, 7, 9, 10, 13, 18, 19, 20), representing 40% of the food supplements analyzed, the percent of declared resveratrol contents ranged between 116% and 234% (Figure 5). In the other six of those 14 food supplements (samples 5, 6, 11, 12, 16, 17), representing 30% of the food supplements analyzed, the percent of the declared resveratrol contents ranged between 5% and 75% (Figure 5). In four food supplements (samples 5, 6, 12, 16), representing 20% of the food supplements analyzed, deviations of determined contents from declared contents showed that determined resveratrol contents were more than 30% lower than declared contents (Figure 6). In two samples (samples 5 and 6), representing 10% of the food supplements analyzed, the deviation of determined content from declared was −95% (Figure 6) as the products contained only 5% of the declared resveratrol content (Figure 5).

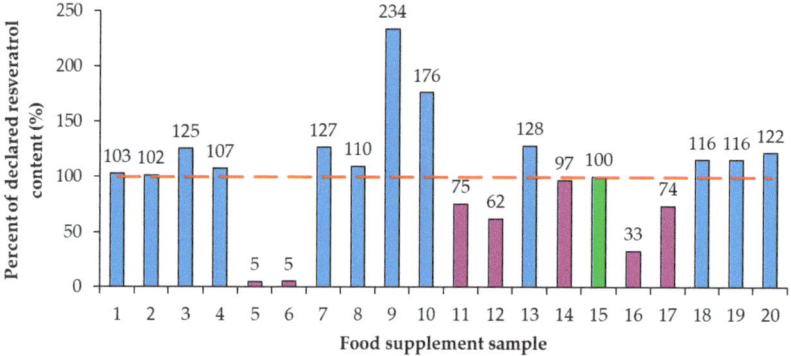

Figure 5. Percent of declared resveratrol content in food supplements.

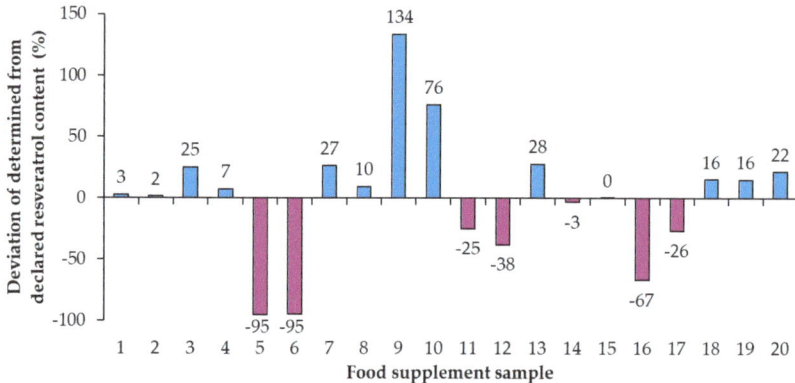

Figure 6. Deviation of determined content from declared content of resveratrol in food supplements.

As evident from the calculated deviations of determined contents from declared contents presented in Figure 5, the determined resveratrol contents for 30% of the food supplements were more than 30% higher/lower than the declared contents. Samples 9 and 10, representing 10% of the food supplements analyzed, had the deviation of the determined from the declared resveratrol content higher than 130% and 70%, respectively (Figure 5). Such deviation can have different consequences for consumers (Figure 5). The declared content of sample 9 was 1 mg, but the determined content was 2.34 mg (Figure 4, Table 2), which means that, although the content declaration was not providing accurate information to the consumer, there is a small likelihood that this could result in adverse health effects for the consumer. The declared content of sample 10 was 100 mg, but the determined content was actually 176 mg (Figure 3, Table 2), which is even higher than the permitted daily intake of 150 mg of *trans*-resveratrol. The determined content in sample 10 poses an even higher risk for the consumer because taking too much resveratrol can lead to health issues (e.g., digestion problems). Therefore, from a food safety perspective, the differences between declared and determined content of resveratrol are not just misinforming consumers, as high concentrations can also result in negative effects on consumer health.

In two other studies of resveratrol in food supplements the authors reported similar deviations of the determined and declared contents [15,16] and also contents (declared and/or determined) higher than 150 mg per unit. In the first study authors analyzed *trans*-resveratrol in 28 food supplements and reported that in 17 food supplements, representing more than 60% of food supplements analyzed, the determined contents were lower than declared contents [15]. Additionally, in the remaining 11 food supplements, representing more than 39% of food supplements analyzed, the determined contents were higher than declared contents [15]. Differences between the declared contents and determined contents were ranging from 24% to 262% [15]. For 17 food supplements the deviations of determined contents from declared contents were up to ±10% [15]. In six food supplement products, representing more than 20% of the food supplements analyzed, the declared and determined contents were higher than 150 mg/unit [15]. In the second study the authors analyzed resveratrol in nine food supplements and found that the determined resveratrol contents were lower in eight samples and higher than the declared contents in one sample [16]. The declared resveratrol contents ranged between 10 and 300 mg per unit, while the determined contents ranged between 3.4 and 147.3 mg per unit. The determined resveratrol contents ranged between 22.8% and 104.7% of the declared contents [16]. Three food supplements, representing 33.3% of the food supplements analyzed, contained less than 60% of the declared contents [16]. The deviation from the declared resveratrol content in one food supplement was 77%. In two food supplements the declared resveratrol contents were higher than 150 mg per unit (250 mg and 300 mg), however, the determined contents were lower than 150 mg per unit (144.9 mg and 147.3 mg) [16]. Surprisingly, a recently published list of products containing 20 to 1400 mg of resveratrol per serving included more than 45% of the products with the declared resveratrol contents higher than 150 mg/unit [17].

Issues of noncompliance of the declared and the determined contents were recently also reported for food supplements claiming to contain folic acid [18], vitamin A [19], vitamin C [19], vitamin E [19] and magnesium [20]. Analyses of 30 folic acid food supplements available on the Polish market revealed that in 29 products, representing 96.6% of food supplements analyzed, the determined contents were lower than the declared [18]. Seventeen food supplements, representing 56.6% of food supplements analyzed, contained less than 80% of the declared folic acid content. Nine food supplements, representing 30% of food supplements analyzed, contained less than 50% of the declared folic acid content [18]. Four food supplements, representing 13.3% of food supplements analyzed, contained less than 3% of the declared content of folic acid [18]. In contrast the analysis of folic acid content in the food supplements sold in Spain [21] showed that the determined content was within a tolerated range with regard to the declared values, which were in accordance with EU regulation requirements. Noncompliances of the declared and determined contents were also found in a study of vitamins A, C and E in 57 food supplements available on the Brazilian market [19]. The determined contents for vitamins A and E were lower than the declared contents in 71% and 50% of food supplements, respectively [19]. In another study of 116 food supplements containing magnesium the authors reported noncompliance of the declared and determined contents for 58.7% of the products analyzed [20]. In only two samples, representing 1.7% of the food supplements analyzed, the declared and determined contents were identical [20].

The results of this study of resveratrol in food supplements and the results of studies performed by other authors for resveratrol or other declared ingredients indicate the need for improved quality control by food supplements producers (including stability studies of the ingredients) as well as more frequent control by regulatory authorities to ensure the reliable declarations for consumers.

3.2. Label Regulatory Compliance

Label regulatory compliance of 20 food supplement products sold on the Slovenian market and claiming to contain resveratrol or *trans*-resveratrol from different sources was evaluated. The origin of resveratrol (Figure 7) was not provided on six products. Most food supplements (12 products) listed Japanese knotweed and some products even specified the plant's rhizomes as the source of resveratrol. The other food supplements listed grapevine (1 product) or dried juice of skins and pips of black grapes (1 product) as the source of resveratrol. The analyzed food supplements were produced by 15 producers (Figure 1), three of which produced more than one product which replicated compliance and noncompliance (errors) across their food labels.

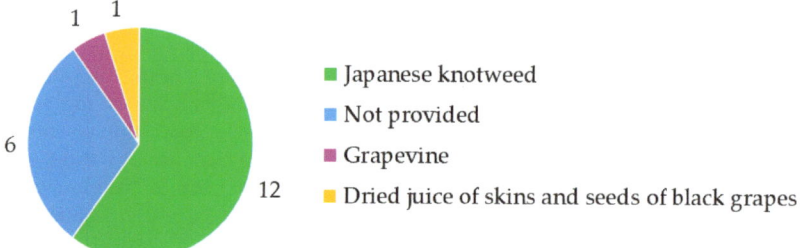

Figure 7. Resveratrol origin declared on food supplements.

3.2.1. Mandatory Food Information

Not all of the 12 mandatory requirements [3] for food information are mandatory for food supplements. The noncompliances noted in the overview of mandatory food information (Figure 8) varied from grammatical mistakes to mistakes that could mislead or negatively influence the consumer.

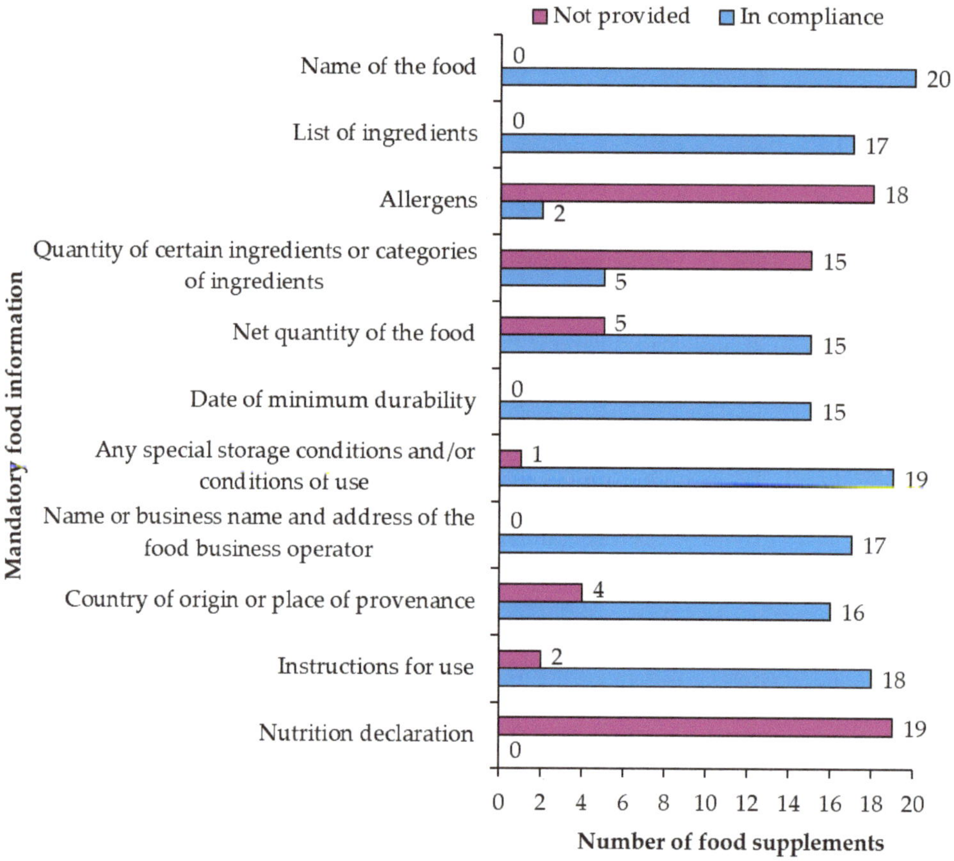

Figure 8. Compliance of mandatory food information on food supplement labels.

Name of the food was written correctly on all 20 food supplement products.

List of ingredients was accurately labeled on 17 food supplement products (1, 2, 5, 6, 7, 8, 9, 10, 11, 12, 13, 14, 16, 17, 18, 19, 20). For most samples the list of ingredients began with a title that included the word "ingredients" followed by a list of ingredients. Lists of ingredients on two samples did not have the word "ingredients" in the title. One sample did not include a list of ingredients, but only listed ingredients "per capsule". Ingredients should be listed in descending order of their mass. Due to lack of information, it was not possible to check if the order was correct (descending) for all the ingredients. For some ingredients (such as vitamins, minerals and resveratrol) the quantities were provided on the labels and it was discovered that these ingredients were not included on the ingredients list according to the descending mass. Labeling of nano materials was compliant with regulatory requirements with the word "(nano)" after the ingredient in both samples (3 and 4). Some lists of ingredients were written in a way that the title "Ingredients" was followed by words "one capsule contains" or "three capsules contain" and then the list of ingredients. There was only one sample where the list of ingredients was unclear and confusing as the list was repeated two times: first the list titled "Ingredients in one capsule" (which included "Japanese knotweed rhizomes extract that contains resveratrol") and second list titled "Ingredients" (which included the whole list of ingredients including "knotweed that contains resveratrol"). Labeling of additives showed a trend of avoiding writing additives with their E-numbers. All additives on all food supplements were correctly labeled with their functional classes and names. Perhaps this trend reflects the consumers dislike of E-numbers that can be connected to bad reputations of some additives. However, writing additives with their names instead of using the E-numbers does not mean that additives are not present in food supplement products. One food supplement even emphasized the information "additive free". On multiple food supplements the adjective "natural" was used when describing the ingredients (e.g., "natural *trans*-resveratrol (from a knotweed species, *Polygonum cuspidatum*)", "natural caramel color", "natural *trans*-resveratrol from Japanese knotweed", "capsule: tapioca gelatin, naturally fermented in pullulan", "natural *trans*-resveratrol", "natural beta-carotene/mixed carotenoids", etc.). The EU legislation is not very clear about the use of the adjective "natural" on food labels, as the term "natural" is only mentioned in cases of flavoring substances (Regulation (EC) No 1334/2008 [22]) and the nutrition claim "natural" [5]. Flavoring substances can be labeled as "natural" if they fulfill the requirements and do not mislead consumers. The nutrition claim "natural" can only be used for natural properties of foods. The current regulation of using the term "natural" on food labels should be improved because there is too much room for consumer confusion and misunderstanding.

Allergens were correctly labeled (e.g., "lecithin (**soy**)" or "**soy** lecithin") on two products (samples 5, 14) and not provided on 17 products. An ingredient ("**fish** oil") was not written correctly, as allergens should be written in a different font (e.g., "fish oil"). There was also some confusion with correctly written ingredient "phytosterols (from **soy**)", which was followed by "Information about allergens: contains soy (emphasized above)". The last statement was not needed, and even if considered as an attempt at voluntary food information, it only confuses the consumer.

Quantity of certain ingredients or categories of ingredients was correct on five products (1, 2, 9, 13, 20) as the quantity of resveratrol was provided in percent in the list of ingredients. The rest of the products did not include this information on their labels, which is alright because this information is only required in case its absence could result in consumers being misled. In most cases, the quantities of ingredients such as vitamins and minerals (when emphasized with a word or image next to the products name) were provided only among the ingredients or in a table of vitamin and mineral content which is compliant with the food supplement regulation [1] and is not regulated as "quantity of ingredients" by food labeling regulation [3].

Net quantity of food is mandatory on all food labels. Net quantity of the food was accurately labeled with appropriate units on 15 products (samples 1, 2, 3, 4, 5, 6, 7, 9, 10, 11, 12, 13, 14, 19, 20) and not included on five products.

Date of minimum durability is mandatory on all food labels, but was properly written on only 15 products (samples 1, 3, 4, 6, 7, 9, 10, 11, 13, 14, 15, 16, 17, 19, 20). Other products had different errors in the writing of the date on the label. The date should be provided with the words "Best before … " when the date includes an indication of the day or "Best before end … " in all other cases followed by the date or the location of the date on the food packaging. An example of an unclear date labeling was "Expiry date (use by Do not consume the enclosed preservative! Leave it in the bottle. Expiry date (Best before end:) and serial number are printed on the bottom of the bottle." On another product the "Best before end" was not written and only the date was printed. There was also a product where the date was written without punctuation ("1023"), which is confusing for the consumers. Even more unclear was the writing on the sample in which the lot or batch number and date were written together with no space or punctuation. Another product had a correctly written date, but the location of the date was not as specified. Yet another product had a correctly written date, but the location of the date was not provided, although required for products where "Best before" is not followed by the date. Although lot numbers (batches of sales units manufactured under almost the same conditions) are not a part of mandatory food information regulation, marketing of foodstuffs requires lot numbers on labels (Directive 2011/91/EU [23]). Lot numbers were provided on 18 products (1, 2, 3, 4, 5, 6, 7, 9, 10, 11, 12, 13, 14, 15, 16, 17, 19, 20).

Special storage conditions and/or conditions of use were provided in accordance with requirements on 19 (samples 2, 3, 4, 5, 6, 7, 8, 9, 10, 11, 12, 13, 14, 15, 16, 17, 18, 19, 20) of 20 food supplements. One sample did not provide this information. Examples of special storage conditions were "store at a temperature up to 25 °C protected from moisture and light", "store in a dry place at room temperature" and "store well closed". Examples of conditions of use included "only for adults", "in case of gastrointestinal unease stop using the product", "not suitable for: pregnant women, breastfeeding mothers and children younger than 12" and "in case of taking immunosuppressants or other prescribed medication consult your doctor about taking this product".

Name or business name and address of the food business operator were correctly labeled on 17 food supplements (samples 1, 2, 5, 6, 7, 8, 9, 10, 11, 12, 13, 14, 15, 17, 18, 19, 20). The irregularities of writing the business name and address included: not writing the complete address, not writing the address at all and writing the town twice instead of the full address.

Country of origin or place of provenance is only strictly mandatory in cases in which the lack of this information could result in misleading consumers. Country of origin was correctly written on 16 (samples 1, 2, 3, 4, 7, 8, 9, 10, 11, 12, 13, 14, 17, 18, 19, 20) and not included on four food supplement products. In most cases this information was provided with the words "Origin", "Produced in" or "Manufactured in". Most products were produced in the UK, France and USA.

Instructions for use were properly provided on 18 food supplements (samples 1, 3, 4, 5, 6, 7, 8, 9, 10, 11, 12, 14, 15, 16, 17, 18, 19, 20) and not included on two food supplements. For sample 14, the product in the form of a powder packet, the instructions were: "put the contents of the packet in a glass or bottle with water (0.2–0.5 L)". Food supplements in the form of capsules or tablets included instructions to take them with liquid (water or juice) and to take them before/during/after a meal in the morning or evening.

Nutrition declaration was not included on 19 of the 20 food supplements. The label of one sample included a nutrition declaration, which was mostly correct, but the energy value units were incorrect.

3.2.2. Voluntary Food Information

Voluntary food information is also regulated [3]. The labels of examined food supplements only included voluntary food information in nine (samples 2, 7, 8, 10, 11, 14, 16, 17, 18) of 20 food supplements (Figure 9).

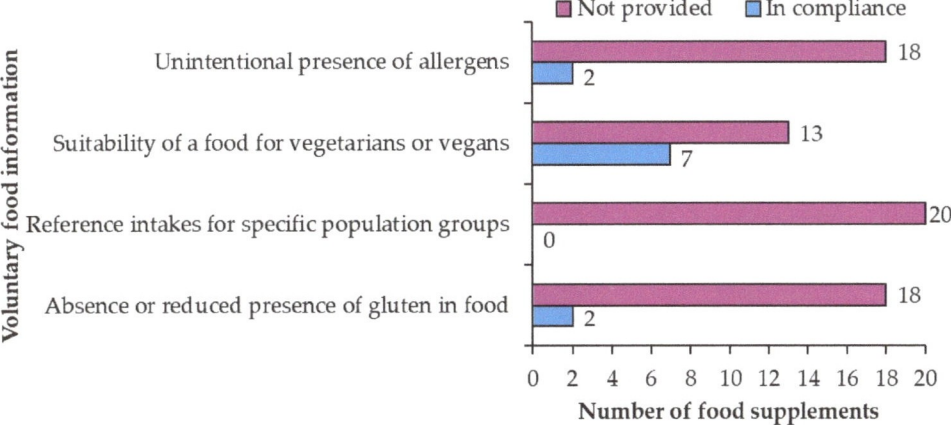

Figure 9. Voluntary food information on food supplement labels.

An **unintentional presence of allergens** was appropriately labeled on two food supplements (samples 2, 11) and not included on the remaining 18. For example, "May contain traces of sulfites." It was noticed that in some cases unintentional presence of allergens was not labeled properly. The irregularities ranged from writing in bold (a different font should only be used for the mandatory labeling of allergens presence) to incorrect use of allergen terminology (for example "nuts" instead of "walnuts").

Suitability of a food for vegetarians or vegans was correctly written on seven products (samples 2, 7, 8, 14, 16, 17, 18) and not provided on 13. One product had the statement about vegetarian/vegan suitability written in English on the original label but was not translated and included on the Slovene label. This is not an irregularity, but it can be confusing for consumers who know both languages and read all the labels.

Reference intakes for specific population groups were not provided on any of the 20 food supplement products.

Absence or reduced presence of gluten in food was correctly labeled on two products (samples 10, 14) as "gluten free". The remaining 18 products did not have this information. The use of "gluten free" is allowed on foods produced in ways that they do not contain gluten. It is also allowed on foods from ingredients that naturally do not contain gluten. This information should not mislead the consumers that the food product has special properties if similar foods also have the same properties [6].

3.2.3. Nutrition and Health Claims

The use of nutrition and health claims (Figure 10) is voluntary [5]. Nutrition claims were only included on one product (sample 10: "salt-free"). Salt content of the product was not included on the label of sample 10. Other resveratrol food supplements also did not contain salt—making "salt-free" a shared property of similar products. The fact that sample 10 is labeled salt-free does not make the products salt content different from similar products. The use of the "salt-free" nutrition claim is permitted if the product does not contain more than 0.005 g of sodium (or the equivalent amount for salt) per 100 g. Therefore, the use of the "salt-free" nutrition claim is misleading. Two more samples had the claim "sugar free" on the original English label, but the Slovenian label did not have this claim.

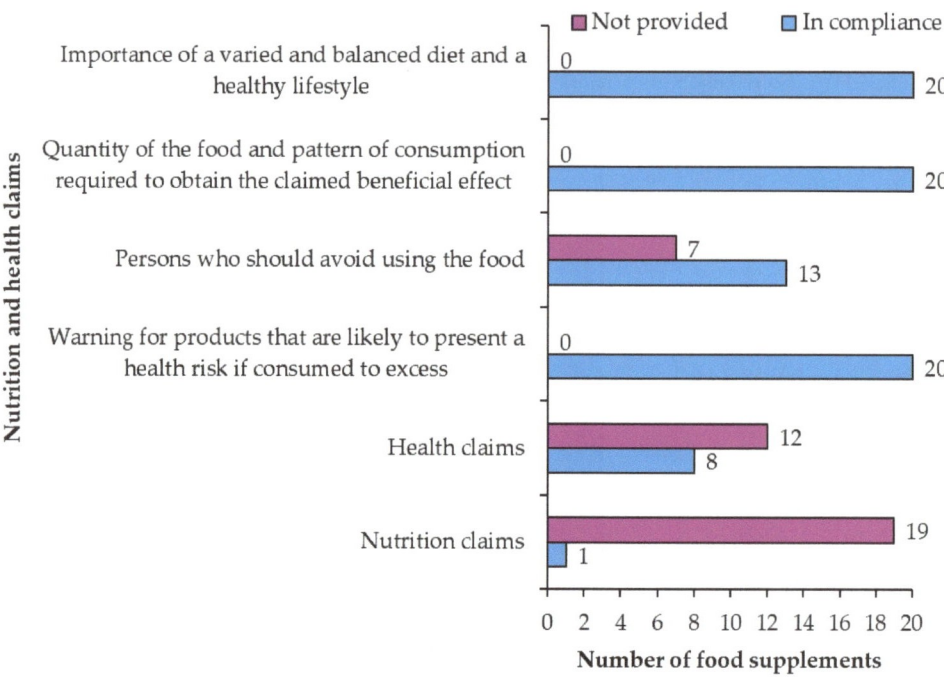

Figure 10. Food supplements with health and nutrition claims.

Health claims were written on eight products (samples 3, 4, 5, 6, 9, 13, 14, 19). Together these eight products contained 74 health claims. Health claims connected the vitamins and minerals in food supplements with the following health effects: protecting cells from oxidative stress, reducing fatigue and exhaustion, functioning of the muscles, heart, nervous and immune system, maintaining vision and healthy bones, releasing energy during metabolism (Table 3).

On some food supplement labels, health claims were written using the same words as on the list of the approved claims [24]. On other products the claims were slightly paraphrased in a way that did not change the meaning of the health claim or the consumer's understanding of the claim. Therefore, it can be concluded that the use of health claims was in compliance with regulatory requirements for all eight samples.

When using nutritional and/or health claims the labels must also include the statements: about the importance of a varied and balanced diet, the amount of food and the required method of consumption and warning about the danger of excessive consumption. The warning for products that are likely to present a health risk if consumed to excess was accurately included on all 20 food supplement labels. A warning for persons who should avoid the food was correctly written on 13 food supplements (samples 2, 3, 4, 5, 6, 8, 10, 12, 13, 16, 17, 18, 19) and not included on the remaining seven food supplements. The labels of all products included the quantity of the food and pattern of consumption required to obtain the benefits claimed as well as the statement regarding the importance of a varied and balanced diet and a healthy lifestyle.

Health claims were also evaluated for regulatory compliance in a study of folic acid food supplements sold in Spain [21]. The results revealed that the food supplements sold in supermarkets fulfilled the requirements for folic acid health claims, while over 14% of food supplements sold online did not fulfill the requirements for folic acid health claims as they contained nonauthorized health claims.

Table 3. Health claims on food supplement labels grouped according to the related nutrients.

Nutrients (Number of Products Using the Health Claim)	Health Claims (Summarized from Commission Regulation (EU) No 432/2012 [24]
Copper (2), zinc (2), manganese (1), selenium (3), vitamin C (3), vitamin E (1)	[Nutrient] contributes to the "protection of cells from oxidative stress."
Magnesium (3), niacin (3), pantothenic acid (3), vitamin B2/riboflavin (3), vitamin B6 (3), vitamin B12 (3), vitamin C (2)	[Nutrient] contributes to the "reduction of tiredness and fatigue."
Calcium (1), potassium (1), magnesium (2), vitamin D (2)	Nutrient] contributes to "normal muscle function."
Thiamine (1)	[Nutrient] contributes to the "normal function of the heart."
Copper (1), zinc (2), folate (2), selenium (1), vitamin B6 (2), vitamin B12 (2), vitamin C (2), vitamin D (3)	[Nutrient] contributes to the "function of the immune system."
Copper (1), biotin (1), iodine (1), potassium (1), magnesium (2), niacin (1), vitamin B1/thiamine (1), vitamin B2/riboflavin (1), vitamin B6 (1), vitamin B12 (1), vitamin C (1)	[Nutrient] contributes to "normal functioning of the nervous system."
Zinc (1)	[Nutrient] contributes to the "maintenance of normal vision."
Calcium (1), vitamin D (1)	[Nutrient] contributes to the "maintenance of normal bones."
Magnesium (1), niacin (1), vitamin B2/riboflavin (1), vitamin B6 (1), vitamin B12 (1)	[Nutrient] contributes to "normal energy-yielding metabolism."

3.2.4. Food Supplements and Novel Foods

According to food supplements regulation [1] products are required to be labeled as "food supplements". All 20 of the examined products fulfilled this requirement (Figure 11). The labels of all 20 products included the information that the products contained resveratrol. Seventeen of these products (samples 2, 3, 4, 5, 6, 8, 9, 11, 12, 13, 14, 15, 16, 17, 18, 19, 20) also included the names of other categories of nutrients while labels of the remaining three products did not include this information (Figure 11). All 20 products were labeled with the following **required warnings** (Figure 11): (1) not to exceed the stated recommended daily dose, (2) that food supplements should not be used as a substitute for a varied diet, and (3) store out of reach of young children. All 20 products also included the information on the portion of product recommended for daily consumption. Five products had unusual labels regarding the recommended daily dose "The recommended daily amount or dose should not be exceeded, unless your doctor has instructed you to do so".

The **amounts of minerals/vitamins** in specified units and as a percentage of the reference values were correctly provided on six (samples 3, 4, 9, 13, 14, 17) and not provided on 10 food supplements (Figure 11). For example, the amount of copper was labeled in mg instead of μg, which should be used according to the regulation [3]. Some samples used the wrong order of ingredients on the list of ingredients not following the descending order of mass.

The **amounts of nutrients/substances** (mainly resveratrol) with nutritional/physiological effect, present in the product and per daily dose were written correctly on all 20 products (Figure 11).

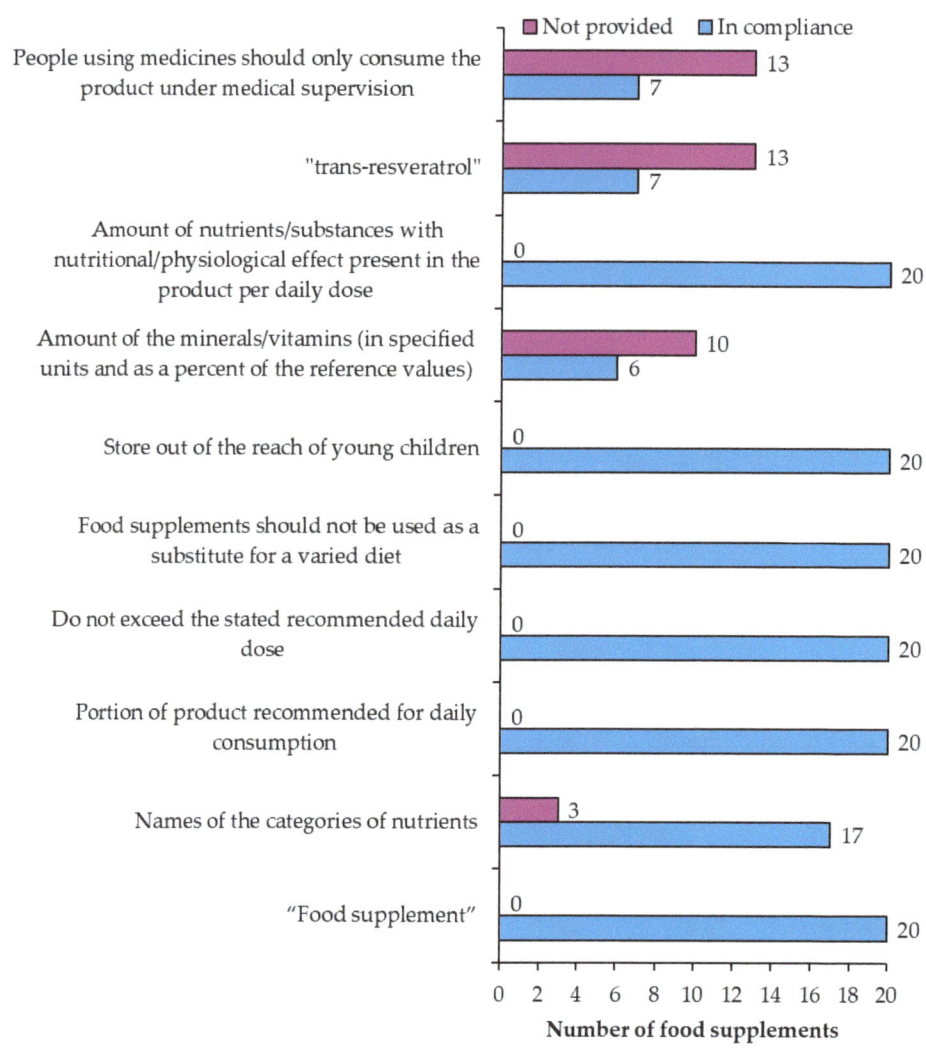

Figure 11. Food supplement information and novel food information on food supplement labels.

The field of **novel food labeling** regulatory [4] compliance proved to be far more challenging than food supplement labeling (Figure 11). The regulation only requires two things for resveratrol food supplements: to be labeled as "*trans*-resveratrol" and to have a warning that people using medicines should only consume the product under medical supervision. Only seven products (samples 1, 2, 7, 8, 11, 17, 18) were labeled to contain "*trans*-resveratrol" and the others usually referred to this compound as only resveratrol (Figure 12). The medical warning about people on medication to take the supplements under a doctor's supervision was only written on seven food supplements (samples 2, 6, 8, 12, 16, 17, 18). In terms of novel food labeling for resveratrol food supplements only four of the products were labeled correctly (samples 2, 8, 17, 18).

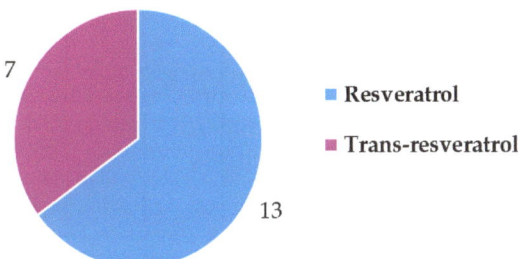

Figure 12. Resveratrol vs. *trans*-resveratrol declarations on food supplement labels.

3.2.5. Other Label Noncompliances

Other noncompliances with the regulation concerning food supplement labeling were also observed such as: typos, use of misleading images, nonauthorized health and nutrition claims as well as overuse of voluntary information.

Typos were a common type of error on food supplement labels. In most cases this included wrong punctuation (swapping periods and commas or incorrect placement of commas and semicolons). On one product words were written in the middle of the date of minimum durability, which made it impossible to read and understand the date. On another product the label included the wrongly spelled word "resveratrol" (it was written "rezervatrol" instead). Such examples may seem innocent, but they can have negative effects on consumers.

Misleading use of photos was observed on several labels. On one product a picture of fruit (apple, pear, lemon and orange slices stacked on top of each other) was placed on the largest side of the cardboard box and while the ingredients did not include these fruits, the manufacturer tried to solve this by writing "The product does not contain the fruit in the picture." next to the photo. Despite this claim, the use of such graphics can mislead consumers. Another product clearly listed Japanese knotweed as the source of resveratrol, but the front of the packaging had an image of mint, which was not listed among the ingredients. This kind of image use could also mislead the consumers. On another product with resveratrol from Japanese knotweed, there was a picture of grapes, which were not present on the list of ingredients.

Another problematic practice was the use of nonauthorized health claims linking food supplements with resveratrol and in some cases also other ingredients with positive health effects. Examples of these claims included: "resveratrol contributes to a healthy cardiovascular system", "natural antioxidant", "preserving youth for smooth skin" and "lignans from flaxseed may support a healthy prostate in aging men".

There were also differences between the information provided on Slovene and English language labels. For example, one product's original label in English language included nonauthorized health claims, which were not translated and included on the Slovenian label. This is both good and bad, because the Slovenian label was in accordance with the regulation regarding health claims, but at the same time consumers knowing both languages could be confused due to the different label contents. There were several other cases in which there were differences between the original (mostly English) and translated (Slovenian) labels. These differences included statements claiming that resveratrol can help to support healthy cardiovascular functions, has cellular anti-aging properties, has the ability to promote a healthy response to biological stress, supports healthy aging, supports antioxidant health, etc. In some cases, these statements were followed by a disclaimer that the statements were not evaluated by the FDA and that the product is not intended to diagnose, treat, cure or prevent any disease.

Statements about not containing certain ingredients were often used. Regulation 1169/2006 [3] permits highlighting special properties of food products, except if similar food products also have the same properties. The use of "lactose free" was not done correctly as its use is only limited to products containing milk or milk products or ingredients. The use of "Lactose free" requires labeling of an actual content of lactose in g/100 g of product. Some food supplement labels claimed not to contain certain ingredients such as: fillers, binders or other excipients, gluten, wheat, lactose, added sugar, sugar, salt starch, soy, milk, lactose, yeast, titanium dioxide, artificial flavorings or colorings.

The labels of some food supplement products included too much voluntary information. Probably the purpose of that was to attract consumers' attention and convince them to purchase the product. However, because these voluntary claims took a larger portion of the label, the legitimacy of using them is questionable as they can confuse the consumer and make it difficult for consumers to access the mandatory food information. Examples of those claims included: descriptions of holistic innovations, procedures for the plant ingredients preparations, comments about research results, etc.

The most important aspect and purpose of food labels in the EU is to provide consumers with understandable information. Clearly the evidence shows that there are still many improvements needed to achieve the goal of clear and comprehensive labeling of food supplements that fulfill all regulatory requirements.

4. Conclusions

Various deviations of the average determined contents of resveratrol from the declared contents were found. Only one of 20 food supplement products analyzed was found to have the same content as declared. Seven products were found to have a lower content of resveratrol and 12 products a higher content of resveratrol. The determined contents ranged from 5% to 234% of declared content. In 40% of the food supplement products analyzed the determined content even exceeded the maximum level (150 mg/day) for *trans*-resveratrol in food supplements set by EU regulation, which can have negative effects on the health of consumers of these food supplements. From a food safety point of view, the differences between declared and determined content of resveratrol in food supplements are concerning.

Resveratrol food supplement labels are very diverse in both style and the information they provide. The results of this label regulatory compliance overview showed that most labels contained the necessary information and that in most aspects labels followed the regulatory requirements for mandatory and voluntary food information, health and nutrition claims as well as food supplement and novel food labeling. However, labels also contained multiple errors (ranging from typos—even resveratrol—to deceptions) that could have different consequences for the consumers as some errors may confuse and misinform them. Particularly concerning were irregularities that were the result of negligence (such as writing the lot number together with the date of minimum durability) and the misleading use of images on the food supplement packaging (e.g., fruit or mint on products that do not contain fruit or mint as well as grapes on a product not made from grapes but Japanese knotweed).

Labels incorrectly provided information about the possible presence of allergenic substances, which could be present due to contamination, as allergenic substances were written in a different font or not represented correctly (e.g., lactose free). The use of too much voluntary information was also a problematic practice as this information took most of the space on the label of some products, which already used very small fonts, making the label information overwhelming and confusing for consumers. Voluntary claims about the absence of certain ingredients (e.g., lactose free, yeast free, salt free, sugar free) were quite common, but in most cases, they were not used appropriately as they referred to ingredients that were not present in any of the food supplement samples. Hence the absence of those ingredients was not a different property (e.g., lactose free or salt free) compared to other similar products. Labels also contained nonauthorized health claims connecting resveratrol and other ingredients with positive health effects (e.g., preserving youth—for smooth skin).

Labels were often translated containing both the original (printed) label and the translated label (on a sticker). In many cases the contents of the original and translated labels were different (e.g., not all information was translated from English to Slovene, which could be confusing for consumers understanding both languages, but in some cases these differences made Slovenian labels compliant with the regulation where English labels were not compliant).

Labels should be improved to reduce the number of truly unnecessary errors and to be fully compliant with the regulatory requirements as well as become more comprehensive for the consumers. Both responsible food business operators and regulatory or inspection bodies should dedicate their attention to improving food supplement labels. There is still a lot of room for improvements. Perhaps it would also be beneficial for regulations to specify some aspects of food labeling in more detail (e.g., use of voluntary claims in relation to scientific evidence or lack thereof and the use of the term "natural"). An increase of minimum font size should be considered by the regulatory body. Present minimum font size and the abundance of text on food supplement labels often result in labels that are extremely difficult to read due to the density of text and use of far too small font size. After all, everyone is a consumer and deserves to have labels with clear information about food supplement products because that helps consumers to choose the right product for them.

Author Contributions: Conceptualization, M.B. and I.V.; methodology, M.B., I.V. and V.G.; validation, M.B., and V.G.; formal analysis, M.B., V.G. and I.V.; investigation, M.B., I.V. and V.G.; resources, I.V.; data curation, M.B., I.V. and V.G.; writing—original draft preparation, M.B., I.V. and V.G.; writing—review and editing, M.B. and I.V.; visualization, M.B.; supervision, V.G. and I.V.; project administration, I.V.; funding acquisition, I.V. All authors have read and agreed to the published version of the manuscript.

Funding: This study was financially supported by the Slovenian Research Agency (research core funding research program P1-0005 "Functional food and food supplements").

Institutional Review Board Statement: Not applicable.

Informed Consent Statement: Not applicable.

Data Availability Statement: The data presented in this study are available on request from the corresponding author.

Acknowledgments: The authors want to express their most sincere gratitude to Merck KGaA, Germany for donating HPTLC plates.

Conflicts of Interest: The authors declare no conflict of interest. The funders had no role in the design of the study; in the collection, analyses, or interpretation of data; in the writing of the manuscript; or in the decision to publish the results.

References

1. Directive 2002/46/EC of the European Parliament and of the Council of 10 June 2002 on the Approximation of the Laws of the Member States Relating to Food Supplements. Available online: https://eur-lex.europa.eu/legal-content/EN/TXT/?uri=CELEX%3A02002L0046-20220930 (accessed on 14 December 2022).
2. European Commission. *2021 Annual Report Alert and Cooperation Network*; Publications Office of the European Union: Luxembourg, 2022. [CrossRef]
3. Regulation (EU) No 1169/2011 of the European Parliament and of the Council of 25 October 2011 on the Provision of Food Information to Consumers. Available online: https://eur-lex.europa.eu/legal-content/EN/TXT/?uri=CELEX%3A02011R1169-20180101 (accessed on 14 December 2022).
4. Commission Implementing Regulation (EU) 2017/2470 of 20 December 2017 Establishing the Union List of Novel Foods in Accordance with Regulation (EU) 2015/2283 of the European Parliament and of the Council on Novel Foods. Available online: https://eur-lex.europa.eu/legal-content/EN/TXT/?uri=CELEX%3A02017R2470-20220829 (accessed on 14 December 2022).
5. Regulation (EC) No 1924/2006 of the European Parliament and of the Council of 20 December 2006 on Nutrition and Health Claims Made on Foods. Available online: https://eur-lex.europa.eu/legal-content/EN/TXT/?uri=CELEX%3A02006R1924-20141213 (accessed on 14 December 2022).
6. Commission Implementing Regulation (EU) No 828/2014 of 30 July 2014 on the Requirements for the Provision of Information to Consumers on the Absence or Reduced Presence of Gluten in Food. Available online: https://eur-lex.europa.eu/eli/reg_impl/2014/828/oj (accessed on 14 December 2022).

7. EU Register of Nutrition and Health Claims Made on Foods (v.3.6). Available online: https://ec.europa.eu/food/safety/labelling_nutrition/claims/register/public/?event=register.home (accessed on 16 August 2022).
8. European Commission Novel Food. Available online: https://food.ec.europa.eu/safety/novel-food_en (accessed on 14 December 2022).
9. Gómez-Maqueo, A.; Escobedo-Avellaneda, Z.; Cano, M.P.; Welti-Chanes, J. Phenolic compounds in food. In *Phenolic Compounds in Food: Characterization and Analysis*; Nollet, M.L.L., Gutierrez-Uribe, J.A., Eds.; CRC Ptrss, Taylor & Francis Group: Boca Raton, FL, USA, 2018.
10. De Angelis, M.; Della-Morte, D.; Buttinelli, G.; Di Martino, A.; Pacifici, F.; Checconi, P.; Ambrosio, L.; Stefanelli, P.; Palamara, A.T.; Garaci, E.; et al. Protective role of combined polyphenols and micronutrients against influenza a virus and SARS-CoV-2 infection in vitro. *Biomedicines* **2021**, *9*, 1721. [CrossRef] [PubMed]
11. Navarro, G.; Martínez Pinilla, E.; Ortiz, R.; Noé, V.; Ciudad, C.J.; Franco, R. Resveratrol and related stilbenoids, nutraceutical/dietary complements with health-promoting actions: Industrial production, safety, and the search for mode of action. *Compr. Rev. Food Sci. Food Saf.* **2018**, *17*, 808–826. [CrossRef] [PubMed]
12. Simonovska, B.; Vovk, I.; Andrenšek, S.; Valentová, K.; Ulrichová, J. Investigation of phenolic acids in yacon (*Smallanthus sonchifolius*) leaves and tubers. *J. Chromatogr. A* **2003**, *1016*, 89–98. [CrossRef] [PubMed]
13. Glavnik, V.; Simonovska, B.; Albreht, A.; Vovk, I. TLC and HPLC screening of *p*-coumaric acid, *trans*-resveratrol, and pterostilbene in bacterial cultures, food supplements, and wine. *J. Planar Chromatogr.-Mod. TLC* **2012**, *25*, 251–258. [CrossRef]
14. Jork, H.; Funk, W.; Fischer, W.R.; Wimmer, H. *Dünnschicht-Chromatographie. Reagenzien und Nachweismethoden, Bd. 1a, Physikalishe und chemische Nach-weismethoden: Grundlagen, Reagenzien I*; Thin-Layer Chromatography; VCH Verlagsgesellschaft: Weinheim, Germany, 1989; ISBN 9783527278343.
15. Omar, J.M.; Yang, H.; Li, S.; Marquardt, R.R.; Jones, P.J.H. Development of an improved reverse-phase high-performance liquid chromatography method for the simultaneous analyses of trans -/ cis-resveratrol, quercetin, and emodin in commercial resveratrol supplements. *J. Agric. Food Chem.* **2014**, *62*, 5812–5817. [CrossRef]
16. Ardelean, F.; Vlase, L.; Mocan, A.M.; Gheldiu, A.M.; Antal, D.S.; Trandafirescu, C.; Marginean, O.; Dragan, S. Dietary supplements with resveratrol, flavonoids and phenolic acids: In-depth HPLC profiling and antioxidant capacity as quality markers. *Rev. Chim.* **2017**, *68*, 401–407. [CrossRef]
17. Khattar, S.; Khan, S.A.; Zaidi, S.A.A.; Darvishikolour, M.; Farooq, U.; Naseef, P.P.; Kurunian, M.S.; Khan, M.Z.; Shamim, A.; Khan, M.M.U.; et al. Resveratrol from dietary supplement to a drug candidate: An assessment of potential. *Pharmaceuticals* **2022**, *15*, 957. [CrossRef]
18. Czarnowska-Kujawska, M.; Klepacka, J.; Zielińska, O.; Samaniego-Vaesken, M. de L. Characteristics of dietary supplements with folic acid available on the Polish market. *Nutrients* **2022**, *14*, 3500. [CrossRef] [PubMed]
19. Abe-Matsumoto, L.T.; Sampaio, G.R.; Bastos, D.H.M. Do the labels of vitamin A, C, and E supplements reflect actual vitamin content in commercial supplements? *J. Food Compos. Anal.* **2018**, *72*, 141–149. [CrossRef]
20. Puścion-Jakubik, A.; Bartosiewicz, N.; Socha, K. Is the magnesium content in food supplements consistent with the manufacturers' declarations? *Nutrients* **2021**, *13*, 3416. [CrossRef] [PubMed]
21. Domínguez, L.; Fernández-Ruiz, V.; Morales, P.; Sánchez-Mata, M.C.; Cámara, M. Assessment of health claims related to folic acid in food supplements for pregnant women according to the european regulation. *Nutrients* **2021**, *13*, 937. [CrossRef] [PubMed]
22. Regulation (EC) No 1334/2008 of the European Parliament and of the Council of 16 December 2008 on Flavourings and Certain Food Ingredients with Flavouring Properties for Use in and on Foods and Amending Council Regulation (EEC) No 1601/91, Regulations (EC) No 2232/96 and (EC) No 110/2008 and Directive 2000/13/EC. Available online: https://eur-lex.europa.eu/legal-content/EN/TXT/?uri=CELEX%3A02008R1334-20220926 (accessed on 14 December 2022).
23. Directive 2011/91/EU of the European Parliament and of the Council of 13 December 2011 on Indications or Marks Identifying the Lot to Which a Foodstuff Belongs (Codification). Available online: https://eur-lex.europa.eu/legal-content/EN/ALL/?uri=celex%3A32011L0091 (accessed on 14 December 2022).
24. Commission Regulation (EU) No 432/2012 of 16 May 2012 Establishing a List of Permitted Health Claims Made on Foods, Other than Those Referring to the Reduction of Disease Risk and to Children's Development and Health. Available online: https://eur-lex.europa.eu/legal-content/EN/TXT/?uri=CELEX%3A02012R0432-20210517 (accessed on 14 December 2022).

Disclaimer/Publisher's Note: The statements, opinions and data contained in all publications are solely those of the individual author(s) and contributor(s) and not of MDPI and/or the editor(s). MDPI and/or the editor(s) disclaim responsibility for any injury to people or property resulting from any ideas, methods, instructions or products referred to in the content.

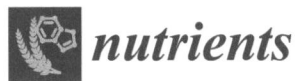

Article

Is the Magnesium Content in Food Supplements Consistent with the Manufacturers' Declarations?

Anna Puścion-Jakubik *,†, Natalia Bartosiewicz † and Katarzyna Socha

Department of Bromatology, Faculty of Pharmacy with the Division of Laboratory Medicine, Medical University of Białystok, Mickiewicza 2D Street, 15-222 Białystok, Poland; natalia_bartosiewicz@wp.pl (N.B.); katarzyna.socha@umb.edu.pl (K.S.)
* Correspondence: anna.puscion-jakubik@umb.edu.pl; Tel.: +48-8574-854-69
† These authors contributed equally to this work.

Abstract: Food supplements (FS) are gaining more and more popularity because they are a quick way to compensate for deficiencies in the diet. Due to their affordable price and easy-to-take form, they are eaten by all age groups and by healthy and sick people. There are many categories of this type of preparations on the market, and FS with magnesium (Mg) are some of the most commonly used. Therefore, the aim of the study was to determine the Mg content in FS and to compare the estimated value with that declared by the manufacturer. The study included 116 FS containing Mg. In order to determine the Mg content, the atomic absorption spectrometry (AAS) method was used. The tested FS were divided in terms of the declared content, pharmaceutical form, chemical form of Mg, composition complexity, and price. It was shown that in the case of 58.7% of the samples, the Mg content was different than the permissible tolerance limits set by the Polish chief sanitary inspectorate, which range from −20% to +45%. It has been estimated that as a result of the differences in the content, the patient may take up to 304% more Mg per day or 98% less than it is stated in the declaration. The above results indicate that the quality and safety of FS should be more closely monitored.

Keywords: magnesium; pharmacy; food supplements; drugstore

1. Introduction

Food supplements (FS) are preparations that are intended to supplement the diet with deficient substances. They contain minerals, vitamins, and other substances that can cause a specific physiological effect, such as fatty acids, amino acids, or probiotics. They come in various pharmaceutical forms, including tablets, capsules, powders, and ampoules. They do not contain medicinal substances, so they cannot be used to treat disease entities [1].

Minerals and vitamins that may be used in FS in Poland are listed in the Regulation of the Minister of Health of 17 September 2018. The minimum amount of vitamins and minerals in a daily portion in FS should not be less than 15% of the reference consumption values. However, maximum acceptable levels are established on the basis of the upper safe levels of consumption, the amounts provided in the diet, and the recommended intake for the population. This value must be safe for the health and life of the consumer [2].

FS are very common, and their popularity and market share are steadily increasing. Data from 2019 indicate that more than half of adults, both in Europe and the US, use FS [3]. According to research by Li et al. (2010), these are more often women than men (38.6% vs. 28.5%), as well as people over 50 (57.4%) and with higher education [4]. This is a consequence of the increased demand for nutrients in these groups. Despite the fact that FS cannot replace a balanced diet, their intake allows them to supplement existing deficiencies. In the elderly, it is particularly important because physiological changes in the body with age and long-term use of many medications make seniors most exposed to nutrient deficiencies.

Our previous research has shown that the use of FS is very widespread. Supplements containing magnesium (Mg) are used by approximately 8% of medical university students [5]. Other data from Poland indicate that FS with Mg account for 7.56% of the market. Preparations with this ingredient are very popular in Poland—about 25.0% of respondents use them. Among the inhabitants of Spain, 13.4% of men take them and among the inhabitants of Germany 18.3% of men and 20.4% of women [6].

The legal regulations governing the FS market in Poland are both national and European requirements. An important legal act is the Food and Nutrition Safety Act of 25 August 2006 [1], Regulation of the Minister of Health of 18 May 2010 amending the regulation on the composition and labeling of FS [7] and the Regulation of the Minister of Health of 17 September 2018, on the composition and labeling of FS [2]. The Regulation of the Minister of Health of 17 September 2018 [2] lists vitamins and minerals and their chemical forms that may be present in supplements. For substances authorized to appear in supplements, which were listed in the above regulation [2], further purity criteria are defined. Dyes and additives should meet the purity requirements specified in Commission Regulation (EU) No 231/2012 of 9 March 2012 [8]. Despite the above-mentioned legal acts being in force, the registration procedures and placing the FS on the market are very simple and only require presentation documentation and packaging design to the chief sanitary inspector. No quality or safety tests are required, which creates a risk that there are low-quality preparations on the market that differ in terms of their composition from the manufacturers' declarations.

Mg is necessary, inter alia, to maintain normal cell function, muscle contraction, including the heart muscle, and conditions nervous excitability [9,10]. Mg deficiency has also been shown to contribute to the development of oxidative stress in obese people [11], disturbances in mineral homeostasis such as Mg may interfere with cancer progression [12], and Mg supplementation may play a beneficial role in controlling asthma by acting as an anti-inflammatory and bronchodilator [13].

The causes of Mg deficiency include: reduced gastrointestinal absorption, loss of Mg from gastrointestinal tract, increased renal loss, excessive sweating, increased requirements (for example in pregnancy), or older age, which disrupts many processes [14].

The above factors prompted us to evaluate the Mg content in FS available on the Polish market, coming from local producers, but also producers known in various European countries. To our knowledge, this is the first study that covers such data as a variety of chemical forms, pharmaceutical forms or preparations at different prices.

2. Materials and Methods

2.1. Materials

Samples of dietary supplements were selected on the basis of previously conducted surveys [5] and on the basis of popularity in the largest chain pharmacies in the country.

Inclusion criteria included: popularity among patients, availability category 'FS', preparations within the expiry date.

The following exclusion criteria were adopted: occasional sales, over-the-counter 'OTC' availability category.

The study included 116 FS purchased in stationary pharmacies as well as online. In order to assess the quality of FS in the best possible way, preparations were selected for the research, which differed in terms of composition, pharmaceutical form, price and, manufacturer. Detailed characteristics of the studied FS are presented in Table S1 in Supplementary Materials.

FS were taken from three different blisters or as three subsamples, analyzed in triplicate (statistically insignificant differences between the determinations) were harvested and tested in 2020–2021.

2.2. Sample Preparation

FS were ground in a vibrating grinder (Testchem, Poland) and weighed into Teflon mineralization vessels of about 0.3 g with an accuracy of 1 mg (exact weights were recorded). Then 4 mL of spectrally pure concentrated (69%) nitric acid (Tracepur, Merck, Darmstadt, Germany) were added. The microwave mineralization process was carried out in a closed system (Berghof, Speedwave, Eningen, Germany), according to the following program:

- Step 1: 170 °C, 10 min, 20 atm., 80% of microwave power;
- Step 2: 190 °C, 10 min, 30 atm., 90% of microwave power;
- Step 3: 210 °C, 10 min, 40 atm., 90% of microwave power;
- Step 4: 50 °C, 18 min, 40 atm., 0% of microwave power.

The obtained mineralizates were quantitatively transferred to polypropylene vessels with deionized water.

2.3. Determination of Mg Content

Mg content was determined by atomic absorption spectrometry (AAS), acetylene-air flame technique with Zeeman background correction. The determination was carried out using the Z-2000 instrument (Hitachi, Tokyo, Japan). Before the analysis, all of the analyzed samples were diluted, depending on the declared content of the tested element. Lanthanum chloride (1% $LaCl_3$, Sigma-Aldrich, Merck, Darmstadt, Germany) was used as the sequestering agent. The assay was performed at a wavelength of 285.2 nm and 7.5 mA current lamps. The concentration was read from the curve prepared using a 1 mg/mL Mg standard solution for AAS (Merck, Germany). The limit of detection (LOD) and limit of quantification (LOQ) were 0.26 mg/kg and 0.78 mg/kg, respectively.

The conducted research did not require the approval of the Bioethics Committee of the Medical University of Bialystok.

2.4. Validation of Method

In order to control the accuracy of the analyses, a certified reference material was used (Simulated Died D, LIVSMEDELS VERKET, National Food Administration, Uppsala, Sweden). The determination was performed before the analysis and after each 10 determinations. All values were within the certified value range (2740–3100 mg/kg). The accuracy (% of error) was 0.67%, and the coefficient of variation V = 1.57%.

2.5. Comparison of Results with the Standards Adopted by the Chief Sanitary Inspectorate in Poland

In accordance with the guidelines adopted by the European Commission in 2012 on establishing tolerance limits for minerals contained on labels, the obtained values were compared with the guidelines adopted by the Commission, amounting to −20 to +45% for FS-containing minerals [15,16].

2.6. Statistical Analyses

Statistica software (Tibco, Palo-Alto, CA, USA) was used for calculations and statistical analyzes. The results are presented as mean (Av.) with standard deviation (SD), minimum (Min), maximum (Max), as well as median (Med.), and lower quartile (Q1), upper quartile (Q3), interquartile range (IQR).

3. Results

The results of the analyses are presented in Tables 1–5. The following classification criteria were used: declared content, pharmaceutical form, chemical form of Mg, amount of minerals (only Mg or multi-component preparations), and price.

Table 1. Magnesium content (mg/portion) in food supplements depending on the declared magnesium content.

Declared Content	n	Mg Content (mg/Portion)					
		Av. ± SD	Min–Max	Med.	Q1	Q3	IQR
Less than 100 mg	49	49.7 ± 38.0	1.5–202.0	40.7	23.7	73.4	49.7
100–200 mg	45	144.9 ± 109.5	7.4–469.6	115.7	66.3	207.2	141.0
Above 200 mg	22	387.0 ± 200.2	39.1–795.7	348.7	249.2	479.2	230.0

Av.—average, IQR—interquartile range, Max—maximum value, Med.—median, Min—minimum value, Q1—lower quartile, Q3—upper quartile, SD—standard deviation.

Table 2. Magnesium content (mg/portion) in food supplements depending on the pharmaceutical form.

Form	n	Mg Content (mg/Portion)					
		Av. ± SD	Min–Max	Med.	Q1	Q3	IQR
Capsules	13	103.8 ± 110.0	1.5–298.5	69.2	22.8	193.0	170.2
Coated tablets	11	68.5 ± 60.4	19.0–202.0	48.0	23.7	77.5	53.8
Dragees	2	78.3 ± 22.7	62.2–94.3	78.3	62.2	94.3	32.1
Effervescent tablets	24	231.2 ± 196.0	4.9–696.9	168.2	78.6	364.2	285.6
Granulates	1	233.1 ± 0.0	-	-	-	-	-
Jelly beans	1	27.5 ± 0.0	-	-	-	-	-
Liquids	7	198.4 ± 120.6	34.0–360.1	219.7	75.4	317.6	242.2
Powders	12	264.2 ± 247.2	22.1–795.7	189.1	81.2	367.4	286.2
Tablets	45	106.8 ± 133.6	5.8–696.5	60.2	31.4	120.8	89.4

Av.—average, IQR—interquartile range, Max—maximum value, Med.—median, Min—minimum value, Q1—lower quartile, Q3—upper quartile, SD—standard deviation.

Table 3. Magnesium content (mg/portion) in food supplements depending on the chemical form.

Chemical Form	n	Mg Content (mg/Portion)					
		Av. ± SD	Min–Max	Med.	Q1	Q3	IQR
Magnesium bisglycinate	6	161.4 ± 103.1	28.5–317.6	154.3	93.8	219.7	126.0
Magnesium carbonate	34	132.2 ± 164.2	5.8–696.9	73.9	40.7	137.8	97.1
Magnesium citrate	35	168.4 ± 201.1	1.5–795.7	79.1	31.5	232.0	200.6
Magnesium glycerophosphate	1	78.8 ± 0.0	-	-	-	-	-
Magnesium hydroxide	2	215.6 ± 263.8	29.1–402.1	215.6	29.1	402.1	373.0
Magnesium lactate	11	45.7 ± 39.4	1.8–129.3	35.4	7.4	77.9	70.5
Magnesium oxide	8	207.6 ± 155.5	18.8–449.4	225.6	52.9	317.9	265.1
Several chemical forms	19	181.2 ± 148.1	22.8–479.2	145.4	61.2	267.6	206.4

Av.—average, IQR—interquartile range, Max—maximum value, Med.—median, Min—minimum value, Q1—lower quartile, Q3—upper quartile, SD—standard deviation.

Table 4. Magnesium content (mg/portion) in food supplements depending on the amount of minerals.

Amount of Minerals	n	Mg Content (mg/Portion)					
		Av. ± SD	Min–Max	Med.	Q1	Q3	IQR
Only magnesium (or vitamin B6)	75	164.8 ± 183.6	1.5–795.7	93.8	34.0	249.2	215.3
Multicomponent preparations	41	124.7 ± 125.6	4.8–469.6	76.4	38.5	188.8	150.2

Av.—average, IQR—interquartile range, Max—maximum value, Med.—median, Min—minimum value, Q1—lower quartile, Q3—upper quartile, SD—standard deviation.

Table 5. Magnesium content in food supplements depending on the price.

Price (PLN)	n	Mg Content (mg/Portion)					
		Av. ± SD	Min–Max	Med.	Q1	Q3	IQR
<10	41	192.1 ± 191.1	13.3–696.9	108.3	35.4	317.6	282.1
10–20	57	112.0 ± 138.8	1.5–795.7	74.4	30.5	129.3	98.7
>20	18	178.4 ± 164.2	22.8–649.8	113.1	71.5	267.6	196.1

Av.—average, IQR—interquartile range, Max—maximum value, Med.—median, Min—minimum value, PLN—currency in force in Poland, Q1—lower quartile, Q3—upper quartile, SD—standard deviation.

In the case of preparations with a declared content below 100 mg of Mg per portion, the highest determined content was 202.0 mg, and the lowest was only 1.5 mg (Table 1).

The second criterion of the division was the criterion of the pharmaceutical form. The formulation with the highest reported content (795.7 mg/portion) was available as a powder to be dissolved in water. The lowest marked values were for supplements available in the form of capsules (1.5 mg/portion), effervescent tablets (4.9 mg/portion), and tablets (5.8 mg/portion).

Most of the studied FS contained Mg in the form of Mg citrate (n = 35) and Mg carbonate (n = 34), while the least contained in the form of hydroxide (n = 2) and glycerophosphate (n = 1). Both the preparation with the lowest determined content of Mg (1.5 mg/portion) and the preparation with the highest determined content (795.7 mg/portion) contained Mg citrate (Table 3).

Out of 116 FS tested, 75 contained only Mg among the minerals. This category includes both the preparation with the lowest determined value (1.5 mg) and the preparation with the highest determined mg content (795.7 mg) (Table 4).

Interestingly, in preparations with a lower price (below PLN 10), the highest mean Mg content was recorded at the level of 192.1 ± 191.1 (Table 5).

The chief sanitary inspectorate, responsible for the quality of FS, allows the deviation of minerals from −20% to +45%. Figure 1 shows the variation in individual samples. It was shown that 58.7% of FS were outside the acceptable range (Figure 1a,b).

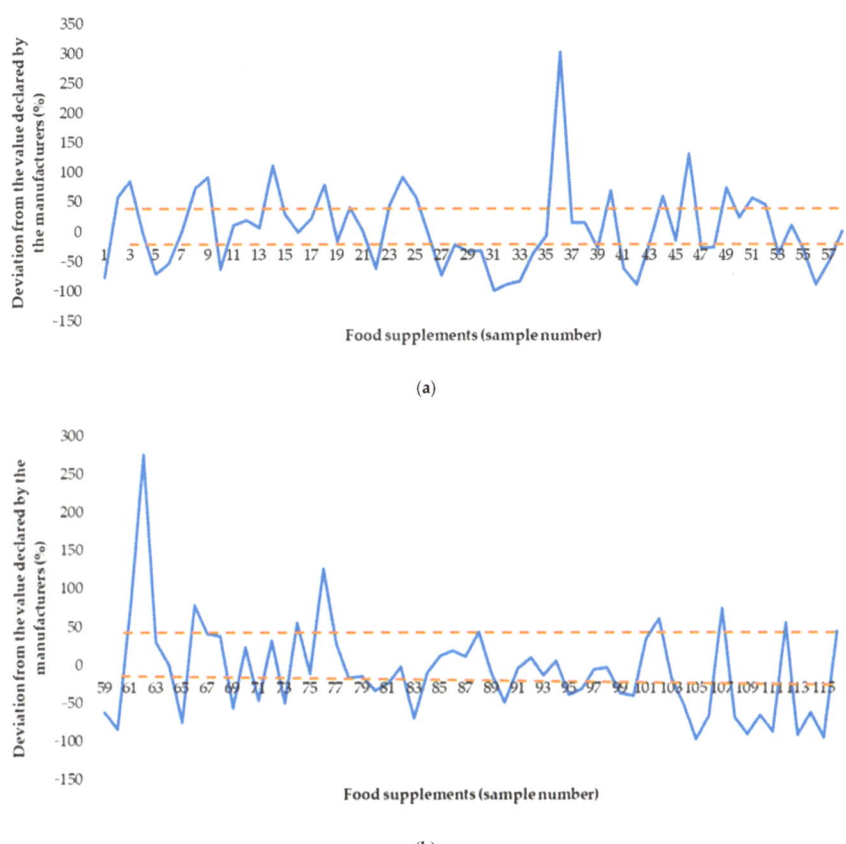

Figure 1. The discrepancy between the declared magnesium content and that determined in dietary supplements (**a**) samples of food supplements from 1 to 58, (**b**) samples of food supplements from 59 to 116.

At a further stage, we also assessed by how many percent the expected value by consumers would differ from the actual value consumed, in accordance with the manufacturer's recommendation, because the tested FS can be taken in amounts greater than just one portion per day. It has been shown that for 54.1% of FS, consumers will consume a lower amount of Mg. For example, for 3.4% it will be 90–100% less than the expected value. Worryingly, in the case of one of the studied FS, consumers, using one portion of the FS each day, will consume as much as 300% more Mg than indicated on the packaging (Figure 2).

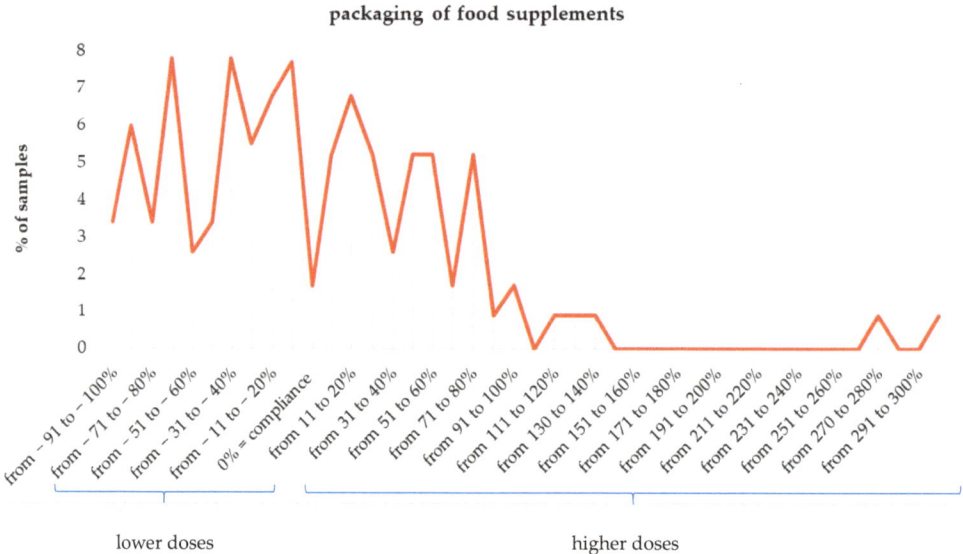

Figure 2. The percentage of food supplements and the difference in the actually taken magnesium dose, resulting from an incorrect declaration of the content.

There were no statistically significant differences ($p > 0.05$) between the previously discussed factors (declaration of Mg content, pharmaceutical form, chemical form, composition, price) and the percentage of samples within the norm, below and above the norm (Table 6).

Table 6. Relationship between factors and percentage of food supplements with normal, below and above normal magnesium levels ($p > 0.05$).

Criterion	Subgroups	n	Below Standard n = 46 (%)	Norm n = 48 (%)	Above Normal n = 22 (%)
Declared content	Less than 100 mg	49	19 (16.4)	24 (20.7)	6 (5.2)
	100–200 mg	45	20 (17.2)	15 (12.9)	10 (8.6)
	Above 200 mg	22	7 (6.0)	9 (7.6)	6 (5.2)
Form	Capsules	13	9 (7.8)	3 (2.6)	1 (0.9)
	Coated tablets	11	5 (4.3)	5 (4.3)	1 (0.9)
	Dragees	2	0 (0.0)	2 (1.7)	0 (0.0)
	Effervescent tablets	24	5 (4.3)	12 (10.3)	7 (6.0)
	Granulates	1	0 (0.0)	0 (0.0)	1 (0.9)
	Jelly beans	1	0 (0.0)	1 (0.9)	0 (0.0)
	Liquids	7	3 (2.6)	3 (2.6)	1 (0.9)
	Powders	12	3 (2.6)	4 (3.4)	5 (4.3)
	Tablets	45	21 (18.1)	18 (15.5)	6 (5.2)

Table 6. Cont.

Criterion	Subgroups	n	Below Standard $n = 46$ (%)	Norm $n = 48$ (%)	Above Normal $n = 22$ (%)
Chemical form	Magnesium bisglycinate	6	2 (1.7)	3 (2.6)	1 (0.9)
	Magnesium carbonate	34	11 (9.5)	15 (12.9)	8 (6.9)
	Magnesium citrate	35	16 (13.8)	12 (10.3)	7 (6.0)
	Magnesium glycerophosphate	1	0 (0.0)	1 (0.9)	0 (0.0)
	Magnesium hydroxide	2	1 (0.9)	0 (0.0)	1 (0.9)
	Magnesium lactate	11	6 (5.2)	5 (4.3)	0 (0.0)
	Magnesium oxide	8	3 (2.6)	4 (3.4)	1 (0.9)
	Several chemical forms	19	7 (6.0)	8 (6.9)	4 (3.4)
Amount of minerals	Only magnesium (or vitamin B6)	75	35 (30.2)	25 (21.6))	15 (12.9
	Multicomponent preparations	41	11 (9.5)	23 (19.8)	7 (6.0)
Price (PLN)	<10	41	16 (13.8)	17 (14.7)	8 (6.9)
	10–20	57	25 (21.6)	22 (18.9)	10 (8.6)
	>20	18	5 (4.3)	9 (7.8)	4 (3.4)

4. Discussion

FS are foodstuffs taken by patients and consumers to supplement existing deficiencies. Their use is not intended to treat or prevent diseases in humans, unlike drugs, and are not required to be subject to detailed qualitative and quantitative research prior to sale, unlike medicinal products. Moreover, their side effects are not monitored rigorously. This generates the need to test their quality. Our research covered more than 100 FS, which may reflect the assortment of the largest pharmacy chains.

As part of the study conducted by the SW RESEARCH agency (2017), a survey was conducted among 807 adults. It was estimated that 72.4% of Poles use FS, and about half of them systematically, i.e., 48%. Worrying is the fact that only 17% consult a doctor or pharmacist before starting supplementation. The most common reasons for taking these preparations were the desire to strengthen the body (55.4%), increase resistance to infections (44.3%), and supplement the daily diet with the missing ingredients (40.7%). Alarmingly, 6% of people argued taking supplements is the current fashion. The respondents declared that during the purchase they were guided by the composition (41.7%), price (38%), their own experience (36.6%), the recommendation of a doctor or pharmacist (34.5%), opinions of other people (25.9%), scientific certificates (16.9%) and other factors (27.7%). Satisfactory is the fact that the most frequent place of purchase was the pharmacy (65%). According to 54.9% of people, taking supplements brought them noticeable benefits, while 41.6% did not notice an effect on their health, while 3.4% were dissatisfied with the effects. In this study, more frequent use of supplements by women (51.7%) than men (48.3%) was observed, as well as among people with higher education (45.5%) [17].

Mg, next to potassium, is the most important intracellular cation. It activates over 300 enzymes. It participates, among others, in neuromuscular conduction, regulation of the body's mineral homeostasis, regulation of blood pressure, insulin metabolism, and muscle contractility. It is a macronutrient necessary for proper functioning, therefore it should be supplied with a balanced diet. A number of factors, including the consumption of highly processed food, contribute to its reduced amount in the diet [18].

It is disturbing that if one of the tested FS is consumed, the patient will be take in 300% more Mg every day than it is stated in the declaration on the packaging. Taking too much of a dose may have side effects. There is no evidence that food-derived Mg can have a negative effect on the body, while in the case of excessive consumption of Mg from various types of supplements or medicinal products, cases of harmful effects have been reported. Since Mg salts are laxative when used in large amounts, osmotic diarrhea may occur. Symptoms also include difficulty breathing, sleep disturbances, changes in heartbeat, muscle weakness and confusion. In extreme cases, when it is accompanied by impaired renal function, serious neurological symptoms may occur, such as, among others, increased axonal excitability threshold, paralysis of the striated and cardiological muscles, including inhibition of heart contractions or prolongation of the QT interval [19]. Serious side effects, including death, were found after children took 2400 mg of Mg, which is three servings of the supplement with the highest content determined in this study [20]. The maximum amount of Mg allowed in FS is 400 mg/day [21], while our study showed almost twice as much Mg in one of the preparations.

The subject of comparing the declared and determined Mg content has so far been rarely discussed in scientific publications. Literature data indicate that the interest of researchers in FS containing Mg is also focused on assessing the safety of their use, due to the presence of potential contaminants [22,23].

It seems necessary to conduct patient education and large-scale campaigns. A 2014 study showed that every fourth Pole was unable to correctly define the definition of a FS. Almost half of the people, as many as 41%, claimed that these products have healing properties, while 31% of people assessed that they were synonymous with vitamins, and 8% that they were synonymous with minerals. Moreover, half of the respondents (50%) believed that they were subject to the same control as drugs [24].

The presence of a large amount of FS on the market makes their control very difficult. As a result of the easy registration process, more and more of them appear on the market. Data from Poland show that from 2007 to 2017, over 29,000 were entered into the register of products in the FS category. In 2016, the chief sanitary inspector received about 600 notifications about the introduction of a new preparation on the market every month [6]. This indicates the need to introduce greater restrictions, preventing the placing on the market of preparation of inappropriate quality.

Ensuring an adequate level of Mg in the body is essential for its proper functioning. The benefits of using it have been reported even in diseases of various pathogenesis, e.g., ulceration [25]. As a result of taking FS of inadequate quality, containing several times the lower doses of Mg than declared by the manufacturer, supplementing the deficiencies may be ineffective, which may result in the lack of the effects expected by patients.

The absorption of Mg is greater from food than from supplements [26–29]. Therefore it is necessary to properly balance the diet so that taking these preparations will not be necessary. However, when it is impossible or when there is an increased demand for this element as a result of other factors, supplementation with high-quality preparations should be used [30,31]. A diet deficient in terms of Mg is quite common. For example, a 2009 study assessed eating habits among people living in Russia, the Czech Republic and Poland. Consumption in line with the recommendations of the standards was shown only in about 65% of the respondents. The highest consumption of this element was among Poles, who consumed 286 mg. Czechs supplied 278 mg and Russians only 97 mg [32].

Such a large discrepancy between the declared values and those actually marked is very surprising. It may result from the improper production process of FS, lack of final product control, and inadequate labeling of the supplement. FS are sold in grocery stores, drugstores, herbal, and medical stores and pharmacies. It seems necessary that FS sold in pharmacies should be subject to greater control, which will improve their quality and increase consumer confidence in this category of food products, sold in a form analogous to drugs.

The limitations of this study are as follows: due to the heterogeneity of FS quality, other batches may have a different Mg content, the study describes the most popular preparations on the market, although the quality of FS produced by niche producers may be different. The limitation is also the large market share of preparations in one pharmaceutical and chemical form. Further research should be based on the assessment of the bioavailability of various Mg compounds and the actual concentration obtained in the blood of patients after FS ingestion.

5. Conclusions

The assessment of the quality of food containing magnesium showed that the declared and actual values in most dietary supplements differed. Only in two samples of the supplements were they identical. Only 41.3% of the tested samples were within the acceptable range of deviations for minerals, in line with the recommendations of the chief sanitary inspectorate. During the intake of food supplements covered by this study by patients, as a result of differences between the declared value and the measured value, the amount of the consumed element may change in the amount from a maximum of 98% less to 304% more than the declared value. Food supplements should be routinely monitored to improve their quality.

Supplementary Materials: The following are available online at https://www.mdpi.com/article/10.3390/nu13103416/s1, Table S1: Characteristics of the studied dietary supplements.

Author Contributions: Conceptualization, A.P.-J.; methodology, K.S., A.P.-J. and N.B.; software, A.P.-J., N.B. and K.S.; validation, K.S. and A.P.-J.; formal analysis, A.P.-J.; investigation, A.P.-J. and K.S.; resources, A.P.-J. and K.S.; data curation, N.B. and A.P.-J.; writing—original draft preparation, A.P.-J. and N.B.; writing—review and editing, K.S.; visualization, A.P.-J. and N.B.; supervision, K.S.; project administration, A.P.-J.; funding acquisition, A.P.-J. All authors have read and agreed to the published version of the manuscript.

Funding: This research was funded by Medical University of Białystok, grant number SUB/2/DN/21/005/2216.

Institutional Review Board Statement: Not applicable.

Informed Consent Statement: Not applicable.

Data Availability Statement: Data are available from the authors.

Conflicts of Interest: The authors declare no conflict of interest.

References and Note

1. The Act of 25 August 2006 on Food and Nutrition Safety. *Journal of Laws 2006 No. 171 Item 1225*, 25 August 2006. (In Polish)
2. Announcement of the Minister of Health of 17 September 2018 on the Publication of the Uniform Text of the Regulation of the Minister of Health on the Composition and Labeling of Dietary Supplements. *Journal of Laws 2018 Item 1951*, 17 September 2018. (In Polish)
3. Costa, J.G.; Vidovic, B.; Saraiva, N.; do Céu Costa, M.; Del Favero, G.; Marko, D.; Oliveira, N.G.; Fernandes, A.S. Contaminants: A dark side of food supplements? *Free Radic. Res.* **2019**, *53* (Suppl. S1), 1113–1135. [CrossRef] [PubMed]
4. Li, K.; Kaaks, R.; Linseisen, J.; Rohrmann, S. Consistency of vitamin and/or mineral supplement use and demographic, lifestyle and health-status predictors: Findings from the European Prospective Investigation into Cancer and Nutrition (EPIC)-Heidelberg cohort. *Br. J. Nutr.* **2010**, *10*, 1058–1064. [CrossRef] [PubMed]
5. Puścion-Jakubik, A.; Kus, K.; Socha, K. Medical university students' perspective on marketing of dietary supplements. *Acta Pol. Pharm.* **2021**, *78*, 205–218. [CrossRef]
6. Suplindex. Available online: https://suplindex.com/wp-content/uploads/2017/10/RAPORT-Suplementy-diety-30.08.2017.pdf (accessed on 10 September 2021).
7. Regulation of the Minister of Health of 18 May 2010 Amending the Regulation on the Composition and Labeling of Dietary Supplements. *Journal of Laws of 2010 No. 91, Item 596*, 18 May 2010. (In Polish)
8. Commission Regulation (EU) No 231/2012 of 9 March 2012 Laying down Specifications for Food Additives Listed in Annexes II and III to Regulation (EC) No 1333/2008 of the European Parliament and of the Council Text with EEA Relevance.
9. Nielsen, F.H. Dietary magnesium and chronic disease. *Adv. Chronic. Kidney Dis.* **2018**, *25*, 230–235. [CrossRef] [PubMed]
10. Van Laecke, S.; Caluwe, R.; Huybrechts, I.; Nagler, E.V.; Vanholder, R.; Peeters, P.; Van Vlem, B.; Van Biesen, W. Effect of magnesium supplements on insulin secretion after kidney transplantation: A randomized controlled trial. *Ann. Transplant.* **2017**, *22*, 524–531. [CrossRef] [PubMed]
11. Morais, J.B.; Severo, J.S.; Santos, L.R.; de Sousa Melo, S.R.; de Oliveira Santos, R.; de Oliveira, A.R.; Cruz, K.J.; do Nascimento Marreiro, D. Role of magnesium in oxidative stress in individuals with obesity. *Biol. Trace Elem. Res.* **2017**, *176*, 20–26. [CrossRef] [PubMed]
12. Mendes, P.M.V.; Bezerra, D.L.C.; Dos Santos, L.R.; de Oliveira Santos, R.; de Sousa Melo, S.R.; Morais, J.B.S.; Severo, J.S.; Vieira, S.C.; do Nascimento Marreiro, D. Magnesium in breast cancer: What is its influence on the progression of this disease? *Biol. Trace Elem. Res.* **2018**, *184*, 334–339. [CrossRef] [PubMed]

13. Abuabat, F.; AlAlwan, A.; Masuadi, E.; Murad, M.H.; Jahdali, H.A.; Ferwana, M.S. The role of oral magnesium supplements for the management of stable bronchial asthma: A systematic review and meta-analysis. *NPJ Prim. Care Respir. Med.* **2019**, *29*, 4. [CrossRef] [PubMed]
14. Schwalfenberg, G.K.; Genius, S.J. The importance of magnesium in clinical healthcare. *Hidawi Sci.* **2017**, *2017*, 4179326. [CrossRef] [PubMed]
15. European Commission; Directorate-General for Health and Consumers. December 2012 Guidance on Setting Tolerance Limits for Labeled Nutrients. Komisja Europejska, Dyrekcja generalna ds. Zdrowia i Konsumentów. Wytyczne z Grudnia 2012 r. w Zakresie Określenia Limitów Tolerancji Dla Składników Odżywczych Wymienionych na Etykiecie. Available online: https://foodsupplementseurope.org/wp-content/themes/fse-theme/documents/publications-and-guidelines/fse-setting-of-tolerances-for-nutrient-values-declared-on-a-label.pdf (accessed on 1 September 2021).
16. Wawrzyniak, A.; Przybyłowicz, K.; Wądołowska, L.; Charzewska, J.; Górecka, D.; Lange, E.; Other Members of the Human Nutrition Science Committee of the Polish Academy of Sciences. Statement of the Committee of Human Nutrition Science of the Polish Academy of Sciences on the use of dietary supplements containing vitamins and minerals by adults. *Rocz Panstw Zakl Hig* **2021**, *77*, 1–6. [CrossRef]
17. SW Research. Available online: https://files.swresearch.pl/raportyPdf/Raport%2364-65-proc-polakow-suplementy-diety-kupuje-w-aptekach.pdf (accessed on 2 May 2021).
18. Jarosz, M.; Rychlik, E.; Stoś, K.; Charzewska, J. *Normy Żywienia Dla Populacji Polski i Ich Zastosowanie*; Narodowy Instytut Zdrowia Publicznego-Państwowy Zakład Higieny: Warsaw, Poland, 2020; pp. 68–437.
19. Institute of Medicine. *Dietary Reference Intakes for Calcium, Phosphorus, Magnesium, Vitamin D, and Fluoride*; The National Academies: Washington, DC, USA, 1997.
20. Kutsal, E.; Aydemir, C.; Eldes, N.; Demirel, F.; Polat, R.; Taspnar, O.; Kulah, E. Severe hypermagnesemia as a result of excessive cathartic ingestion in a child without renal failure. *Pediatr. Emerg. Care* **2007**, *23*, 570–572. [CrossRef] [PubMed]
21. Resolution No. 19/2019 of the Team for Diet Supplements of 13 December 2019 on Expressing an Opinion on the Maximum Dose of Magnesium in the Recommended Daily Dose in Dietary Supplements. In Polish, Uchwała nr 19/2019 Zespołu do Spraw Suplementów Diety z Dnia 13 Grudnia 2019 r. w Sprawie Wyrażenia Opinii Dotyczącej Maksymalnej Dawki Magnezu w Zalecanej Dziennej Porcji w Suplementach Diety. Available online: https://gis.gov.pl/wp-content/uploads/2019/05/uchwa%C5%82a-19-2019-Magnez.pdf (accessed on 9 September 2021).
22. Moniakowska, A.; Dzierwanowska, A.; Strumińska-Parulska, D. On uranium 234U and 238U radionuclides in calcium and magnesium supplements and the potential effective radiation dose assessment to the consumers. *Food Addit. Contam. Part B Surveill* **2019**, *12*, 175–181. [CrossRef] [PubMed]
23. Strumińska-Parulska, D.I. ^{210}Pb in magnesium dietary supplements. *Isot. Environ. Health Stud.* **2017**, *53*, 111–115. [CrossRef] [PubMed]
24. TNS Polska. Available online: https://www.rynekzdrowia.pl/Farmacja/Badanie-TNS-jedna-czwarta-ankietowanych-sadzi-ze-suplementu-nie-mozna-przedawkowac,139554,6.html (accessed on 23 April 2021).
25. Afzali, H.; Jafari Kashi, A.H.; Momen-Heravi, M.; Razzaghi, R.; Amirani, E.; Bahmani, F.; Gilasi, H.R.; Asemi, Z. The effects of magnesium and vitamin E co-supplementation on wound healing and metabolic status in patients with diabetic foot ulcer: A randomized, double-blind, placebo-controlled trial. *Wound Repair. Regen.* **2019**, *27*, 277–284. [CrossRef] [PubMed]
26. Blancquaert, L.; Vervaet, C.; Derave, W. Predicting and testing bioavailability of magnesium supplements. *Nutrients* **2019**, *11*, 1663. [CrossRef] [PubMed]
27. Schuchardt, J.P.; Hahn, A. Intestinal absorption and factors influencing bioavailability of magnesium—An update. *Curr. Nutr. Food Sci.* **2017**, *13*, 260–278. [CrossRef] [PubMed]
28. Jahnen-Dechent, W.; Ketteler, M. Magnesium basics. *Clin. Kidney J.* **2012**, *5* (Suppl. S1), i3–i14. [CrossRef]
29. Graham, L.; Caesar, J.; Burgen, A. Gastrointestinal absorption and excretion of Mg^{28} in man. *Metabolism* **1960**, *9*, 646–659. [PubMed]
30. Gröber, U.; Schmidt, J.; Kisters, K. Magnesium in prevention and therapy. *Nutrients* **2015**, *7*, 8199–8226. [CrossRef] [PubMed]
31. Kunachowicz, H. *Tabele Składu i Wartości Odżywczej Żywności*; PZWL Wydawnictwo Lekarskie: Warsaw, Poland, 2017.
32. Boylan, S.; Welch, A.; Pikhart, H.; Malyutina, S.; Pajak, A.; Kubinova, R.; Bragina, O.; Simonova, G.; Stepaniak, U.; Gilis-Januszewska, A.; et al. Dietary habits in three Central and Eastern European countries: The HAPIEE study. *BMC Public Health* **2009**, *9*, 439. [CrossRef] [PubMed]

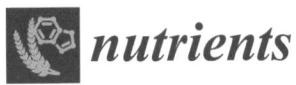

Article

Micronutrients in Food Supplements for Pregnant Women: European Health Claims Assessment

Laura Domínguez *, Virginia Fernández-Ruiz and Montaña Cámara

Nutrition and Food Science Department, Faculty of Pharmacy, Complutense University of Madrid (UCM), Plaza Ramón y Cajal, s/n, E-28040 Madrid, Spain; vfernand@ucm.es (V.F.-R.); mcamara@ucm.es (M.C.)
* Correspondence: ladoming@ucm.es

Abstract: Micronutrients play a critical role in pregnant women, a vulnerable group with higher nutritional requirements. The first strategy to achieve adequate micronutrients intake should always be through a healthy and balanced diet. In the case where the diet is not enough to meet these requirements, food supplements should be prescribed under supervision to complement the diet, and these products must bear reliable information about the declared nutritional contents and health benefits. Based on the data provided by the Coordinated System of Fast Interchange of Information (SCIRI) and to know the current national situation, this work addresses the assessment of the content and the adequacy of health claims related to some micronutrients (vitamin C, vitamin B_9, iron, copper, manganese, zinc, calcium, magnesium) contained in food supplements for pregnant women commercialized in Spain. Analytical results coincided with the declared values and were covered by the ranges of tolerances, and samples met the requirements to use health claims. Although the samples could even include more claims, manufacturers could have selected those which either best addressed pregnant women's conditions or best aligned with marketing intentions. This study confirms an adequate use of health claims in food supplement samples, which could be interesting for strengthening consumers' confidence in the benefits shown in the labeling and for encouraging the use of health claims as a useful tool for making better-informed purchasing decisions.

Keywords: micronutrient; food supplement; health claim; labeling; European legislation

1. Introduction

Food supplements are concentrated sources of micronutrients (vitamins, minerals) with a nutritional and positive physiological effect that are commercialized in different dose forms (e.g., capsules, pills, sachets of powder, etc.) [1–3], and they are intended to complement diet, improve health status, or even reduce the risk of some diseases [4–6].

In 2022, a survey conducted in 14 European Member States, including Spain, revealed that almost 9 in 10 European consumers had taken food supplements in their lives, and the great majority of them (93%) had done it in the past year [7]. Baladia et al. (2021) performed a comprehensive market study on the consumption of these products by the Spanish population (18–65 years), and the results demonstrated that 70% of the studied Spanish sample (N = 2630) took at least one food supplement during a specific period in 2020, with the most used (63%) being the ones containing vitamins and minerals. Vitamin C (31%) and magnesium, calcium, iron, zinc, and copper (6–13%) are the most frequently present vitamins and minerals in these food supplements [8].

Pregnant women are a vulnerable group of population whose nutritional requirements are high. The diet before and during pregnancy is a crucial element for the optimal development and growth of the fetus, as the nutritional status of pregnant women directly influences the size of the placenta, which is the main connection link with the fetus, as well as cell proliferation and differentiation [9–12].

A healthy diet is assumed to cover all nutritional needs; however, sometimes, diets are not very well equilibrated to provide enough amounts of some micronutrients such

Citation: Domínguez, L.; Fernández-Ruiz, V.; Cámara, M. Micronutrients in Food Supplements for Pregnant Women: European Health Claims Assessment. *Nutrients* **2023**, *15*, 4592. https://doi.org/10.3390/nu15214592

Academic Editor: George Moschonis

Received: 13 October 2023
Revised: 25 October 2023
Accepted: 27 October 2023
Published: 28 October 2023

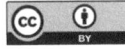

Copyright: © 2023 by the authors. Licensee MDPI, Basel, Switzerland. This article is an open access article distributed under the terms and conditions of the Creative Commons Attribution (CC BY) license (https://creativecommons.org/licenses/by/4.0/).

as vitamins (folic acid; vitamins C, D, B_1, B_2, B_6) and minerals (calcium, magnesium, iron, zinc, copper, manganese, etc.) with important health benefits. Thus, their daily intake must be reinforced through supplementation to avoid micronutrient deficiencies [9–14].

Folic acid is probably the most crucial micronutrient before and during pregnancy. Folic acid deficiency is related to the appearance of anemia, complications during pregnancy, and serious health problems in the fetus such as intrauterine growth restriction, premature birth, low birth weight, neural tube defects, and other fetal malformations [15,16]. Neural tube defects are the most common congenital anomalies that cause severe disability and infant mortality. Up till now, scientific evidence has shown that an adequate folic acid supplementation ($\geq$400 µg/day) before and during the first weeks of pregnancy can reduce the risk of neural tube defects in the fetus in up to 46% of cases [9,10].

Iron deficiency is the most common micronutrient deficiency during pregnancy that provokes anemia [17]. According to the World Health Organization (WHO), 40% of pregnant women around the world suffer anemia because of an inappropriate daily intake of this mineral. Iron supplementation during pregnancy is, therefore, considered essential [14]. Calcium is another fundamental mineral as its deficiency can cause a low birth weight and negatively affect bone mineral content in children [13]. In addition, low calcium intake is associated with the onset of preeclampsia, a pregnancy-specific multi-systemic disorder that provokes hypertension and proteinuria in pregnant women, and it is considered a leading cause of maternal mortality globally [18,19]. Antenatal calcium supplementation is also recommended by the WHO as it can prevent approximately one-half of preeclampsia cases in accordance with the scientific literature [14]. Zinc and copper are also considered indispensable micronutrients during pregnancy. A moderate maternal zinc deficiency may cause alterations in protein synthesis and cellular replication, which could affect fetal development and lead to malformations and a low birth weight [13,20]. Low serum levels of copper in pregnant women are linked to a premature rupture of membranes, weak amniotic membrane, and spontaneous abortion [21]. Turan et al. (2019) observed that miscarriage rates were significantly higher in pregnant women with lower serum copper concentrations (30–35%) [22], whereas optimum levels of this mineral at 15 weeks of gestation could reduce spontaneous abortion [23]. Maternal supplementation with vitamin C has been widely studied to elucidate its potential health benefits as it has been suggested that it could decrease the risk of appearance of maternal anemia and other complications such as preeclampsia and intrauterine growth restriction [24,25]. Along with iron, zinc, and copper, vitamin C is included in the United Nations International Multiple Micronutrient Antenatal Preparation (UNIMMAP), an established formulation that is recommended by the WHO and contains 15 micronutrients (vitamins and minerals) to provide pregnant women and their offspring with a healthy start to life [14]. Regarding magnesium, scientific evidence suggests that this mineral has a significant role in glucose metabolism, and low serum concentrations have been associated with gestational diabetes mellitus. This mineral could also have a protective role against pregnancy inflammation through the inhibition of nitric oxide synthase enzyme [26].

Apart from these micronutrients, there are other important vitamins needed during pregnancy. Vitamin D is considered to play an important role in bone metabolism through calcium regulating and maintaining phosphate homeostasis. Vitamin D deficiency in pregnant women, above all during the winter months, could increase the risk of preeclampsia, gestational diabetes mellitus, and preterm birth, among others [27,28]. To avoid this deficiency, the WHO and FAO recommend a vitamin D intake of 5 µg (200 IU) per day for pregnant women [27]. Vitamins B_1, B_2, and B_6 are important in different functions of the nervous system. During pregnancy, these vitamins could contribute to the development of fetus brain and nerves. Likewise, vitamins B_2 and B_6 could reduce the risk of developing preeclampsia and prevent a low birth weight, respectively [29–31].

Pregnant women must be adequately informed about the beneficial effects provided by the consumption of food supplements containing the previously mentioned micronutrients. To protect this vulnerable group of population from misunderstandings and misinformation, health claims included in the labeling of these products must be based on strong scientific evidence and be clear and comprehensible. Thus, pregnant women can rely on those health benefits and make well-informed choices [6,32].

In order to guarantee a constant vigilance of any risk potentially associated with food supplements that could affect the health status of consumers, including pregnant women, Spain counts on with the Coordinated System of Fast Interchange of Information (SCIRI). In a period of seven years (2015–2021), the national network SCIRI reported several notifications regarding food supplements, and most of them were due to an incorrect labeling, including health claims. In fact, in 2021, the notifications related to food supplements were 11 times higher than in 2015 [33].

Based on these alarming data provided by SCIRI reports and with a view to having a clear overview of the current national situation, the objective of the present work is to assess the content and the adequacy of health claims related to micronutrients of food supplements for pregnant women commercialized in the Spanish market according to the European regulation. A prior literature search was carried out by the authors in order to know the state of the art about this matter. To the authors' knowledge, no scientific articles regarding the evaluation of health claims related to certain micronutrients in food supplements for pregnant women were found. Thus, this study could be useful to widen the knowledge in this particular research perspective, which combines two different areas that are narrowly interconnected (chemical analysis and legislation).

2. Materials and Methods

In order to verify the adequacy of information regarding health benefits in food supplements for pregnant women, only micronutrients showing health claims in the labeling of these products were considered in this study; that is, vitamin C, vitamin B_9 (folic acid), iron, copper, manganese, zinc, calcium, and magnesium. Due to the importance of folic acid in pregnancy, the authors published one study in 2021, which was only focused on this micronutrient [6]. With a view to having a more complete overview of this topic, folic acid results are summarized and included in the present work. Other compounds, such as vitamin D, vitamin B_1, vitamin B_2, etc., are not addressed in this study and are not chemically analyzed because of the lack of related health claims in the labeling of samples.

2.1. Micronutrients' Health Claims Approved in the European Union (EU)

An updated review of the health claims approved for vitamin C, vitamin B_9 (folic acid), iron, copper, manganese, zinc, calcium, and magnesium was carried out using the official European Register of nutrition and health claims made on food and food supplements (https://ec.europa.eu/food/safety/labelling_nutrition/claims/register/public/?event=register.home, accessed on 18 June 2023) [34]. The following search filters were used in the European register platform: "claims status: authorised", "type of claim: Art. 13 and Art. 14(1)(a)", "EFSA Opinion reference: all", "Legislation: all". Use conditions established for each approved health claim were reviewed as well.

2.2. Spanish Market Research and Sample Selection

A market research of food supplements for pregnant women with health claims related to micronutrients was completed by consulting 10 national food establishments with a high market share in Spain. In addition, the online purchasing platforms used by these establishments were reviewed to provide a detailed overview of the food supplements offered. Sample selection for analysis was performed through the application of three inclusion criteria: (1) food supplements with a clear and unequivocal indication about the target population (pregnant women) in their labeling; (2) food supplements for pregnant women containing micronutrients in their nutritional composition; and (3) food supplements with health claims related to micronutrients.

2.3. Chemical Analysis of Micronutrient Contents in Samples

Vitamin C, folic acid, iron, copper, manganese, zinc, calcium, and magnesium were subject to health claims in food supplement samples; thus, they were chemically analyzed in the laboratory.

2.3.1. Vitamin C: L-Ascorbic Acid

In food matrices, vitamin C can be presented in the forms of L-Ascorbic Acid (AA) (reduced form) and L-Ascorbic Acid Dehydro (DHA) (oxidized form) [35,36]. Although both forms have the same vitamin activity, it is the reduced form that is used commercially [37]. Hence, vitamin C was determined in the form of AA in the food supplement samples. The determination of vitamin C was performed through an extraction in an acid medium, followed by a quantification using a reverse phase in HPLC-UV detection as described by Sánchez-Mata et al. (2000) [38]. An adequate amount of the food supplement samples was weighed, and 25 mL of 4.5% (w/v) metaphosphoric acid was added. With the aid of a magnetic stirrer (P-Selecta, Asincro), the mixture was shaken for at least 15 min until it dissolved at room temperature and was protected from direct light. The resulting extract was filtered through Albet paper filter No. 1242 (Merck Life Science S.L.U., Madrid, Spain) and collected in an Erlenmeyer flask (Labbox Labware, S.L., Premia de Dalt, Barcelona, Spain). The extract was filtered again with a 0.45 μm Millex PVDF membrane filter (Merck Millipore, Burlington, MA, USA) into a vial and was injected into the chromatographic equipment to quantify it [35]. The calibration curve was plotted daily from a stock solution of AA in metaphosphoric acid, with a final concentration of 0.4 mg/mL. The results were expressed in mg AA/100 g. Figure 1 shows the chromatographic equipment and conditions as well as the calibration curve and one example of the chromatograms obtained for vitamin C analysis.

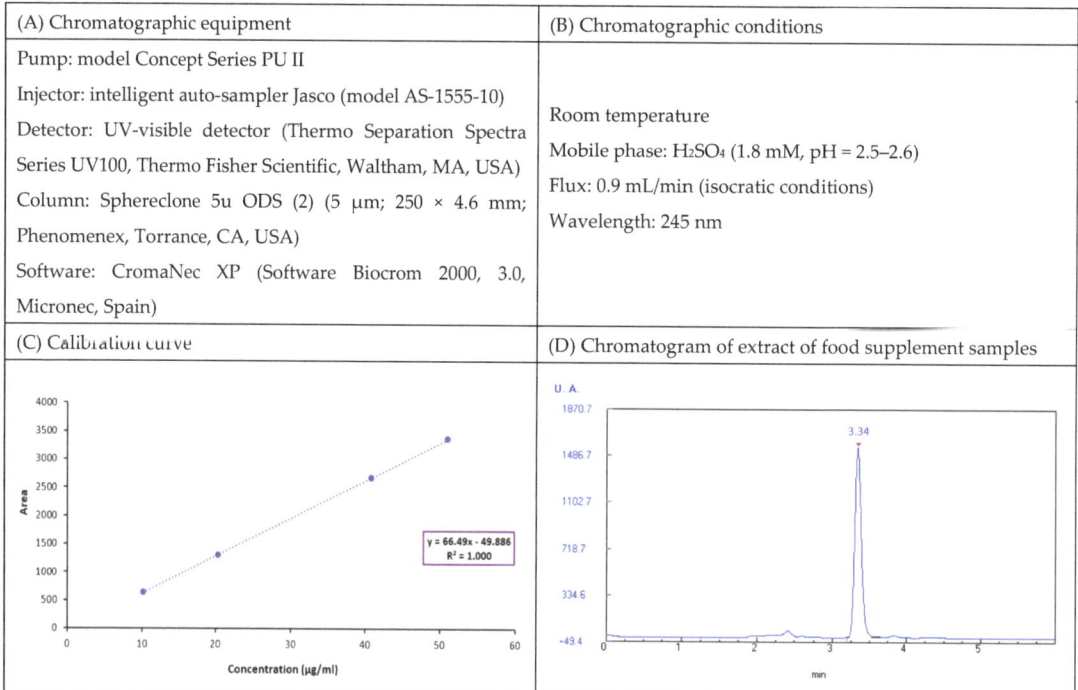

Figure 1. Description of vitamin C determination: (**A**) Chromatographic equipment; (**B**) Chromatographic conditions used in this study; (**C**) Calibration curve; (**D**) Chromatograms obtained for extract of samples containing ascorbic acid through HPLC-UV-visible.

2.3.2. Vitamin B$_9$ (Folic Acid)

Folic acid content was determined in the selected food supplement samples following the method previously published by the authors, being fully described in Domínguez et al. (2021) [6].

2.3.3. Micro- and Macrominerals

The determination of the micro- and macrominerals was carried out following the AOAC 930.05 procedure [39]. From each food supplement, 0.5 g was weighted in porcelain round-bottomed dishes and was subjected to incineration in a microwave oven (Carbolite Furnaces, model CSF 1100; Neuhausen, Germany) from room temperature to 450 °C until white ashes were obtained. Ashes were gravimetrically quantified [40].

Microminerals (Fe, Cu, Mn, Zn) present in ashes were extracted in an acid mixture prepared with 1 mL of HCl:H$_2$O (50% v/v) and 1 mL of HNO$_3$:H$_2$O (50% v/v). The solution was filtered by using an Albert® No. 145 ashless filter (Merck Life Science S.L.U., Madrid, Spain) and collected in a volumetric flask, which was made up to 25 mL with distilled water. The resulting extracts were measured through Atomic Absorption Spectroscopy (AAS) (Analyst 200 Perkin Elmer equipment, Perkin Elmer, Waltham, MA, USA) at the specific wavelength for each mineral and using standard solutions for calibration purposes.

An additional 1/10 (v/v) dilution was completed in La$_2$O$_3$ (5.864%, w/v) for the macrominerals' determination (Ca, Mg). As in the case of microminerals, these solutions were measured through AAS. The results of the micro- and macrominerals were expressed as mg/100 g [39].

2.3.4. Statistical Analysis

Two batches of each food supplement sample were analyzed in triplicate. Data were statistically assessed by comparing both batches of each sample through Tukey's HSD Test with a level of statistical significance of α = 0.05. Statgraphics Plus 5.1 software was used for statistical analysis.

For a better understanding, Figure 2 graphically describes the experimental design followed in the present work.

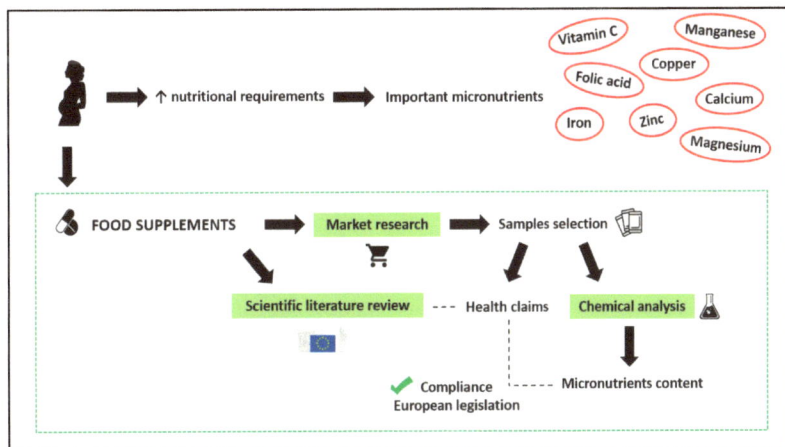

Figure 2. Experimental design to evaluate the adequacy of health claims related to micronutrients of food supplements for pregnant women commercialized in the Spanish market.

3. Results and Discussion

3.1. Health Claims Approved in the EU for Analyzed Micronutrients

As shown in Table 1, the micronutrient with the highest number of approved health claims was zinc (18 declarations), followed by vitamin C (15), magnesium (10), copper (8), calcium (8), and iron (7). On the contrary, manganese had the lowest number of authorized health claims (4). Most of the selected micronutrients have been scientifically demonstrated to be able to contribute to a normal energy-yielding metabolism, the immune and nervous systems, as well as to protecting cells from oxidative stress caused by the reactive species of oxygen (ROS) [34].

Table 1. Approved health claims referring to vitamin C, vitamin B_9 (folic acid), iron, copper, manganese, zinc, calcium, and magnesium in food supplements according to the European regulation [34].

Micronutrients	Health Claims (N°)	Approved Claims
Vitamin C	15	Vitamin C contributes to maintaining the normal functions of the immune system during and after intense physical exercise; normal collagen formation for the normal function of blood vessels, bones, cartilage, gums, skin, teeth; normal energy-yielding metabolism; functioning of the nervous system; psychological function; function of the immune system; protection of cells from oxidative stress; reduction of tiredness and fatigue; regeneration of the reduced form of vitamin E. Vitamin C increases iron absorption.
Vitamin B_9	8	Folate contributes to maternal tissue growth during pregnancy, normal amino acid synthesis, blood formation, homocysteine metabolism, psychological function, function of the immune system, reduction of tiredness and fatigue. Folate has a role in the process of cell division.
Iron	7	Iron contributes to normal cognitive function, energy-yielding metabolism, formation of red blood cells and hemoglobin, oxygen transport in the body, function of the immune system, reduction of tiredness and fatigue. Iron has a role in the process of cell division.
Copper	8	Copper contributes to maintenance of normal connective tissues, energy-yielding metabolism, functioning of the nervous system, hair pigmentation, iron transport in the body, skin pigmentation, function of the immune system, protection of cells from oxidative stress.
Manganese	4	Manganese contributes to normal energy-yielding metabolism, formation of connective tissue, maintenance of normal bones, protection of cells from oxidative stress.
Zinc	18	Zinc contributes to normal acid–base metabolism, carbohydrate metabolism, cognitive function, DNA synthesis, fertility and reproduction, macronutrient metabolism, metabolism of fatty acids, metabolism of vitamin A, protein synthesis. Zinc contributes to the maintenance of normal bones, hair, nails, skin, testosterone levels in the blood, vision, function of the immune system. Zinc contributes to the protection of cells from oxidative stress. Zinc has a role in the process of cell division.
Calcium	8	Calcium contributes to normal blood clotting, energy-yielding metabolism, muscle function, neurotransmission, function of digestive enzymes. Calcium is needed for the maintenance of normal bones and teeth. Calcium has a role in the process of cell division and specialization.
Magnesium	10	Magnesium contributes to reduction of tiredness and fatigue, electrolyte balance, normal energy-yielding metabolism, functioning of the nervous system, muscle function, protein synthesis, psychological function, maintenance of normal bones and teeth. Magnesium has a role in the process of cell division.

To use these health claims, food supplements must meet the use conditions particularly established for each nutrient, that is, to be a "Source of [name of vitamin] and/or [name of mineral]", which means that samples must provide at least 15% of the Nutrient Reference Values (NRVs) of each nutrient supplied by 100 g of the food supplement in question [41,42]. Table 2 provides the minimum content that food supplements must have to include those health claims in their labeling, presentation, and/or advertising.

Table 2. Use conditions for health claims related to vitamin C, vitamin B_9, iron, copper, manganese, zinc, calcium, and magnesium in the food supplement samples according to the European regulation [41,42].

Micronutrients	NRV	Required Amount to Use the Claim (15% NRV)
Vitamin C	80 mg	12 mg/100 g
Vitamin B_9	200 µg	30 µg/100 g
Fe	14 mg	2.1 mg/100 g
Cu	1 mg	0.15 mg/100 g
Mn	2 mg	0.3 mg/100 g
Zn	10 mg	1.5 mg/100 g
Ca	800 mg	120 mg/100 g
Mg	375 mg	56.25 mg/100 g

NRV = Nutrient Reference Values.

3.2. Spanish Market Search and Samples Selection

A Spanish market search of food supplements for pregnant women containing micronutrients was carried out, with a result of 81 food supplements. The majority (86.5%) were commercialized through online purchasing platforms used by the 10 selected establishments, whereas only 13.5% were found in situ (physical establishments). A total of 4 food supplements met the inclusion criteria, and they were named as the S1, S2, S3, and S4 samples.

3.3. Micronutrients Content and Assessment of the Application of Health Claims in Selected Samples

3.3.1. Vitamin C

Only the S1 and S4 samples included ascorbic acid in their formulation. As shown in Table 3, batches 1 and 2 of both food supplements showed similar mean values of vitamin C, and no statistically significant differences were found between batches of the same sample. Total mean value of the S1 and S4 samples coincided with the values included in their composition labeling. According to the European Guidance document published in 2012 by the European Commission regarding the setting of tolerances for nutrient values declared on a label [43], it can be assumed that the analyzed food supplements fulfilled the established requirements as the declared values of ascorbic acid were within the ranges of tolerance (RTs) calculated for each food supplement (Table 3).

Table 3. Assessment of the tolerances established for vitamin C in the food supplement samples pursuant to the European Guidance document [43].

Sample	Analytical Value (mg/sachet)	Declared Value (mg/sachet)	Range of Tolerances (RT) (mg/sachet)
S1	127.385 ± 6.179 [a] 111.804 ± 7.347 [a] $\bar{x}$ = 119.595 ± 11.017	110	87.600–165.600
S4	217.856 ± 7.307 [a] 233.815 ± 7.451 [a] $\bar{x}$ = 225.836 ± 11.285	225	179.600–338.100

In each column, [a] means statistically significant differences ($p < 0.05$) compared through Tukey's HSD Test.

Regarding the application of health claims, only the S1 sample showed the following health claim: "Vitamin C contributes to the normal function of the immune system", although both food supplements contained the minimum amount of vitamin C (12 mg/100 g) required to include in their labeling the 15 health claims approved for this micronutrient.

3.3.2. Vitamin B$_9$ (Folic Acid)

As previously reported by the authors [6], all food supplement samples contained folic acid in their nutritional composition. Analytical results of this micronutrient coincided with the declared values in the labeling of samples, and they were covered by the ranges of tolerance (RTs) calculated for each food supplement following the European Guidance document [43] (Table 4).

Table 4. Assessment of the tolerances established for vitamin C in the food supplement samples [6] pursuant to the European Guidance document [43].

Sample	Analytical Value Range (mg/sachet)	Declared Value (mg/sachet)	Range of Tolerances (RT) (mg/sachet)
S1	499.63–519.47	500	399.60–750.60
S2	399.12–418.06	400	390.03–600.60
S3	426.27–432.77	400	396.25–600.60
S4	211.60–229.78	200	159.60–300.60

Regarding health claims, all food supplements (S1, S2, S3, and S4) showed in their labeling at least one health claim approved for folic acid, and they contained more than the 15% NRV (30 µg/100 g) necessary to use them according to the European regulation in force [41,42].

3.3.3. Micro- and Macro-Elements

Regarding the mineral content, mean values of both micro- and macro-elements were similar between batches of the same food supplement samples. No statistically significant differences were found (Table 5).

Table 5. Mean values of the micro- and macro-elements contents analyzed in food supplement samples. Results expressed as mg/sachet.

	Fe	Cu	Mn	Zn	Ca	Mg
S1 sample						
Batch 1	4.856 ± 0.017 [a]	0.954 ± 0.003 [a]	0.070 ± 0.007 [a]	5.205 ± 0.019 [a]	393.016 ± 5.528 [a]	182.486 ± 3.213 [a]
Batch 2	4.864 ± 0.021 [a]	0.931 ± 0.004 [a]	0.072 ± 0.007 [a]	5.227 ± 0.019 [a]	387.441 ± 3.835 [a]	177.360 ± 2.145 [a]
Mean	4.860 ± 0.005	0.942 ± 0.017	0.071 ± 0.001	5.216 ± 0.016	390.228 ± 3.942	179.923 ± 3.625
S2 sample						
Batch 1	0.047 ± 0.005 [a]	0.026 ± 0.000 [a]	0.025 ± 0.002 [a]	0.038 ± 0.003 [a]	1.285 ± 0.038 [a]	0.036 ± 0.003 [a]
Batch 2	0.049 ± 0.002 [a]	0.024 ± 0.002 [a]	0.025 ± 0.002 [a]	0.039 ± 0.002 [a]	1.396 ± 0.136 [a]	0.039 ± 0.002 [a]
Mean	0.048 ± 0.002	0.025 ± 0.001	0.025 ± 0.000	0.038 ± 0.000	1.340 ± 0.079	0.038 ± 0.002
S3 sample						
Batch 1	0.017 ± 0.000 [a]	0.014 ± 0.001 [a]	2.009 ± 0.130 [a]	10.791 ± 0.524 [a]	1.010 ± 0.100 [a]	0.090 ± 0.006 [a]
Batch 2	0.015 ± 0.000 [a]	0.015 ± 0.001 [a]	2.032 ± 0.096 [a]	10.560 ± 0.393 [a]	1.053 ± 0.103 [a]	0.078 ± 0.001 [a]
Mean	0.705 ± 0.066	0.014 ± 0.000	2.020 ± 0.016	10.675 ± 0.163	1.031 ± 0.030	0.084 ± 0.008
S4 sample						
Batch 1	6.123 ± 0.060 [a]	0.555 ± 0.012 [a]	0.989 ± 0.030 [a]	6.033 ± 0.224 [a]	200.358 ± 1.456 [a]	153.869 ± 6.987 [a]
Batch 2	6.153 ± 0.096 [a]	0.550 ± 0.009 [a]	1.000 ± 0.037 [a]	6.011 ± 0.210 [a]	200.213 ± 6.087 [a]	148.602 ± 8.524 [a]
Mean	6.138 ± 0.021	0.553 ± 0.003	0.995 ± 0.008	6.022 ± 0.016	200.286 ± 0.102	151.236 ± 3.724

In each column, [a] means statistically significant differences ($p < 0.05$) compared through Tukey's HSD Test.

On the one hand, the Scientific Committee on Food (SCF) and the Panel on Dietetic Products, Nutrition and Allergies (NDA) of the European Food Safety Authority (EFSA) established maximum levels of the total chronic intake of different micronutrients (zinc, calcium, and magnesium, among others) that are unlikely to pose a risk of adverse health effects in humans, which are called tolerable Upper intake Levels (ULs). Different ULs were set according to the age/life-stage group (children, teenagers, adults, pregnant and lactating women). In this case, mean values obtained for zinc, calcium, and magnesium in all food supplement samples were lower than the ULs set for pregnant women (UL zinc = 25 mg/day; UL calcium = 2500 mg/day; UL magnesium = 250 mg/day). No UL had yet been established for iron, copper, and manganese, as sufficient and/or adequate scientific evidence is not available to derive ULs [44–46].

On the other hand, to verify if the selected food supplements complied with the requirements established by the European Guidance document, the authors calculated the ranges of tolerances (RT) for those minerals whose content was available in the labeling of each sample. As shown in Table 6, all analytical values were included within the RT.

Table 6. Assessment of ranges of tolerance (RT) established for those minerals whose contents are available in the labeling of each selected samples according to the European Guidance document [43]. Results expressed as mg/sachet product.

Mineral	Analytical Value (mg/sachet)	Declared Value (mg/sachet)	Range of Tolerances (RT) (mg/sachet)
Fe			
S1 sample	4.855–4.865	5	4–7.25
S4 sample	6.117–6.159	6	4.8–8.7
Cu			
S1 sample	0.925–0.959	1	0.8–1.45
S4 sample	0.550–0.555	0.5	0.4–0.725
Mn			
S3 sample	2.004–2.036	2	1.6–2.9
S4 sample	0.987–1.003	1	0.8–1.45
Zn			
S1 sample	5.200–5.232	5	4–7.25
S3 sample	10.512–10.838	10	8–14.5
S4 sample	6.006–6.038	6	4.8–8.7
Ca			
S1 sample	386.286–394.17	400	320–580
S4 sample	200.184–200.388	200	160–290
Mg			
S1 sample	176.298–183.548	180	144–261
S4 sample	147.512–154.960	150	120–217.5

Regarding health claims, all declarations shown in the labeling of these food supplements fulfilled the strict requirements and use conditions established by the European regulation [41,42].

Focusing on the micro-elements, the S1 sample showed three health claims related to Fe (iron contributes to the normal "formation of red blood cells and haemoglobin" and "function of the immune system"; "iron has a role in the process of cell division"), whereas the S4 sample included only one claim referring to children's development and health ("iron contributes to normal cognitive development of children"). Both samples could include the seven health claims approved for this mineral as they met the specific use conditions. The S2 and S3 samples did not fulfill these conditions, as their Fe mean values were below the legal limit required to use these health claims (2.1 mg Fe/100 g food supplement).

Only the S1 sample included one health claim referring to Cu in its label ("copper contributes to the normal function of the immune system"), avoiding the use of the other seven authorized health claims. The S2, S3, and S4 samples did not include any Cu health claim, although they could have included a claim due to their Cu content.

Concerning Zn, the labeling of the S1 sample showed 3 health claims (zinc contributes to the normal "fertility and reproduction" and "function of the immune system"; "zinc has a role in the process of cell division") out of the 18 authorized ones. The S3 sample included only one health claim ("zinc contributes to the normal fertility and reproduction"), whereas the S4 sample did not make any declaration, although its Zn mean value was above the necessary limit to use those claims (1.5 mg Zn/100 g food supplement).

The S3 sample is the only food supplement which included one health claim referring to Mn ("Manganese contributes to the protection of cells from oxidative stress") out of the four approved ones. The analytical results showed that the S1, S2, and S4 samples could make use of these health claims; however, no Mn claims appeared in their labeling, presentation, and/or advertisement.

Finally, the analytical data obtained for macro-elements in the present study showed that the S1 and S4 samples were able to use 8 and 10 health claims approved for Ca and Mg, respectively, in their labeling. However, the S1 sample included two health claims authorized for Ca ("calcium is needed for the maintenance of normal bones"; "calcium has a role in the process of cell division and specialization") and one for Mg ("magnesium has a role in the process of cell division"), while the S4 sample only made one claim referring to children's development and health in relation to the Ca content ("calcium is needed for normal growth and development of bone in children").

4. Conclusions

Reliable information about the declared nutritional contents and the benefits promised by the health claims shown in the labeling of food supplements with micronutrients is crucial for vulnerable groups of the population, such as pregnant women. All analytical results of micronutrients (vitamin C, vitamin B_9, iron, copper, manganese, zinc, calcium, and/or magnesium) contained in the food supplements selected from the Spanish market coincided with the declared values in their labeling and were within the ranges of tolerance (RTs) established by the European Guidance document published by the European Commission. The zinc, calcium, and magnesium contents in samples were lower than the tolerable upper intake levels established for pregnant women in accordance with scientific deliberations of the Scientific Committee on Food and the EFSA Panel on Dietetic Products, Nutrition and Allergies. In addition, the food supplements analyzed in the present study met all the specific requirements for using the health claims shown in their labeling. Although the samples could use more health claims than the ones already included in their labeling, the manufacturers could have selected those health claims which either best addressed the physiological conditions of this group of population or which best aligned with marketing intentions. Although it would have been interesting to address the chemical analysis of other compounds in the laboratory, this study could be useful to verify the adequate use of health claims related to some micronutrients in the labeling of food supplements as well as to contribute to consumer protection by confirming the inclusion of reliable information about the health benefits provided by the consumption of these products. In addition, the results of the present work could be interesting for strengthening consumers' confidence, particularly pregnant women, in the benefits shown in the labeling of food supplements and to encourage them to consider these health claims as a useful tool for making better-informed purchasing decisions.

Author Contributions: Conceptualization, V.F.-R. and M.C.; Funding acquisition, M.C.; Investigation, L.D., V.F.-R. and M.C.; Methodology, L.D., V.F.-R. and M.C.; Supervision, V.F.-R. and M.C.; Validation, V.F.-R. and M.C.; Writing—original draft, L.D.; Writing—review and editing, L.D., V.F.-R. and M.C. All authors have read and agreed to the published version of the manuscript.

Funding: The authors thank the support from UCM ALIMNOVA Research Group (Ref.: GRFN14/22). Laura Domínguez is grateful for her PhD grant (UCM-Santander; Ref.: CT42/18-CT43/18).

Institutional Review Board Statement: Not applicable.

Informed Consent Statement: Not applicable.

Data Availability Statement: Not applicable.

Conflicts of Interest: The authors declare no conflict of interest.

References

1. European Food Safety Authority (EFSA). Food Supplements—Introduction. Available online: https://www.efsa.europa.eu/en/topics/topic/food-supplements (accessed on 26 June 2023).
2. European Commission. Food Supplements. Available online: https://ec.europa.eu/food/safety/labelling_nutrition/supplements_en (accessed on 20 June 2023).
3. European Parliament and Council of the European Union. Directive 2002/46/EC of the European Parliament and of the Council of 10 June 2002 on the approximation of the laws of the Member States relating to food supplements. *Off. J. Eur. Union* **2002**, *L183*, 51. Available online: http://eur-lex.europa.eu/legal-content/EN/ALL/?uri=CELEX:32002L0046 (accessed on 21 June 2023).
4. Cámara, M.; Fernández-Ruiz, V.; Domínguez, L.; Cámara, R.M.; Sánchez-Mata, M.C. Global Concepts and Regulations in Functional Foods. In *Functional Foods, Series of Bioprocessing in Food Science*; Chhikara, N., Panghal, A., Chaudhary, G., Eds.; Wiley, Scrivener Publishing LLC: Beverly, MA, USA, 2022; pp. 511–554.
5. Domínguez, L.; Fernández-Ruiz, V.; Cámara, M. The frontier between nutrition and pharma: The international regulatory framework of functional foods, food supplements and nutraceuticals. *Crit. Rev. Food Sci. Nutr.* **2019**, *60*, 1738–1746. [CrossRef] [PubMed]
6. Domínguez, L.; Fernández-Ruiz, V.; Morales, P.; Sánchez-Mata, M.C.; Cámara, M. Assessment of Health Claims Related to Folic Acid in Food Supplements for Pregnant Women According to the European Regulation. *Nutrients* **2021**, *13*, 937. [CrossRef]
7. Ipsos. Europeans' Attitudes towards Food Supplements. Available online: https://www.ipsos.com/en/nutrition-pill-europeans-attitudes-towards-food-supplements (accessed on 25 June 2023).
8. Baladia, E.; Moñino, M.; Martínez-Rodríguez, R.; Miserachs, M.; Picazo, O.; Fernández, T.; Morte, V.; Russolillo, G. *Uso de Suplementos Nutricionales en la Población Española. Uso de Complementos Alimenticios, Alimentos para Grupos Específicos (Usos Médicos Especiales y Deportivos) y Productos a Base de Extractos de Plantas en Población Española: Un Estudio Transversal*; Fundación MAPFRE: Madrid, Spain, 2021; ISBN 978-84-9844-782-8.
9. Koletzko, B.; Cremer, M.; Flothkötter, M.; Graf, C.; Hauner, H.; Hellmers, C.; Kersting, M.; Krawinkel, M.; Przyrembel, H.; Röbl-Mathieu, M.; et al. Diet and Lifestyle Before and During Pregnancy—Practical Recommendations of the Germany-wide Healthy Start—Young Family Network. *Geburtsh Frauenheilk* **2018**, *78*, 1262–1282. [CrossRef] [PubMed]
10. Meija, L.; Rezeberga, D. Proper Maternal Nutrition during Pregnancy Planning and Pregnancy: A Healthy Start in Life Recommendations for Health Care Professionals—The Experience from Latvia. Recommendations for Health Care Specialists. 2017. Available online: https://www.euro.who.int/en/health-topics/disease-prevention/nutrition/publications/2017/propermaternal-nutrition-during-pregnancy-planning-and-pregnancy-a-healthy-start-in-life-2017 (accessed on 17 June 2023).
11. United Nations International Children's Emergency Fund (UNICEF). *UNICEF Programming Guidance. Maternal Nutrition Prevention of Malnutrition in Women before and during Pregnancy and while Breastfeeding*; Nutrition Guidance Series; UNICEF: New York, NY, USA, 2022.
12. U.S. Department of Health and Human Services. Nutrition During Pregnancy to Support a Healthy Mom and Baby. Available online: https://health.gov/news/202202/nutrition-during-pregnancy-support-healthy-mom-and-baby (accessed on 20 October 2023).
13. World Health Organization (WHO). *Good Maternal Nutrition. The Best Start in Life*; WHO Regional Office for Europe: Copenhagen, Denmark, 2016; ISBN 978-92-890-5154-5.
14. World Health Organization (WHO). *WHO Antenatal Care Recommendations for a Positive Pregnancy Experience. Nutritional Interventions Update: Multiple Micronutrient Supplements during Pregnancy*; World Health Organization: Geneva, Switzerland, 2020; ISBN 978-92-4-000778-9.
15. Brown, B.; Wright, C. Safety and efficacy of supplements in pregnancy. *Nutr. Rev.* **2019**, *78*, 813–826. [CrossRef] [PubMed]
16. World Health Organization (WHO). Daily Iron and Folic Acid Supplementation during Pregnancy. Available online: https://www.who.int/tools/elena/interventions/daily-iron-pregnancy (accessed on 21 October 2023).
17. Michael, K.; Georgieff, M.D. Iron Deficiency in Pregnancy. *Am. J. Obstet. Gynecol.* **2020**, *223*, 516–524. [CrossRef]
18. Omotayo, M.O.; Dickin, K.L.; O'Brien, K.O.; Neufeld, L.M.; De Regil, L.M.; Stoltzfus, R.J. Calcium supplementation to prevent preeclampsia: Translating guidelines into practice in low-income countries. *Adv. Nutr.* **2016**, *7*, 275–278. [CrossRef]
19. World Health Organization (WHO). Calcium Supplementation during Pregnancy to Reduce the Risk of Pre-Eclampsia. Available online: https://www.who.int/tools/elena/interventions/calcium-pregnancy (accessed on 21 October 2023).
20. Iqbal, S.; Ali, I. Effect of maternal zinc supplementation or zinc status on pregnancy complications and perinatal outcomes: An umbrella review of meta-analyses. *Heliyon* **2021**, *7*, e07540. [CrossRef]
21. Gohari, H.; Khajavian, N.; Mahmoudian, A.; Bilandi, R.R. Copper and zinc deficiency to the risk of preterm labor in pregnant women: A case control study. *BMC Pregnancy Childbirth* **2023**, *23*, 366. [CrossRef]
22. Turan, K.; Arslan, A.; Uçkan, K.; Demir, H.; Demir, C. Change of the levels of trace elements and heavy metals in threatened abortion. *J. Chin. Med. Assoc.* **2019**, *82*, 554–557. [CrossRef]

23. Parisi, F.; Di Bartolo, I.; Savasi, V.M.; Cetin, I. Micronutrient supplementation in pregnancy: Who, what and how much? *Obstet. Med.* **2019**, *12*, 5–13. [CrossRef]
24. Rumbold, A.; Ota, E.; Nagata, C.; Shahrook, S.; Crowther, C.A. Vitamin C supplementation in pregnancy. *CDSR* **2015**, *9*, CD004072. [CrossRef]
25. World Health Organization (WHO). Vitamin C Supplementation in Pregnancy. Systematic Review Summary. Available online: https://www.who.int/tools/elena/review-summaries/vitaminsec-pregnancy{-}{-}vitamin-c-supplementation-in-pregnancy (accessed on 21 October 2023).
26. Prabhu, K.; Dastidar, R.G.; Aroor, A.R.; Rao, M.; Poojari, V.G.; Varashree, B.S. Micronutrients in Adverse Pregnancy Outcomes. *F1000Research* **2022**, *11*, 1369. [CrossRef]
27. WHO. *Guideline: Vitamin D Supplementation in Pregnant Women*; World Health Organization: Geneva, Switzerland, 2012.
28. World Health Organization (WHO). Vitamin D Supplementation during Pregnancy. Available online: https://www.who.int/tools/elena/interventions/vitamind-supp-pregnancy (accessed on 21 October 2023).
29. American Pregnancy Association. Roles of Vitamin B in Pregnancy. Available online: https://americanpregnancy.org/healthy-pregnancy/pregnancy-health-wellness/vitamin-b-pregnancy/ (accessed on 15 September 2023).
30. Ballestín, S.S.; Campos, M.I.G.; Ballestín, J.B.; Bartolomé, M.J.L. Is Supplementation with Micronutrients Still Necessary during Pregnancy? A Review. *Nutrients* **2021**, *13*, 3134. [CrossRef]
31. World Health Organization (WHO). Vitamin B6 Supplementation during Pregnancy. Available online: https://www.who.int/tools/elena/interventions/vitaminb6-pregnancy (accessed on 21 October 2023).
32. Domínguez, L.; Fernández-Ruiz, V.; Cámara, M. An international regulatory review of food health-related claims in functional food products labeling. *J. Funct. Foods* **2020**, *68*, 103896. [CrossRef]
33. Agencia Española de Seguridad Alimentaria y Nutrición (AESAN). Informes del Sistema Coordinado de Intercambio de Información (SCIRI). Available online: https://www.aesan.gob.es/AECOSAN/web/seguridad_alimentaria/subseccion/SCIRI.htm (accessed on 13 July 2023).
34. European Commission. EU Register of Nutrition and Health Claims Made on Food. Available online: http://ec.europa.eu/food/safety/labelling_nutrition/claims/register/public/?event=register.home (accessed on 18 June 2023).
35. Sánchez-Mata, M.C.; Cabrera Loera, R.D.; Morales, P.; Fernández-Ruiz, V.; Cámara, M.; Díez Marqués, C.; Pardo-de-Santayana, M.; Tardío, J. Wild vegetables of the Mediterranean area as valuable sources of bioactive compounds. *Genet. Resour. Crop Evol.* **2012**, *59*, 431–443. [CrossRef]
36. Domínguez, L.; Dorta, E.; Maher, S.; Morales, P.; Fernández-Ruiz, V.; Cámara, M.; Sánchez-Mata, M.C. Potential Nutrition and Health Claims in Deastringed Persimmon Fruits (*Diospyros kaki* L.), Variety 'Rojo Brillante', PDO 'Ribera del Xúquer'. *Nutrients* **2020**, *12*, 1397. [CrossRef]
37. Kaur, R.; Nayyar, H. Ascorbic Acid: A Potent Defender Against Environmental Stresses. *Antioxid. Redox Signal.* **2014**, 235–287. [CrossRef]
38. Sánchez-Mata, M.C.; Cámara-Hurtado, M.; Diez-Marques, C.; Torija-Isasa, M.E. Comparison of HPLC and spectrofluorimetry for vitamin C analysis of green beans. *Eur. Food Res. Technol.* **2000**, *210*, 220–225. [CrossRef]
39. Latimer, G.W. *Official Methods of Analysis of AOAC International*, 21st ed.; AOAC International: Gaithersburg, MD, USA, 2019.
40. Fernández-Ruiz, V.; Olives, A.I.; Cámara, M.; Sánchez-Mata, M.C.; Torija, M.E. Mineral and trace elements content in 30 accessions of tomato fruits (*Solanum lycopersicum* L.) and wild relatives (*Solanum pimpinellifolium* L., *Solanum cheesmaniae* L. Riley, and *Solanum habrochaites* S. Knapp & D.M. Spooner). *Biol. Trace Elem. Res.* **2010**, *141*, 329–339. [CrossRef]
41. European Parliament and Council of the European Union. Regulation (EC) No 1924/2006 of the European Parliament and of the Council of 20 December 2006 on nutrition and health claims made on food. *Off. J. Eur. Union* **2006**, *L404*, 9. Available online: http://eurlex.europa.eu/legal-content/EN/ALL/?uri=CELEX%3A02006R1924-20121129 (accessed on 21 June 2023).
42. European Parliament and Council of the European Union. Regulation (EU) No 1169/2011 of the European Parliament and of the Council of 25 October 2011 on the provision of food information to consumers, amending Regulations (EC) No 1924/2006 and (EC) 1925/2006 of the European Parliament and of the Council, and repealing Commission Directive 87/250/EEC, Council Directive 90/496/EEC, Commission Directive 1999/10/EC, Directive 2000/13/EC of the European Parliament and of the Council, Commission Directives 2002/67/EC and 2008/5/EC and Commission Regulation (EC) No 608/2004. *Off. J. Eur. Union* **2011**, *L304*, 18. Available online: http://eur-lex.europa.eu/legal-content/EN/TXT/?uri=CELEX:32011R1169 (accessed on 19 June 2023).
43. European Commission. Guidance Document for Competent Authorities for the Control of Compliance with EU Legislation on Regulation (EU) No 1169/2011, Council Directive 90/496/EEC and Directive 2002/46/EC with Regard to the Setting of Tolerances for Nutrient Values Declared on a Label. Available online: https://ec.europa.eu/food/safety/labelling_nutrition/labelling_legislation/nutrition-labelling_en (accessed on 17 June 2023).
44. European Food Safety Authority (EFSA). Tolerable Upper Intake Levels for Vitamins and Minerals. Scientific Committee on Food Scientific Panel on Dietetic Products, Nutrition and Allergies. 2006. Available online: https://www.efsa.europa.eu/sites/default/files/efsa_rep/blobserver_assets/ndatolerableuil.pdf (accessed on 21 June 2023).

45. European Food Safety Authority (EFSA). Scientific Opinion on the Tolerable Upper Intake Level of Calcium. *EFSA J.* **2012**, *10*, 2814. [CrossRef]
46. European Food Safety Authority (EFSA). Overview on Tolerable Upper Intake Levels as derived by the Scientific Committee on Food (SCF) and the EFSA Panel on Dietetic Products, Nutrition and Allergies (NDA). Summary of Tolerable Upper Intake Levels. 2018. Available online: https://www.efsa.europa.eu/sites/default/files/assets/UL_Summary_tables.pdf (accessed on 21 June 2023).

Disclaimer/Publisher's Note: The statements, opinions and data contained in all publications are solely those of the individual author(s) and contributor(s) and not of MDPI and/or the editor(s). MDPI and/or the editor(s) disclaim responsibility for any injury to people or property resulting from any ideas, methods, instructions or products referred to in the content.

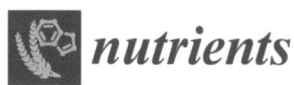

Article

Characteristics of Dietary Supplements with Folic Acid Available on the Polish Market

Marta Czarnowska-Kujawska [1,*], Joanna Klepacka [1], Olga Zielińska [1] and María de Lourdes Samaniego-Vaesken [2]

[1] Department of Commodity and Food Analysis, The Faculty of Food Sciences, University of Warmia and Mazury in Olsztyn, 10-726 Olsztyn, Poland
[2] USP-CEU Group of Excellence "Nutrition for Life", ref: E02/0720, Department of Health and Pharmaceutical Sciences, Faculty of Pharmacy, Universidad San Pablo-CEU, CEU Universities, Montepríncipe Urbanization, 28660 Boadilla del Monte, Spain
* Correspondence: marta.czarnowska@uwm.edu.pl; Tel.: +48-89-524-5276

Abstract: One way of increasing folate status, especially in a state of increased demand (e.g., women of childbearing age), is dietary supplementation with folic acid (FA). The dietary supplements market in Poland shows a controversial situation and, for many reasons (the ease of placing them on the market, the lack of control of chemical composition), the possibility of inaccurate information provided on the supplement's label arises. We questioned whether FA supplements available in Poland are indeed complying with regulations and if they could actually improve folate status amongst the target population groups consuming them. Almost 500 products containing FA were identified and available for sale in pharmacies, all of them including specific information provided by manufacturers on the packaging, such as the amount of FA, their intended use and daily dosage. HPLC analysis of FA content in 30 randomly purchased supplements exposed that in four of the tested products, FA content was less than 4% of the declared value (DV). Another 11 samples exposed that the difference with declared FA content varied from 25% up to 80% of the DV. The obtained results are in agreement with the ones from inspections previously conducted on the Polish dietary supplements market and indicate the urgent need to implement improvements in the notification system as well as the monitorization of these product's authenticity.

Keywords: folic acid; dietary supplements; HPLC; food authenticity; neural tube defects; pregnancy

1. Introduction

The present work was inspired by the results of the Report on the Polish dietary supplements market presented by the Polish Supreme Audit Office in 2017. An inspection conducted between 2014 and 2016 showed that the safety level of dietary supplements was not sufficiently provided [1,2]. Directive 2002/46/EC of the European Parliament and of the Council of 10 June 2002 [3] defines "food supplements" as "foodstuffs the purpose of which is to supplement the normal diet and which are concentrated sources of nutrients or other substances with a nutritional or physiological effect, alone or in combination, marketed in dose form, namely forms such as capsules, pastilles, tablets, pills and other similar forms, sachets of powder, ampoules of liquids, drop dispensing bottles, and other similar forms of liquids and powders designed to be taken in measured small unit quantities". It emphasizes that in order to ensure a high level of protection for consumers, the products that will be placed on the market must be safe and bear adequate and appropriate labeling [3]. Meanwhile, in the conclusions from the Report by Polish authorities [1], the food supplements market was identified as a key risk area, inadequately assessed and supervised by the State institutions responsible for food safety. It was found that not only was the supervision over the health quality of dietary supplements ineffective, but the nutritional education concerning these products was also insufficiently implemented. This is

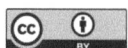

mainly due to the deficient legislative solutions enforcing the introduction and advertising of supplements to the market [1,2]. Currently, a supplement can be placed on the market only after declaring its composition to the health authorities, the Chief Sanitary Inspectorate (GIS) in Poland, through a so-called "notification" [4]. According to the Supreme Audit Office, theoretically, there are chances that the product that is initially placed on the market will be tested, but in practice, the scale of the market exceeds the current control capabilities of the Sanitary Inspections. Controls carried out by the Inspection concern only a part of the market and the control procedures might even take up to several years to complete. In many cases, commercialized dietary supplements are not tested at all [1,2]. It seems that the dynamic expansion of the dietary supplements market does not go hand in hand with the development of effective tools for their control.

The inspection of the Supreme Audit Office showed that amongst dietary supplement sales, including online and also in pharmacies in addition to reliable preparations, there were also adulterated food supplements, containing, for example, prohibited substances from the psychoactive list, or stimulants structurally similar to amphetamines, which can act like drugs [1]. Moreover, testing the samples of supplements to compare their actual content with the composition declared on the product label showed an inappropriate quality, as the samples in question did not display the properties declared by the manufacturers [1]. Consequently, can consumers trust that the supplements they buy actually contain bioactive substances, such as vitamins, minerals, proteins, phytochemicals, antioxidants, etc., in the amounts declared on the product packaging?

Dietary supplements containing folic acid (FA) are a relevant case of study due to their popularity amongst women of reproductive or childbearing age: those who are either planning a pregnancy or those who are already pregnant. In 1991, the randomized trial performed by the Medical Research Council (MRC) Vitamin Study Research Group [5] demonstrated that FA supplementation starting before pregnancy could prevent neural tube defects (NTDs) in the fetus. Anencephaly and spina bifida are two of the most common and serious congenital malformations recognized as NTDs; these severe conditions are incapacitant to the newborn and even incompatible with life [6]. Unfortunately, NTDs affect approximately one in a thousand pregnancies in Europe [7] and at present, most FA supplements available to women of childbearing age are formulated to contain the recommended daily allowance (RDA) of 400 µg per dose [8]. The aim of the current study was to evaluate the assortment of folic acid dietary supplements available on the Polish market and the assessment of their FA content in selected dietary supplements by using a validated HPLC technique.

2. Materials and Methods

2.1. Folic Acid Supplements Database

The analysis of the Polish market of dietary supplements containing FA was conducted based on the assortment available on the websites of two of the largest pharmacy retailers [9,10]. Data were collected throughout May 2022, and it was based on the information provided by the manufacturers of supplements on pharmacy's websites. Only those dietary supplements available for sale and with complete information about the product were included in our study. Products were characterized on the basis of their composition, the amount of FA declared per dose (declared value (DV)), the form of occurrence, intended use, price per package and unit. Dose was defined as one tablet, effervescent tablet, capsule, or jelly; and in the case of powdered supplements, one sachet, the weight of which is indicated on the packaging by the manufacturer, and in the case of liquid supplements, the portion per milliliters (mL). In summary, the compiled information included only those dietary supplements that were available for purchase with comprehensive information about the product.

2.2. Materials and Reagents

Test materials comprised a total of thirty dietary supplements containing FA, of which eight were single-ingredient supplements containing only FA, twelve were multi-ingredient supplements containing other vitamins and bioactive ingredients, and ten were multi-ingredient liquid supplements. All tested products were chosen based on their positioning on the website of one of the largest pharmacy retailers in Poland. After weighing, supplements in the form of tablets were crushed and thoroughly ground in a mortar, those in capsule form were dissolved in an extraction buffer while stirring on a magnetic stirrer, and liquid supplements were added directly to centrifugal flasks after mixing.

Folic acid standard was obtained from Sigma Aldrich (St. Louis, MO, USA) and prepared as described by Konings [11]. Acetonitrile used for analysis was of HPLC grade, while other chemicals were of analytical grade. Water was purified in the Mili-Q system (Millipore; Vienna, Austria).

2.3. Sample Preparation and Folic Acid Quantification

Samples were analyzed in triplicate. Supplements which were in the form of tablets and capsules were weighed in an amount corresponding to the weight of a single tablet or capsule; samples in liquid form in the amount of 10 mL were poured into 30 mL centrifuge flasks (30-mL PPCO Oak Ridge PPCO Nalgene centrifuge tube; Rochester, NY, USA). Then, 20 mL of an extraction buffer (0.1 M phosphate buffer, pH 7.0, with 1% (w/v) sodium ascorbate and 0.1% (v/v) 2-mercaptoethanol) were added and shaken (2500 rpm/10 s Vortex 4 basic IKA Vortex 4 basic; Staufen, Germany). After boiling in a water bath for 15 min and cooling in ice, samples were centrifuged twice at 12,000 rpm/4 °C/20 min (MPW-350R; Warsaw, Poland). Each time, supernatants were collected in 50-mL amber volumetric flasks filled up with the extraction buffer. The extract was filtered through filter paper, flushed with nitrogen, and then stored until HPLC analysis at −70 °C.

Sample purification using solid phase extraction (SPE) and HPLC analysis were carried out as previously described [12]. In short, the chromatographic separation of FA was carried using the Shimadzu Nexera-i LC-2040 C plus HPLC system (Shimadzu Co.; Kyoto, Japan) and the C18 LC column (150 × 4.6 mm, 3 µm, Luna 100 Å; Phenomenex; Torrance, CA, USA). Briefly, conditions for binary gradient elution, with 30 mM phosphoric acid buffer (pH 2.3) and acetonitrile used as the mobile phases were as follows: starting with 6% (v/v) acetonitrile maintained isocratically for the first 5 min, then raised linearly to 25% within 20 min. Separation time—42 min; the flow rate—0.4 mL/min; injection volume—20 µL; column temperature—25 °C. Peaks in the samples were identified based on standard retention time. Quantification of FA was based on UV detection (290 nm) using the external multilevel ($n = 8$) calibration curve with the linear range of 2 ng/mL–9 µg/mL (correlation coefficient >0.9996). The variation obtained between the replicates for each analyzed sample was lower than 10%. Recovery tests were performed by adding known amounts of FA before the extraction with the mean recovery ($n = 4$) obtained at the level of 92% ± 7. The repeatability of the analytical procedure was checked on different extraction days.

3. Results and Discussion

3.1. Market Analysis of Folic Acid Supplements

Folate, also known generically as vitamin B9, is a water-soluble vitamin which naturally occurs in many foods, such as green leafy vegetables, eggs, liver, legumes, grains and nuts [13–15]. Folic acid (FA) is the synthetic form of folate used for food fortification and in dietary supplements; other synthetic forms include L-methylfolate calcium and (6S)-5-methyltetrahydrofolate glucosamine [16]. The generic term 'folate' includes both natural folates from food sources and the synthetic form, FA. Folates cannot be synthesized by the body and must, therefore, be provided in the diet [13–15]. The daily recommendations for folate intake depend on age, gender and physiological condition and are higher for pregnant and lactating women (Table 1). According to the Polish Society of Gynecologists and Obstetricians Guidelines, women of childbearing age planning a pregnancy should additionally use folate supplementation for a period of at least twelve weeks prior to conception and continue throughout pregnancy, the postpartum period and breastfeeding [17]. It is estimated that the effective absorption in the digestive tract of dietary folates does not exceed 50%. Meanwhile, the absorption of synthetic FA from a dietary supplement can reach up to 100%. Considering the differences of folate bioavailability from different sources, the dietary folate equivalents (DFE) equivalence was established, where 1 µg DFE is equal to 1 µg of dietary folates = 0.6 µg of FA from fortified foods or dietary supplements consumed with foods = 0.5 µg of FA from dietary supplements taken on an empty stomach [18].

Table 1. Polish standards for the recommended daily allowance (RDA) and adequate intake (AI) for folates.

Gender and Age	Folate Equivalent (µg/day)	
	RDA	AI
Infants		
0–6 months		65
7–11 months		80
Children		
1–3	150	
4–6	200	
7–9	300	
Teenagers		
10–12	300	
13–18	400	
Adults		
19–75	400	
Pregnant women	600	
Lactating	500	

Based on Jarosz et al., 2017 [8].

In the current situation of low folate status observed in Europe, dietary supplementation with FA is commonly recommended, especially in those states of increased demand [19]. FA is crucial in DNA replication and repair, methylation and synthesis of nucleotides, as well as in the metabolism of other vitamins and amino acids [20]. Low folate status in all population groups has been linked to a number of health problems, such as megaloblastic anemia, increased cardiovascular risk and colorectal cancer, as well as neurocognitive decline in the elderly [21–25]. Maternal folate deficiency is associated, as already mentioned, with a higher risk of NTDs, in addition to cleft lip and palate and Down's syndrome [26]. Moreover, other complications of pregnancy such as miscarriages, inhibition of intrauterine growth and pre-eclampsia may occur more frequently [27,28]. Data analysis indicates that in Poland, daily folate intakes in adults is at an average level of 110–352 µg per day, while among young non-pregnant women it is approximately 127–315 µg per day. Folate intakes among those aged sixty and above was 133–284 µg per day [29]. Moreover, results from a national survey conducted in the UK between 2008 and 2017 showed that around 90% of childbearing aged women had a folate status below the level recommended to reduce the risk of NTDs. In addition, an estimated 28% of girls and 15% of boys aged 11 to 18 years and 7% of adults had low blood folate levels, which increases their risk of anemia [30].

Meanwhile, in Poland, the market of dietary supplements, including those containing FA, is developing very dynamically, which is undoubtedly influenced by their widespread advertising [1,31]. It is estimated that, currently, over 65% of Poles use dietary supplements, most often without consulting a doctor or pharmacist. The most popular are vitamin and mineral preparations. There are already nearly 30,000 entities producing and selling dietary supplements, and the market value is estimated at EUR 1.25 billion [32]. According to the Act of 25 August 2006 on food and nutrition safety, dietary supplements and fortified foods are subjected to the obligation to notify the Chief Sanitary Inspectorate of their initial placement on the market [4]. According to a register run by the Sanitary Inspectorate, in 2020, the highest number of more than 14,500 notifications of supplements with declared addition of FA was recorded, and it was more than 58% of all notified products that year (Figure 1) [31]. These numbers, however, indicate the products notified, but it remains unknown how many of them were actually placed on the market, how many and after how long were they withdrawn from sale by the manufacturer.

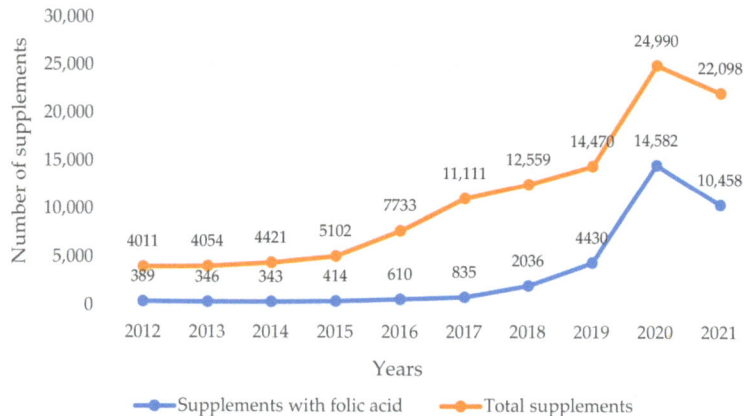

Figure 1. Number of supplements with the notification of the first appearance on the market in the years 2012–2021 based on Chief Sanitary Inspectorate data [30].

Consumer opinion polls conducted in Poland show that pharmacies are the most frequent place for purchasing supplements, and account for 65% of sales [32,33]. Based on the analysis of assortment available in the two largest pharmacy retailers in Poland (May 2022), 470 dietary supplements with FA were available for sale [9,10]. Most of these were multi-ingredients products containing, often, other vitamins and minerals (94.5%). Nonetheless, only 26 supplements (5.5%), were mono-ingredient and contained only FA. The most popular form of supplements with FA addition were tablets (36.4%) and capsules (35.7%). Less than 10% of evaluated products were in the form of effervescent tablets, in liquid and powder. Other formats, such as lozenges, jellybeans, lollipops and soluble gums, constituted only 6.4%. Most of the analyzed products were intended for adults to supplement their daily diet with vitamins and minerals. The second most numerous group were products intended for pregnant women, breastfeeding women or those planning pregnancy (Table 2). The vast majority of available supplements (85.7%) contained FA in the form of pteroylglutamic acid (PGA). However, as regulated by the Polish Minister of Health in the area of the composition and labeling of dietary supplements [34], FA can be also added in the form of L-methylfolate calcium and (6S)-5-methyltetrahydrofolate glucosamine salt. The main differences between these chemical forms used as salts in supplement formulation are related to their bioavailability, or proportion of the ingested folate that is accessible and absorbed in the intestinal lumen and is therefore available for metabolic processes or storage [35]. Their metabolic use and fate in the one-carbon (monocarbon) metabolism where they exert their essential functions is related to nucleotide synthesis and red blood cell formation, amongst others [13,35]. PGA was considered to have the highest bioavailability, but currently research has shown that also L-methylfolate calcium and (6S)-5-methyltetrahydrofolate glucosamine can have a similar absorption rate [16]. In the analyzed assortment, 67 supplements contained the methyl folate form alone or in combined addition with PGA. The use of this form of folates, naturally occurring in the blood plasma, results from the controversy related to the potential adverse effects of excessive consumption of synthetic FA, such as masking low status of vitamin B12. A further possible risk is the unknown long-term effect of synthetic PGA not metabolized in the body [36,37]. The amount of FA in analyzed supplements ranged from 12 µg to as high as 2 mg in one dose. The most numerous were supplements with the declared FA content (DV) of 200 µg per dose (29.8%) and 400 µg per dose (26.6%). In twelve products (2.5%), FA was in the amount of 600 µg per dose; in seventeen supplements (3.6%)—800 µg per dose. One analyzed supplement had a declared FA content of 1 mg per dose, which is the considered maximum safe intake of FA from supplements per day [38], and one contained as much as 2 mg of FA. Moreover, according to the Resolution No. 7/2019 [39], the Polish Chief Sanitary Inspectorate's Dietary Supplements Panel, which is a consultative and advisory body of the Chief Sanitary Inspector in Poland, set the maximum amount of FA in the recommended daily dose at 600 µg for adults and 800 µg in supplements designed for pregnant women. For dietary supplements containing ≥800 µg of FA, it is recommended that the warning: "pregnant women should consult a doctor before use" should appear on the label. Within the analyzed assortment, only three products followed the recommendation, not including those supplements with the highest declared folate content of 1 mg and 2 mg. As a comparison, in the FA dietary market analysis from 2012 [40], 326 supplements with FA were found and similarly to our results; most of them were in the form of multi-ingredients products, in the form of tablets and capsules. More than half of the supplements contained from 200 to 400 µg FA in one dose. Similarly at that time, the most numerous group were products intended for use by adults in order to supplement their daily diet and intended for women planning to be or already pregnant. Additionally, the presence of L-methylfolate calcium was declared only in two supplements, while the others contained PGA [40].

Table 2. Indications for the use of dietary supplements containing folic acid provided by the manufacturers on product packaging.

Intended Use	No. of Products	Declared Folic Acid Content (µg per Dose)	
		Min-Max	Mode *
For adults			
Supplementation of the daily diet	164	16–1000	200
Proper heart function, maintenance of normal cholesterol levels and homocysteine metabolism	29	30–600	200
Promotes proper vision	6	100–400	200
Increased physical and mental effort	19	40–400	200
Supporting the functioning of the nervous system, supporting the work of the brain	11	200–400	200
For women			
For women (general)	21	100–400	200
For women planning and/or pregnant and breastfeeding	76	100–800	400
Better condition of skin, hair and nails	28	25–600	200
For women over 50 and going through menopause	12	20–400	400
For men	18	133–400	200
For children	36	12.5–300	100
For the elderly	14	100–400	100

* mode—the most common amount of folic acid (µg per dose).

3.2. Folic Acid Content Analysis

As previously mentioned, such a large offer of easily available dietary supplements, including those with FA, raises the question of their quality and authenticity. Table 3 presents the results of the analysis of FA content in thirty purchased supplements determined using an HPLC technique. In all thirty tested samples, except for one, the differences in the content of FA were related to a lower content than the manufacturer's declared value (DV). The first category were eight supplements containing only FA with a dose of 400 µg. All supplements in this category were intended, as clearly stated on the product packaging, for women planning pregnancy or already pregnant. One product had the information that was also intended for smokers, elderly people, women who use oral contraceptives and people who abuse alcohol—all groups characterized as being deficient in FA. In three out of eight one-ingredient supplements, the difference between the determined and the declared vitamin content did not exceed 10%. Conversely, in another different five, the difference ranged from 20% to almost 28%.

Table 3. Folic acid (FA) content determined and declared in the tested dietary supplements.

Product No.	Determined FA Content	Declared FA Content (DV [1])	Difference with the Declared FA Content
	One-ingredient supplements (µg per tablet, capsule)		[%]
1	296.5[2] ± 8.4	400	25.9
2	374.6 ± 9.3	400	6.4
3	374.5 ± 10.8	400	6.4
4	290.4 ± 22.7	400	27.4
5	292.5 ± 20.5	400	26.9
6	361.1 ± 2.9	400	9.7
7	320.2 ± 26.6	400	20.0
8	304.0 ± 14.7	400	24.0
	Multi-ingredients supplements (µg per tablet, capsule)		[%]
9	3.8 ± 0.3	400	99.1
10	339.2 ± 13.5	400	15.2
11	327.2 ± 20.4	400	18.2
12	3.6 ± 0.2	400	99.1
13	193.9 ± 9.1	600	67.7
14	314.7 ± 28.1	400	21.3
15	371.6 ± 48.4	600	38.1
16	209.9 ± 8.57	400	47.5
17	258.2 ± 1.79	400	35.5
18	250.4 ± 6.8	300	16.5
19	195.2 ± 8.94	200	2.4
20	167.3 ± 2.56	200	16.4
	Multi-ingredients liquid supplements (µg per portion mL)		[%]
21	204.1 ± 7.7	200	+2.0
22	10.7 ± 0.7	30	64.4
23	87.8 ± 3.4	180	51.2
24	173.4 ± 4.1	200	13.3
25	80.6 ± 3.1	100	19.4
26	65.1 ± 0.9	147	55.7
27	1.2 ± 0.1	50	97.5
28	184.1 ± 17.9	200	8.0
29	1.2 ± 0.1	169	99.3
30	57.9 ± 1.0	290	80.0

[1] DV: Folic acid content declared by manufacturers or declared value. Results are presented as the mean of three replicates ± standard deviation.

Multi-ingredient supplements in the form of tablets, capsules or liquids contained mainly other vitamins apart from FA, even over twenty, and over a dozen different minerals with an exact specification of their amount in one dose on the label [9,10]. In the category of multi supplements in tablets and capsules, declared FA content ranged from 200 to 600 µg per dose. In two out of twelve supplements, determined FA content contained no more than 4 µg despite declaring 400 µg (Table 3). Unfortunately, these were vitamin complexes intended for women planning pregnancy. In the next four products, differences with the declared FA content were at the level of 35–68%, and in another four, from 16% to 21%. Only one supplement (No. 19 in this category) had a vitamin content similar to that specified on the packaging by the manufacturer. In the last category of multi-ingredient supplements in liquid, declared FA content was given in the recommended portion (in mL) and ranged from 30 to 290 µg per dose. The tested products in this category were intended primarily for seniors and adults who want to "improve their vitality, strength and energy". In this group, two supplements out of ten, No. 21 and No. 28, had similar FA content to that declared. Unfortunately, in two supplements the difference between content determined and specified on the label reached 97.5% for No. 27, and 99.3% for No. 29. In the next four supplements in this group, it was determined that over half of products showed less FA than declared.

Based on the conducted market analysis, there are nearly 500 FA-containing supplements available in pharmacies, a large number of which theoretically would cover the daily requirements of this vitamin. More than 30 years have passed since the publication of the study that revolutionized modern day supplementation strategies, confirming that the majority of NTDs could be prevented with FA supplementation before conception and in the first trimester of pregnancy [5]. Meanwhile, according to EUROCAT's (the European network of population-based registries for the epidemiological surveillance of congenital anomalies) Special Reports, no progress in preventing NTDs in Europe was observed since then [7]; but there is still an on-going debate whether this remains the best strategy for increasing folate status. A serious disadvantage of this approach seems to be the lack of knowledge of proper daily diet supplementation with FA. As estimated, in Europe, half of pregnancies are unplanned. Meanwhile, NTDs occur in the first four weeks of pregnancy when most women do not know that they are pregnant. Even in planned pregnancies, many mothers do not take FA supplements to increase folate status before conception and for first twelve week of pregnancy [7,38], and the percentage of women who do, however, take dietary supplements at the right time, cannot be sure whether they obtain an authentic product with the amount of FA declared on the supplement label, as confirmed by the results of our study. The problem, therefore, appears to be more complex.

According to the Polish Society of Gynecologists and Obstetricians Guidelines, during supplementation, preparations with a documented composition and effect should be taken into account [17]. Consumers can purchase FA in the form of an over-the-counter drug in a dosage of, for example, 400 µg [9,10]. However, these are not as popular as commonly advertised supplements. Another strategy to increase the FA intake across the population is to introduce the obligation to fortify certain foods with the synthetic form of this vitamin: mandatory fortification of wheat flour has been implemented in the United States of America (USA) since 1998, and at present, more than 80 countries worldwide share this public health measure; nevertheless, none of them belong to the European Union (EU) [41]. Mandatory fortification has proved to be a better strategy for its widespread distribution across the population from children to adults, as long as wheat flour is consumed; but this measure has also been called a "double-edged sword strategy", as excessive FA intakes could promote certain types of cancer amongst non-targeted population groups (e.g., the elderly) [42]. Conversely, a recent metanalysis by Moazzen et al. found no significant incidence of overall colorectal cancer risk in the population consuming FA [43].

FA, as the synthetic form of B9 folate vitamers, shows a higher bioavailability and, thus, a greater potential for improving folate status [44]. In a recent review by Garret and Bailey [45], the authors underlined that large-scale, mandatory FA fortification is an evidence-based intervention that effectively reduces the prevalence of NTDs, and that it is still underutilized in low- and middle-income countries and should be a main component of public health strategies targeted at NTD prevention.

While European countries remain reluctant to introduce widespread mandatory fortification of cereal flours such as wheat flour, the market of FA voluntary fortified foods is also developing towards offering, for instance, cereal-based products (e.g., ready-to-eat breakfast cereals) and fruit and vegetable juices with the addition of synthetic FA. However, recent studies on FA voluntary fortified products in Europe already indicated the problem of their authenticity. Results demonstrate that both too little or too much uncontrolled addition of the vitamin might be a common practice of manufacturers [46,47]. However, the most important, and at the same time safe and effective, strategy for all population groups—to increase natural folate intake—cannot be forgotten and undervalued [48]. The consumption of naturally occurring folate-rich food should be promoted and be a basic element of a combined strategy with supplemental folate; namely, the Mediterranean diet includes many food groups which are excellent sources of folates and of other health-promoting nutrients, with the potential to reduce chronic disease risk [48,49]. Data analysis of Sicińska and Wyka [29] showed that among the Polish population, the main sources of dietary folate were vegetables and bread, while using FA supplements was declared by 18–25% of young non-pregnant women aged 18–35, and merely 13–14% of the elderly.

4. Conclusions

There is a strong need for a combined strategy to promote folate intake increase in various population groups. Education on the proper intake of FA supplements, especially in women of childbearing age, and the promotion of foods naturally rich in folates, should be at the basis of this strategy. However, neither the strategy of using dietary supplements, nor increasing consumption of foods enriched with FA, will bring the expected results unless these products are authentic and comply with declared values.

The conducted studies on FA supplements confirmed the urgent need to introduce legislative changes which will allow greater control of the dietary supplements market by Sanitary Inspections. An effective control system to confirm the authenticity of supplements initially placed on the market and already available on sale, as well as an efficient withdrawal procedure of adulterated products are needed. Increasing notification fees and fines for placing products on the market in which actual composition is different than that declared on the label, can help protect the consumer from unfair practice.

Author Contributions: M.C.-K. performed the experiment, methodology and validation, data analysis, review and writing—original draft preparation, project administration and funding acquisition; J.K., review and editing, project administration and funding acquisition; O.Z., data analysis and editing, methodology; M.d.L.S.-V., writing—review and editing, supervision. All authors have read and agreed to the published version of the manuscript.

Funding: This project was financially supported by the Minister of Education and Science under the program entitled "Regional Initiative of Excellence" for the years 2019–2022, Project No. 010/RID/2018/19, amount of funding 12.000.000 PLN.

Institutional Review Board Statement: Not applicable.

Informed Consent Statement: Not applicable.

Data Availability Statement: Data is contained within the article.

Conflicts of Interest: The authors declare no conflict of interest.

References

1. The Polish Supreme Audit Office. Admission to Trading of the Dietary Supplements. Information about the Control Result. LLO.430.002.2016. Evidence Number 195/2016/P/16/078/LLO. 2017, pp. 1–61. Available online: https://www.nik.gov.pl/plik/id,13031,vp,15443.pdf (accessed on 16 April 2022). (In Polish)
2. The Polish Supreme Audit Office. (Un)controlled Dietary Supplements. 2022. Available online: https://www.nik.gov.pl/aktualnosci/niekontrolowane-suplementy-diety.html (accessed on 16 April 2022). (In Polish)
3. Directive 2002/46/EC of the European Parliament and of the Council of 10 June 2002 on the Approximation of the Laws of the Member States Relating to Food Supplements. Available online: https://eur-lex.europa.eu/legal-content/EN/TXT/?uri=CELEX:32002L0046 (accessed on 16 April 2022).
4. Act of August 25, 2006 on Food and Nutrition Safety. Available online: https://lexlege.pl/ustawa-o-bezpieczenstwie-zywnosci-i-zywienia/ (accessed on 9 July 2022). (In Polish).
5. MRC Vitamin Study Research Group. Prevention of neural tube defects: Results of the Medical Research Council Vitamin Study. *Lancet* **1991**, *338*, 131–137. [CrossRef]
6. WHO. *Guideline: Optimal Serum and Red Blood Cell Folate Concentrations in Women of Reproductive Age for Prevention of Neural Tube Defects*; World Health Organization: Geneva, Switzerland, 2015.
7. An Official Website of the European Union. Folic Acid and Neural Tube Defects. Available online: https://eu-rd-platform.jrc.ec.europa.eu/eurocat/prevention-and-risk-factors/folic-acid-neural-tube-defects_en (accessed on 8 July 2022).
8. Jarosz, M.; Stoś, K.; Przygoda, B.; Matczuk, E.; Stolińska-Fiedorowicz, H.; Kłys, W. Vitamins. In *Standards for the Population of Poland*; Jarosz, M., Ed.; IŻŻ: Warsaw, Poland, 2017; pp. 166–170. Available online: https://ncez.pl/upload/normy-net-1.pdf (accessed on 1 June 2022). (In Polish)
9. DOZ.pl. Available online: https://www.doz.pl/ (accessed on 1 May 2022).
10. Apteka Gemini. Available online: https://gemini.pl/ (accessed on 1 May 2022).
11. Konings, E. Validated liquid chromatographic method for determining folates in vegetables, milk powder, liver, and flour. *J. AOAC Int.* **1999**, *82*, 119–127. [CrossRef] [PubMed]
12. Czarnowska-Kujawska, M.; Draszanowska, A.; Gujska, E.; Klepacka, J.; Kasińska, M. Folate Content and Yolk Color of Hen Eggs from Different Farming Systems. *Molecules* **2021**, *26*, 1034. [CrossRef] [PubMed]
13. Gregory, J.F. Chemical and nutritional aspects of folate research, analytical procedures, methods of folate synthesis, stability, and bioavailabilty of dietary folates. *Adv. Nutr.* **1989**, *33*, 1–101. [CrossRef]
14. Dang, J.; Arcot, J.; Shrestha, A. Folate retention in selected processed legumes. *Food Chem.* **2000**, *68*, 295–298. [CrossRef]
15. Delchier, N.; Herbig, A.L.; Rychlik, M.; Renard, C.M.G.C. Folates in fruits and vegetables: Contents, processing and stability. *Compr. Rev. Food Sci. Food Saf.* **2016**, *15*, 506–528. [CrossRef]
16. Saldanha, L.G.; Dwyer, J.T.; Haggans, C.J.; Mills, J.L.; Potischman, N. Perspective: Time to resolve confusion on folate amounts, units, and forms in prenatal supplements. *Adv. Nutr.* **2020**, *11*, 753–759. [CrossRef]
17. Bomba-Opoń, D.; Hirnle, L.; Kalinka, J.; Seremak-Mrozikiewicz, A. Folate supplementation during the preconception period, pregnancy and puerperium. Polish Society of Gynecologists and Obstetri0cians Guidelines. *Ginekol. Pol.* **2017**, *88*, 633–636. [CrossRef]
18. Institute of Medicine. *Food and Nutrition Board. Dietary Reference Intakes: Thiamin, Riboflavin, Niacin, Vitamin B6, Folate, Vitamin B12, Pantothenic Acid, Biotin, and Choline*; National Academy Press: Washington, DC, USA, 1998. [CrossRef]
19. Dhonukshe-Rutten, R.A.M.; de Vries, J.H.M.; de Bree, A.; van der Put, N.; van Staveen, W.A.; de Groot, L.C.P.G.M. Dietary intake and status of folate and vitamin B12 and their association with homocysteine and cardiovascular disease in European populations. *Eur. J. Clin. Nutr.* **2009**, *63*, 18–30. [CrossRef]
20. Arnesen, E.; Refsum, H.; Bonaa, K.H.; Ueland, P.M.; Forde, O.H.; Nordrehaug, J.E. Serum total homocysteine and coronary heartdisease. *Int. J. Epidemiol.* **1995**, *24*, 704–709. [CrossRef]
21. Morris, M.S.; Jacques, P.F.; Rosenberg, I.H.; Selhub, J. Folate and vitamin B-12 status in relation to anemia, macrocytosis, and cognitive impairment in older, Americans in the age of folic acid fortification. *Am. J. Clin. Nutr.* **2007**, *85*, 193–200. [CrossRef] [PubMed]
22. Wang, X.; Qin, X.; Demirtas, H.; Li, J.; Mao, G.; Huo, Y. Efficacy of folic acid supplementation in stroke prevention: A meta-analysis. *Lancet* **2007**, *369*, 1876–1882. [CrossRef]
23. Choi, S.W.; Mason, J.B. Folate and carcinogenesis: An integrated scheme. *J. Nutr.* **2000**, *130*, 129–132. [CrossRef] [PubMed]
24. Selhub, J.; Jacques, P.F.; Wilson, P.W.F.; Rush, D.; Rosenberg, I.H. Vitamin status and intake as primary determinants of homocysteinemia in an elderly population. *JAMA* **1993**, *270*, 2693–2698. [CrossRef] [PubMed]
25. Rampersaud, G.C.; Bailey, L.B.; Kauwell, G.P.A. Folate: Relationship to colorectal and cervical cancer. Review and recommendations for practitioners. *J. Am. Diet Assoc.* **2002**, *102*, 1273–1282. [CrossRef]
26. Bean, L.J.; Allen, E.G.; Tinker, S.W.; Hollis, N.D.; Locke, A.E.; Druschel, C.; Hobbs, C.A.; O'Leary, L.; Romitti, P.A.; Royle, M.H.; et al. Lack of maternal folic acid supplementation is associated with heart defects in Down syndrome: A report from the National Down Syndrome Project. *Birth Defects Res. A Clin. Mol. Teratol.* **2011**, *91*, 885–893. [CrossRef]
27. Li, Z.; Ye, R.; Zhang, L.; Li, H.; Liu, J.; Ren, A. Folic acid supplementation during early pregnancy and the risk of gestational hypertension and preeclampsia. *Hypertension* **2013**, *61*, 873–879. [CrossRef]

28. Wen, S.W.; Guo, Y.; Rodger, M.; White, R.R.; Yang, Q.; Smith, G.N.; Perkins, S.L.; Walker, M.C. Folic Acid Supplementation in Pregnancy and the Risk of Pre-Eclampsia-A Cohort Study. *PLoS ONE* **2016**, *11*, e0149818. [CrossRef]
29. Sicińska, E.; Wyka, J. Spożycie folianów w Polsce na podstawie piśmiennictwa z ostatnich 10 lat (2000-2010). Folate intake in Poland on the basis of literature from the last ten years (2000–2010). *Roczn. PZH* **2011**, *62*, 247–256. (In Polish)
30. National Diet and Nutrition Survey Results from 2008 to 2017 Assessing Time and Income Trends for Diet, Nutrient Intake and Nutritional Status for the UK. Available online: https://www.gov.uk/government/statistics/ndns-time-trend-and-income-analyses-for-years-1-to-9 (accessed on 1 June 2022).
31. Chief Sanitary Inspectorate. Food Safety and Nutrition Department. Register of Products Subjected to the Notification of the First Placing to the Market. Available online: https://powiadomienia.gis.gov.pl/ (accessed on 9 July 2022). (In Polish)
32. Raport. Polacy a Suplementy Diety. Report. Poles and Dietary Supplements. Supplementation Habits. 2022. Available online: https://pulsmedycyny.pl/67-proc-polakow-zazywa-suplementy-diety-blisko-polowa-nie-konsultuje-tego-z-zadnym-specjalista-raport-1148877 (accessed on 10 July 2022). (In Polish).
33. Dziedziński, M.; Goryńska-Goldmann, E.; Kobus-Cisowska, J.; Szczepaniak, O.; Marciniak, G. Problem nadkonsumpcji suplementów diety przez Polaków. The problem of overconsumption of supplements by Poles. *Intercathedra* **2019**, *3*, 235–242.
34. Journal of Laws 2018 Item 1951. Announcement of the Minister of Health of 17 September 2018 on the Publication of the Uniform Text of the Regulation of the Minister of Health on the Composition and Labeling of Dietary Supplements. Available online: https://www.infor.pl/akt-prawny/DZU.2018.199.0001951,rozporzadzenie-ministra-zdrowia-w-sprawie-skladu-oraz-oznakowania-suplementow-diety.html (accessed on 15 August 2022).
35. McNulty, H.; Pentieva, K. Folate bioavailability. *Proc. Nutr. Soc.* **2004**, *63*, 529–536. [CrossRef] [PubMed]
36. Sweeney, M.R.; McPartlin, J.; Scott, J. Folic acid fortification and public health: Report on threshold doses above which unmetabolised folic acid appear in serum. *BMC Public Health* **2007**, *7*, 41. [CrossRef] [PubMed]
37. Altic, L.; McNulty, H.; Hoey, L.; McAnena, L.; Pentieva, K. Validation of Folate-Enriched eggs as a functional food for improving folate intake in consumers. *Nutrients* **2016**, *8*, 777. [CrossRef]
38. The UK Government. Proposal to Add Folic Acid to Flour: Consultation Document. 2021. Available online: https://www.gov.uk/government/consultations/adding-folic-acid-to-flour/proposal-to-add-folic-acid-to-flour-consultation-document (accessed on 9 July 2022).
39. No. 7/2019 of the Team for Dietary Supplements of June 11, 2019 on Expressing an Opinion on the Maximum Dose of Folic Acid in the Recommended Daily Dose in Dietary Supplements. Available online: https://www.gov.pl/web/gis/zespol-do-spraw-suplementow-diety (accessed on 11 August 2022). (In Polish)
40. Sicinska, E.; Wasik, M. Suplementy diety jako dodatkowe źródło kwasu foliowego. Dietary supplements as additional sources of folic acid. *Bromat. Chem. Toxicol. XLV* **2012**, *2*, 152–158. (In Polish)
41. Kancherla, V.; Botto, L.D.; Rowe, L.A.; Shlobin, N.A.; Caceres, A.; Arynchyna-Smith, A.; Zimmerman, K.; Blount, J.; Kibruyisfaw, Z.; Ghotme, K.A.; et al. Preventing birth defects, saving lives, and promoting health equity: An urgent call to action for universal mandatory food fortification with folic acid. *Lancet Glob. Health* **2022**, *10*, e1053–e1057. [CrossRef]
42. Kim, Y. Folate: A magic bullet or a double edged sword for colorectal cancer prevention? *Gut* **2006**, *55*, 1387–1389. [CrossRef]
43. Moazzen, S.; Dolatkhah, R.; Tabrizi, J.S.; Shaarbafi, J.; Alizadeh, B.Z.; de Bock, G.H.; Dastgiri, S. Folic acid intake and folate status and colorectal cancer risk: A systematic review and meta-analysis. *Clin. Nutr.* **2018**, *37*, 1926–1934. [CrossRef]
44. Blakley, R. *The Biochemistry of Folic Acid and Related Pteridines*; North-Holland Publishing Company: Amsterdam, The Netherlands, 1969; Volume 13.
45. Garrett, G.S.; Bailey, L.B. A public health approach for preventing neural tube defects: Folic acid fortification and beyond. *Ann. N. Y. Acad. Sci.* **2018**, *1414*, 47–58. [CrossRef]
46. Samaniego-Vaesken, M.L.; Alonso-Aperte, E.; Varela-Moreiras, G. Voluntary fortification with folic acid in Spain: An updated food composition database. *Food Chem.* **2016**, *193*, 148–153. [CrossRef]
47. Gujska, E.; Michalak, J.; Czarnowska, M. Effect of storage time and temperature on the stability of folic acid and folate in selected fruit and fruit and vegetable juices. *Zywn. Nauka. Technol. Jakosc.* **2013**, *6*, 130–138. (In Polish) [CrossRef]
48. Rampersaud, G.C.; Kauwell, G.P.; Bailey, L.B. Folate: A key to optimizing health and reducing disease risk in the elderly. *J. Am. Coll. Nutr.* **2003**, *22*, 1–8. [CrossRef] [PubMed]
49. Finglas, P.M.; de Meer, K.; Molloy, A.; Verhoef, P.; Pietrzik, K.; Powers, H.J.; van der Straeten, D.; Jägerstad, M.; Varela-Moreiras, G.; van Vliet, T.; et al. Research goals for folate and related B vitamin in Europe. *Eur. J. Clin. Nutr.* **2006**, *60*, 287–294. [CrossRef] [PubMed]

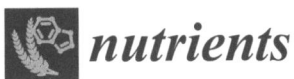

Article

Assessment of Health Claims Related to Folic Acid in Food Supplements for Pregnant Women According to the European Regulation

Laura Domínguez *, Virginia Fernández-Ruiz, Patricia Morales, María-Cortes Sánchez-Mata and Montaña Cámara

Nutrition and Food Science Department, Pharmacy Faculty, Complutense University of Madrid (UCM), Plaza Ramón y Cajal, s/n, E-28040 Madrid, Spain; vfernand@farm.ucm.es (V.F.-R.); patmoral@ucm.es (P.M.); cortesm@farm.ucm.es (M.-C.S.-M.); mcamara@ucm.es (M.C.)
* Correspondence: ladoming@ucm.es; Tel.: +34-923941802; Fax: +34-913941799

Abstract: Pregnant women are a vulnerable group with increased nutritional requirements. The daily intake of folic acid, a crucial vitamin for embryonic development, must be reinforced through supplementation, as sometimes diets are not well equilibrated. As consumers increasingly rely on food supplements, it is vital to properly inform them about the health benefits provided by supplements' consumption to ensure their safe use. The objective of this work was to assess the compliance level of health claims related to folic acid in food supplements commercialized in Spain according to the European regulation. Authors performed (1) a review of health-related claims approved for folic acid in Europe, (2) a market research of food supplements commercialized in Spain with those claims, and (3) a selection of food supplements for chemical analysis in the lab to assess these claims. The results showed that nine health-related claims are currently approved for folic acid in Europe. The analytical results for folic acid content in the selected samples were consistent with the declared values and within the tolerance ranges established in the European Guidance document. All samples included accurate dosages and met the legal requirements (European Regulations 1924/2006, 432/2012, 1169/2011) for all approved claims for folic acid.

Keywords: food supplement; folic acid; pregnancy; food safety; health claims; nutrition

Citation: Domínguez, L.; Fernández-Ruiz, V.; Morales, P.; Sánchez-Mata, M.-C.; Cámara, M. Assessment of Health Claims Related to Folic Acid in Food Supplements for Pregnant Women According to the European Regulation. *Nutrients* **2021**, *13*, 937. https://doi.org/10.3390/nu13030937

Academic Editor: Rima Obeid

Received: 23 December 2020
Accepted: 12 March 2021
Published: 14 March 2021

Publisher's Note: MDPI stays neutral with regard to jurisdictional claims in published maps and institutional affiliations.

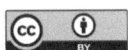

Copyright: © 2021 by the authors. Licensee MDPI, Basel, Switzerland. This article is an open access article distributed under the terms and conditions of the Creative Commons Attribution (CC BY) license (https://creativecommons.org/licenses/by/4.0/).

1. Introduction

Food supplements are concentrated sources of nutrients (vitamins and minerals) or other substances (e.g., amino acids) with a nutritional or physiological effect, which are aimed at supplementing the normal diet for a specific period of time to reduce the risk of a specific disease [1–3].

The consumption of food supplements is increasing in Europe. In 2016, more than the 25% of the European population consumed food supplements to complement the habitual diet or maintain an adequate health status [4]. This percentage greatly increases up to 59.4% for pregnant women [5,6], a specific group of the population whose nutritional requirements (especially micronutrients such as folic acid) are increased [7–9]. According to the EuroPrevall Birth Cohort, a multi-center study carried out in nine European countries, the most commonly used food supplements by European pregnant women are those with folic acid, and Spain is the country with the highest consumption of food supplements (97.8% of Spanish pregnant women) [10,11].

1.1. Food Supplements' Safety: An Overview of the State of the Art

The European Directive 2002/46/EC (last amendment in 2017) establishes a list of vitamins, minerals, and their sources allowed for use in food supplements [12], although safety dosage limits have yet to be established.

Food supplements could involve risks for consumer's health. As an example, Brown and Wright (2019) carried out an extensive literature review focused on the key functions of folic acid during pregnancy as well as on the efficacy and safety of food supplements for pregnant women. The results concluded that high dosages (>1000 µg/day) of folic acid could provoke undesirable modifications in fetus neurodevelopment or even the appearance of side effects (diabetes, thyroid disorders, allergies, etc.) [13].

Food supplements are included in the Rapid Alert System for Food and Feed (RASFF) [14]. In the last five years (1 January 2015–31 December 2019), the RASFF received 848 notifications related to food supplements in Europe. The second cause of these notifications was the overdose of vitamins and minerals (87/463 notifications, that is, 18.8 %). Apparently there were no alerts regarding folic acid in the studied period [15].

1.2. Health-Related Claims of Food Supplements: Regulatory Framework in Europe and Its Implications for Consumers Health

Consumers should be properly informed about the health benefits provided by the consumption of food supplements in order to ensure their safe use [16–19]. According to the European Consumer Organization (Bureau European des Unions de Consommateurs, BEUC), one of the most important issues regarding consumers' misunderstanding is related to the health claims made in food supplements' labeling, presentation, and/or advertising [4,18].

Only those claims based on sound and independent scientific evidence are allowed to be included in food supplements labeling [20,21]. This ensures that all consumers (above all those considered the most vulnerable, e.g., pregnant women) can trust the health benefits claimed by these products and make well-informed food supplement choices [22–24]. Health claims referring to the reduction of disease risk and to children's development and health must undergo a more complex assessment and authorization process.

Spain counts on a Coordinated System of Fast Interchange of Information (SCIRI), a national network that ensures a constant vigilance of any risk related to food products that could affect consumer health. Within five years (1 January 2014–31 December 2018), the SCIRI has received several notifications regarding food supplements, and most of them were due to an incorrect labeling, including claims. In this five-year period, the notifications related to food supplements more than the doubled, increasing from 5.2% to 12.8%, [25].

Considering the worrying situation and the impact that it can have on consumers' health and, most importantly, on at-risk groups of the population like pregnant women, the objective of the present work is to analyze and verify the level of compliance of the health claims related to folic acid in food supplements commercialized in the Spanish market according to the European regulation. To accomplish this goal, the authors performed the following tasks. First, a scientific literature review focused on the health-related claims approved for folic acid by the European regulation. Second, a market research of food supplements commercialized in the Spanish market with those health-related claims. Third, a selection of food supplements for pregnant women, which were subjected to subsequent laboratory chemical analysis to evaluate the appropriateness of the health-related claims included in their labeling, presentation, and/or advertisement.

2. Materials and Methods

2.1. Scientific Literature Review

In a first step, a detailed and in-depth study of the regulatory framework regarding health-related claims was conducted. An up-to-date review focused on the above-mentioned claims which are currently approved for folic acid was performed based on public information included in the European Register of nutrition and health claims made for food and food supplements (Available on: https://ec.europa.eu/food/safety/labelling_nutrition/claims/register/public/?event=register.home) (accessed on 22 December 2020). The search filters used were the following: "claims status: authorised", "type of claim: Art. 14(1)(a) and Art. 13", "EFSA Opinion reference: all", "Legislation: all" [24].

2.2. Food Supplements Market Research

Second, a comprehensive search of the food supplements commercialized in the Spanish market, labelled with any of the approved health-related claims for folic acid, was carried out. This task was performed in two phases: the first one consisted of a preliminary search through the official online purchasing platforms used by 10 food establishments with a high market share in Spain and other e-commerce companies. Besides, an in situ search in the above-mentioned national establishments was performed. Information of both online and in situ searches was checked and verified by all authors and provided them a wide and detailed overview of the state of the art regarding food supplements marketed with health claims related to folic acid. Table S1 includes the designed template used to compile information about food supplements products and health-related claims included in their labeling, presentation, and/or advertisement.

2.3. Analytical Determination of Folic Acid

Third, the chemical analysis of the selected food supplements consisted in the determination of the content of folic acid. The term "folic acid" or "vitamin B_9" includes vitamers with an equivalent biological activity. There are other terms in the literature that are interchangeably used to refer to folic acid, such as "folate(s)", "folacin", and "pteroylmonoglutamic acid" (PteGlu). The chemical structure of folic acid includes a pteridine ring, a residue of p-aminobenzoic acid, and a residue of glutamic acid, all of them linked by a methylene bridge and an amide bond. All the folate derivatives have this main chemical structure called "pteroylmonoglutamic acid" and differs from each other by their oxidation status, the substituents of the pteridine ring, and the number of glutamate residues that are linked to the p-aminobenzoglutamate residue by a peptide bond, the most frequent being mono-, penta- and hexa-glutamates. As folic acid is only synthesized by microorganisms and plants, humans depend on several dietary sources for its intake. Folic acid is naturally presented in food matrices as polyglutamates, which are not directly absorbable by the organism. These polyglutamates must be hydrolyzed in the intestinal mucosa by enzymes to obtain monomer units. Only one of these monomer units, i.e., tetrahydrofolate monoglutamate (THF-monoglutamate), is bioavailable and absorbable by the human organism. Once absorbed, THF-monoglutamate is transformed to 5-methyl-THF-monoglutamate (5-MTHF-monoglutamate), the biologically active vitamer.

The method for folic acid extraction was adapted from the one used by Morales et al. (2015) [26]. The determination of both vitamers was carried out by extraction in a buffer medium and quantification through High-Performance Liquid Chromatography (HPLC) with fluorescence detection for 5-MTHF-monoglutamate vitamer and UV–visible detection for pteroylmonoglutamic acid. In a Falcon tube, 1 g of each food supplement sample was weighed and 10 mL of $NaH_2PO_4 \cdot 2H_2O$ phosphate buffer (100 Mm, pH = 4.4) was added. The resulting mixture was subjected to (1) agitation for 30 minutes in the dark and at a temperature of 80 °C in a magnetic stirrer (Selecta, Spain) and (2) subsequent sonication (30 min, t = 50 °C) in an ultrasonic bath (Selecta, Spain). These conditions were finally considered optimal to achieve the complete dissolution of the granules after testing other solvents. A methanol–distilled water (50:50) mixture, NaH_2PO_4/Na_2HPO_4 buffer (0.1 mol/L; pH = 9), and $Na_2HPO_4 \cdot 2H_2O$ phosphate buffer (100 mM; pH = 7) were tested according to different extraction methods proposed by Matias et al. (2014) and Morales et al. (2015) [26,27]. These solvents, including the eventually selected one ($NaH_2PO_4 \cdot 2H_2O$ phosphate buffer; 100 mM; pH = 4.4), were tested at different temperatures (0 °C, 50 °C, and 80 °C) and stirring times (30 and 60 min).

The resulting solution was centrifuged at 7000 revolutions per minute (rpm) for 15 min. The centrifuge used was a Universal 320 model (Hettich Zentrifugen, Kirchlengern, Germany). The supernatant liquid obtained was filtered through a Millex PVDF 0.45 μm filter into a vial, prior injection for identification and quantification by HPLC. Figure S1 shows the characteristics of the chromatographic equipment as well as the conditions used in the determination of each vitamer of folic acid.

Statistical Analysis

The analyzed food supplement samples contained one of the two following vitamers of folic acid: 5-MTHF-monoglutamate and pteroylmonoglutamic acid. Two batches of each sample were analyzed in triplicate. The data obtained were statistically evaluated through T Student's t test, using $\alpha = 0.05$ as the level of statistical significance. The software used for carrying out the above-mentioned statistical analysis was Statgraphics Plus 5.1.

3. Results and Discussion

3.1. Scientific Literature Review of Health-Related Claims Approved for Folic Acid in the European Regulation

According to the European Database "EU Register of nutrition and health claims made on foods", there are nine claims currently approved in the European regulation: eight health claims and one "Reduction of disease risk" claim [24]. As it is shown in Table 1, the "Reduction of disease risk" claim is referred to supplemental folic acid intake and it is only allowed in the labeling, presentation, and/or advertising of food supplements. The other health claims are related to folate content in both foods and food supplements that are considered a "Source of folate" in accordance with the requirements established in the Annexes of Regulation (EC) N° 1924/2006 and Regulation (EU) N° 1169/2011 [18,19].

Table 1. Health-related claims approved for folic acid according to the European regulation.

Model Claim	European Food Safety Authority (EFSA) Opinion Reference
Health claims	
"Folate contributes to maternal tissue growth during pregnancy"	[28]
"Folate contributes to normal amino acid synthesis"	[29]
"Folate contributes to normal blood formation"	[28]
"Folate contributes to normal homocysteine metabolism"	[28]
"Folate contributes to normal psychological function"	[29]
"Folate contributes to the normal function of the immune system"	[28]
"Folate contributes to the reduction of tiredness and fatigue"	[29]
"Folate has a role in the process of cell division"	[28,29]
Use conditions: Food and food supplements which are at least a "Source of folate" according to the requirements established in the Annex to Regulation (EC) N° 1924/2006	
Reduction of disease risk claim	
"Supplemental folic acid intake increases maternal folate status. Low maternal folate status is a risk factor in the development of neural tube defects in the developing fetus"	[30]
Use conditions: Food supplements that provide at least 400 µg of folic acid/day. The target population is women of child-bearing age, and the beneficial effect is obtained with a supplemental folic acid daily intake of 400 µg for at least one month before and up to three months after conception	

3.2. Food Supplements Market Research Results

A comprehensive search of the food supplements commercialized in the Spanish market was carried out. As it is shown in Table 2, 81 food supplements with health-related claims attributed to folic acid were found. The great majority (86.4%) was marketed through online supermarkets' platforms and other e-commerce companies. All food supplements sold in physical supermarkets were adequately labeled in terms of health-related claims, whereas 14.3% of the food supplements marketed through online supermarkets' platforms and e-commerce companies showed at least one health claim not included in the positive list established by the European Regulation (Regulations (EC) 1924/2006, (EC) No 432/2012, and (EU) No 1169/2011) [18,19,31]. Some examples of the unapproved health claims shown in the labeling, presentation, and/or advertisement of those food supplements were the following: "folic acid contributes to normal cognitive function", "folic acid helps the protection of cells from oxidative stress", "folates contribute to the maintenance of normal regulation of the organism", and "folates contribute to the normal functioning of the nervous system". This percentage (14.3%) is in line with the last value published by the SCIRI (12.8%) that reflects the alerts regarding food supplements in Spain mainly caused by an incorrect labeling, as it was previously mentioned.

Table 2. Summary of the folic acid food supplements directed to pregnant women found in the Spanish market.

Source	Total Number	Food Supplements with Approved Health Claims Related to Folic Acid	Food Supplements with Unapproved Health Claims Related to Folic Acid
In situ purchase	11	11	0
Online purchase	70	60	10

3.3. Sample Selection for Chemical Analysis

Among the 71 food supplements correctly labeled (in terms of health-related claims), samples were selected for chemical analysis in the lab. The selection criteria were (1) food supplements directed to pregnant women, with a clear and unequivocal indication about this specific target population in their labeling, presentation, and/or advertisement, (2) the inclusion of the "Reduction of disease risk" claim approved for folic acid, and (3) the inclusion of other health claims related to vitamins and/or minerals that contribute to the maintenance of an adequate health status of pregnant women. All the above-mentioned claims had to be approved by the European regulation and included in the positive list.

The application of the first and second inclusion criteria resulted in a first selection of 12 food supplements, as they were directed to pregnant women and included the "Reduction of disease risk" claim referred to folic acid in their labeling, presentation, and/or advertisement. Taking into account the third inclusion criterion, and as it is shown in Table 3, four food supplements were selected that strictly met all the established inclusion criteria. These four food supplements were commercialized through online platforms and were dosed in sachets to be suspended in water. Interestingly, only two of them included health claims related to folic acid in addition to the "Reduction of disease risk" claim referred to this compound.

Table 3. Application of the inclusion criteria to select food supplements samples containing folic acid that were subject to chemical analysis (FS1, FS2, FS3, and FS4).

	Inclusion Criterion 1 Target Population: Pregnant Women	Inclusion Criterion 2 "Reduction of Disease Risk" Claim Referred to Folic Acid	Inclusion Criterion 3 Health Claims Related to Vitamins and Minerals
Total	71	12	4
FS1	✔	✔	23 health claims Vitamins: B_6, B_9, B_{12}, C, D Minerals: Cu, Fe, Zn, Ca, Mg, Se, I
FS2	✔	✔	4 health claims Vitamins: B_9, D
FS3	✔	✔	2 health claims Minerals: Mn, Zn
FS4	✔	✔	5 health claims Vitamins: D Minerals: Fe, Ca, I

Inclusion criterion 1: food supplements directed to pregnant women; inclusion criterion 2: food supplements with the "Reduction of disease risk" claim approved for folic acid; inclusion criterion 3: food supplements with health claims related to vitamins and/or minerals which contribute to the maintenance of an adequate health status of pregnant women. (✔) symbol means requirement fulfilled.

According to the information shown in the label, FS1 was the product with the highest content of folic acid (500 µg pteroylmonoglutamic acid/sachet), whereas FS4 declared the lowest one (200 µg 5-MTHF-monoglutamate/sachet). FS2 and FS3 samples had both a declared value of 400 µg pteroylmonoglutamic acid/sachet.

3.4. Analytical Determination of Folic Acid and Assessment of the Level of Compliance of Its Health-Related Claims

Immediately after reception, selected food supplement samples commercialized in a granular form (FS1, FS2, FS3, and FS4) were stored in a cool, dry place away from heat and direct light, as recommended in the package leaflet so to preserve the nutritional composition. Two batches of each sample (FS1, FS2, FS3, and FS4) were analyzed in triplicate in order to evaluate the appropriateness of the health-related claims of folic acid, that is, the compliance with the specific use conditions of each claim in the labeling, appearance, and/or presentation of food supplements. For the analysis, folic acid standards were kept and prepared following the recommended storage and handling conditions provided by the manufacturer, and reagent blanks were prepared regularly and measured together with the samples in order to monitor the trueness of the data obtained.

Figure S2 includes the chromatograms obtained in the analysis of folic acid vitamers (5-MTHF-monoglutamate and pteroylmonoglutamic acid).

To comply with the Regulation and to avoid consumers' misleading, the content of folic acid in the analyzed samples should not deviate substantially from the declared values shown in the labeling. The analytical mean values of all samples were slightly higher than the declared value in the labeling. It is difficult that these products maintain the exact declared value during their shelf-life period due to the high degradation rate of folic acid, that depends on storage conditions (temperature, humidity, light exposure) and storage time. In all analyzed samples, the folic acid content of the batches 1 and 2 were similar, with no statistically significant differences.

Tolerance for nutrient values (vitamins and minerals) declared in the labeling of food supplements was consensually agreed upon by the European Commission and the representatives of the Member States, and a Guidance document was published for competent authorities for the control of compliance with EU legislation on Regulation (EU) No 1169/2011, Council Directive 90/496/EEC and Directive 2002/46/EC. It is important to note that this Guidance cannot be considered as an official interpretation of the European legislation, as this right is reserved to the relevant judicial authorities [32].

The application of tolerance covers one important factor related to food safety, as it sets the maximum contents of certain vitamins and minerals whose excessive intake could provoke important adverse effects [32]. According to the above-mentioned European Guidance, the values of folic acid declared for our samples met the requirements, as they did not deviate from the Range of Tolerance (RT) calculated for each food supplement (Table 4).

Table 4. Assessment of the tolerance established for folic acid in the food supplements samples according to the Guidance document for competent authorities for the control of compliance with EU legislation with regard to the setting of tolerances for nutrient values declared in the labeling of food supplements.

Food Supplement Sample	Value Declared in the Labeling (µg/sachet)	Range of Tolerance (RT) (µg/sachet)	Analytical Value (µg/sachet)
FS1	500	399.60–750.60	509.55 ± 9.92
FS2	400	390.03–600.60	408.59 ± 9.47
FS3	400	396.25–600.60	429.52 ± 3.25
FS4	200	159.60–300.60	220.69 ± 9.09

The eight health claims approved for folic acid (see Table 1) can only be declared in those products which are at least a "Source of folate" (Regulations (EC) No 1924/2006 and (EU) No 1169/2011), that is, a minimum content of 15% of the Nutrient Reference Value (NRV) of folic acid is supplied by 100 g of product (NRV of folic acid = 200 µg/100 g; 15% NRV = 30 µg/100 g) [18,19,31].

As it was mentioned in Section 3.3 and in Table 3, only the FS1 and FS2 samples included health claims related to folic acid. FS1 showed three health claims ("Folate contributes to maternal tissue growth during pregnancy", "Folate has a role in the process of cell division", and "Folate contributes to the normal function of the immune system"). FS2 included two health claims in its labeling, presentation, and/or advertisement ("Folate has a role in the process of cell division" and "Folate contributes to the normal homocysteine metabolism"). The "Reduction of disease risk" claim ("Supplemental folic acid intake increases maternal folate status. Low maternal folate status is a risk factor in the development of neural tube defects in the developing fetus") can only be used in the labeling of those food supplements that provide a daily intake of 400 µg of folic acid. All samples (FS1, FS2, FS3, and FS4) reported the "Reduction of disease risk" claim in their labeling (see Table 3). According to the results of the present work, the analyzed food supplements met the legal requirements and could legitimately include the nine health-related claims of folic acid (eight health claims and 1 "Reduction of disease risk" claim) approved by the European regulation. Although the FS4 sample contained 200 µg folic acid/sachet, it fulfilled the requirement of the "Reduction of disease risk" claim, as its labeling advised pregnant women to take two sachets per day (that is, a daily intake of 400 µg folic acid).

Finally, in Table 5, we summarize the assessment process of the level of compliance of the health-related claims of folic acid in each food supplement sample that we carried out in the present work.

Table 5. Summary of the assessment process of health-related claims of folic acid in each sample. FS1, FS2, and FS3 samples recommended in their labeling to take 1 sachet/day (500 µg folic acid/day for FS1 and 400 µg folic acid/day for FS2 and FS3), whereas the FS4 sample recommended 2 sachets/day (that is, 400 µg folic acid/day); all food supplements met the legal requirement established in the European regulation.

Sample	Declared Value (Labeling)	Analytical Value (µg/sachet)	Health Claims — Legal Requirement to Use the Claims	Reduction of Disease Risk Claim — Legal Requirement to Use the Claim
FS1	500 µg/sachet 1 sachet = 14 g	509.55 ± 9.92	Food supplements must be a "Source of folate", that is, 15% of the Nutrient Reference Value (NRV) of folic acid is supplied by 100 g NRV of folic acid = 200 µg/100 g 15% NRV = 30 µg/100 g	Food supplements must provide at least 400 µg of folic acid/day.
FS2	400 µg/sachet 1 sachet = 4.02 g	408.59 ± 9.47		
FS3	400 µg/sachet 1 sachet = 2.3 g	429.52 ± 3.25		
FS4	200 µg/sachet 1 sachet = 6 g	220.69 ± 9.09		

Further studies with a higher number of samples commercialized in other markets within the European Union are needed to allow a better picture of the state of the art of this issue.

4. Conclusions

Consumers deserve high-quality and safe food supplements that bear reliable information and fulfill the health effects promised by the health-related claims reported in their labeling. This is particularly important for pregnant women, who usually take food supplements with folic acid, for its crucial role in embryonic development and formation of the fetal tissues.

Our analytical results of folic acid were consistent with the declared values shown in the labeling of the corresponding food supplements and within the ranges of tolerance according to the European Guidance. Taking into account our analytical results, it can be concluded that all food supplement samples met the legal requirements (Regulations (EC) 1924/2006, (EC) No 432/2012 and (EU) No 1169/2011) for reporting the nine claims approved for folic acid (eight health claims and one "Reduction of disease risk" claim). Interestingly, all samples could include more health claims referred to folic acid than the ones already declared in their labeling; however, the manufacturers could have selected claims that they believe best address the particular situation and physiological conditions of pregnant women.

Supplementary Materials: The following are available online at https://www.mdpi.com/2072-6643/13/3/937/s1, Figure S1: Chromatographic equipment and HPLC conditions used in this study for the determination of folic acid vitamers, Figure S2: Chromatograms obtained for 5-MTHF-monoglutamate (measured by HPLC-fluorescence) and pteroylmonoglutamic acid (measured by HPLC-UV), Table S1: Designed template used to compile information from Spanish market research.

Author Contributions: Conceptualization, V.F.-R. and M.C.; Funding acquisition, M.C.; Investigation, L.D., V.F.-R., and M.C.; Methodology, L.D., V.F.-R., P.M., M.-C.S.-M., and M.C.; Supervision, V.F.-R., L.D., and M.C.; Validation, V.F.-R., P.M., M.-C.S.-M., and M.C.; Writing—original draft, L.D.; Writing—review and editing, V.F.-R., P.M., M.-C.S.-M., and M.C. All authors have read and agreed to the published version of the manuscript.

Funding: This research was funded by UCM ALIMNOVA Research Group ref: 951505 and Project OTRI Art. 83 ref: 252-2017, UCM-Fundación Sabor y Salud. Laura Domínguez acknowledges her PhD grant (UCM-Santander; Ref: CT42/18-CT43/18).

Institutional Review Board Statement: Not applicable.

Informed Consent Statement: Not applicable.

Conflicts of Interest: The authors declare no conflict of interest.

References

1. European Parliament and Council of the European Union. Directive 2002/46/EC of the European Parliament and of the Council of 10 June 2002 on the approximation of the laws of the Member States relating to food supplements. *Off. J. Eur. Union* **2002**, *L183*, 51. Available online: http://eur-lex.europa.eu/legal-content/EN/ALL/?uri=CELEX:32002L0046 (accessed on 21 December 2020).
2. European Food Safety Authority (EFSA). Food Supplements—Introduction. Available online: https://www.efsa.europa.eu/en/topics/topic/food-supplements (accessed on 20 December 2020).
3. Domínguez Díaz, L.; Fernández-Ruiz, V.; Cámara, M. The frontier between nutrition and pharma: The international regulatory framework of functional foods, food supplements and nutraceuticals. *Crit. Rev. Food Sci. Nutr.* **2019**, *60*, 1738–1746. [CrossRef] [PubMed]
4. Bureau Européen des Unions de Consommateurs (BEUC). *Food Supplements. Challenges & Risks for Consumers*; BEUC-X-2016-092; BEUC Publications: Brussels, Belgium, 2016.
5. Funnell, G.; Naicker, K.; Chang, J.; Hill, N.; Kayyali, R. A cross-sectional survey investigating women' information sources, behaviour, expectations, knowledge and level of satisfaction on advice received about diet and supplements before and during pregnancy. *BMC Pregnancy Childbirth* **2018**, *18*, 182. [CrossRef] [PubMed]
6. Jun, S.; Gahche, J.J.; Potischman, N.; Dwyer, J.T.; Guenther, P.M.; Suader, K.A.; Bailey, R.L. Dietary Supplement Use and Its Micronutrient Contribution During Pregnancy and Lactation in the United States. *Obstet. Gynecol.* **2020**, *135*, 623–633. [CrossRef] [PubMed]
7. World Health Organization (WHO). *Good Maternal Nutrition. The Best Start in Life*; WHO Regional Office for Europe: Copenhagen, Denmark, 2016; ISBN 978 92 890 5154 5.
8. Koletzko, B.; Cremer, M.; Flothkötter, M.; Graf, C.; Hauner, H.; Hellmers, C.; Kersting, M.; Krawinkel, M.; Przyrembel, H.; Röbl-Mathieu, M.; et al. Diet and Lifestyle Before and During Pregnancy—Practical Recommendations of the Germany-wide Healthy Start—Young Family Network. *Geburtsh Frauenheilk* **2018**, *78*, 1262–1282. [CrossRef] [PubMed]
9. Meija, L.; Rezeberga, D.; Proper Maternal Nutrition during Pregnancy Planning and Pregnancy: A Healthy Start in Life Recommendations for Health Care Professionals—The Experience from Latvia. Recommendations for Health Care Specialists; 2017. Available online: https://www.euro.who.int/en/health-topics/disease-prevention/nutrition/publications/2017/proper-maternal-nutrition-during-pregnancy-planning-and-pregnancy-a-healthy-start-in-life-2017 (accessed on 17 December 2020).
10. Ducker, G.S.; Rabinowitz, J.D. One-Carbon Metabolism in Health and Disease. *Cell Metab.* **2017**, *25*, 27–42. [CrossRef] [PubMed]

11. Oliver, E.M.; Grimshaw, K.E.C.; Schoemaker, A.A.; Keil, T.; McBride, D.; Sprikkelman, A.B.; Ragnarsdottir, H.S.; Trendelenburg, V.; Emmanouil, E.; Reche, M.; et al. Dietary Habits and Supplement Use in Relation to National Pregnancy Recommendations: Data from the EuroPrevall Birth Cohort. *Matern. Child Health J.* **2014**, *18*, 2408–2425. [CrossRef] [PubMed]
12. European Commission. Food Supplements. Available online: https://ec.europa.eu/food/safety/labelling_nutrition/supplements_en (accessed on 18 December 2020).
13. Brown, B.; Wright, C. Safety and efficacy of supplements in pregnancy. *Nutr. Rev.* **2020**, *78*(10), 813–826. [CrossRef] [PubMed]
14. European Commission. RASFF—Food and Feed Safety Alerts. Available online: https://ec.europa.eu/food/safety/rasff_en (accessed on 12 December 2020).
15. European Commission. RASFF Portal. Available online: https://webgate.ec.europa.eu/rasff-window/portal/?event=searchResultList&StartRow=1 (accessed on 18 December 2020).
16. National Food Institute—Technical University of Denmark (DTU). Many Danes Take Dietary Supplements although Few Need Them. Available online: https://www.food.dtu.dk/english/news/2016/03/many-danes-take-dietary-supplements-although-few-need-them?id=f9017469-c293-4f28-bd71-163a491a4ae8 (accessed on 15 December 2020).
17. German Federal Institute for Risk Assessment (BfR). German Test Suggests "Many" Vitamin Supplements Exceed Safe Dose Limits. Available online: https://www.nutraingredients.com/Article/2017/09/07/German-test-suggests-many-vitamin-supplements-exceed-safe-dose-limits?utm_source=copyright&utm_medium=OnSite&utm_campaign=copyright (accessed on 16 December 2020).
18. European Parliament and Council of the European Union. Regulation (EC) No 1924/2006 of the European Parliament and of the Council of 20 December 2006 on nutrition and health claims made on food. *Off. J. Eur. Union* **2006**, *L404*, 9. Available online: http://eurlex.europa.eu/legal-content/EN/ALL/?uri=CELEX%3A02006R1924-20121129 (accessed on 22 December 2020).
19. European Parliament and Council of the European Union. Regulation (EU) No 1169/2011 of the European Parliament and of the Council of 25 October 2011 on the provision of food information to consumers, amending Regulations (EC) No 1924/2006 and (EC) 1925/2006 of the European Parliament and of the Council, and repealing Commission Directive 87/250/EEC, Council Directive 90/496/EEC, Commission Directive 1999/10/EC, Directive 2000/13/EC of the European Parliament and of the Council, Commission Directives 2002/67/EC and 2008/5/EC and Commission Regulation (EC) No 608/2004. *Off. J. Eur. Union* **2011**, *L304*, 18. Available online: http://eur-lex.europa.eu/legal-content/EN/TXT/?uri=CELEX:32011R1169 (accessed on 22 December 2020).
20. Domínguez Díaz, L.; Fernández-Ruiz, V.; Cámara, M. An international regulatory review of food health-related claims in functional food products labeling. *J. Funct. Foods* **2020**, *68*, 103896. [CrossRef]
21. Domínguez Díaz, L.; Dorta, E.; Maher, S.; Morales, P.; Fernández-Ruiz, V.; Cámara, M.; Sánchez-Mata, M.C. Potential Nutrition and Health Claims in Deastringed Persimmon Fruits (*Diospyros kaki* L.), Variety 'Rojo Brillante', PDO 'Ribera del Xúquer'. *Nutrients* **2020**, *12*, 1397. [CrossRef] [PubMed]
22. Getov, I.N.; Lebanova, H.; Grigorov, E. Food supplements—marketing and health claims analysis. *Arch. Balk. Med Union* **2011**, *46*, 26–29. [CrossRef]
23. U.S. Pharmacopeia (USP). Ensuring the Quality of Dietary Supplements. OTH430F_2016-02. 2016. Available online: https://www.usp.org/sites/default/files/usp/document/about/public-policy/public-policy-dietary-supplements.pdf (accessed on 18 December 2020).
24. European Commission. EU Register of Nutrition and Health Claims Made on Food. Available online: http://ec.europa.eu/food/safety/labelling_nutrition/claims/register/public/?event=register.home (accessed on 18 December 2020).
25. Agencia Española de Seguridad Alimentaria y Nutrición (AESAN). Informes del Sistema Coordinado de Intercambio de Información (SCIRI). Available online: http://www.aecosan.msssi.gob.es/AECOSAN/web/seguridad_alimentaria/subseccion/SCIRI.htm (accessed on 15 December 2020).
26. Morales, P.; Fernández-Ruiz, V.; Sánchez-Mata, M.C.; Cámara, M.; Tardío, J. Optimization and Application of FL-HPLC for Folates Analysis in 20 Species of Mediterranean Wild Vegetables. *Food Anal. Methods* **2015**, *8*, 302–311. [CrossRef]
27. Matias, R.; Ribeiro, P.R.S.; Sarraguça, M.C.; Lopes, J.A. A UV spectrophotometric method for the determination of folic acid in pharmaceutical tablets and dissolution tests. *Anal. Methods* **2014**, *6*, 3065. [CrossRef]
28. European Food Safety Authority (EFSA). Scientific Opinion on the substantiation of health claims related to folate and blood formation, homocysteine metabolism, energy-yielding metabolism, function of the immune system, function of blood vessels, cell division, and maternal tissue growth during pregnancy pursuant to Article 13(1) of Regulation (EC) No 1924/2006. *EFSA J.* **2009**, *7*, 1213. Available online: https://efsa.onlinelibrary.wiley.com/doi/pdf/10.2903/j.efsa.2009.1213 (accessed on 22 December 2020).
29. European Food Safety Authority (EFSA). Scientific Opinion on the substantiation of health claims related to folate and contribution to normal psychological functions, maintenance of normal vision, reduction of tiredness and fatigue, cell division and contribution to normal amino acid synthesis pursuant to Article 13(1) of Regulation (EC) No 1924/2006. *EFSA J.* **2010**, *8*, 1760. Available online: https://efsa.onlinelibrary.wiley.com/doi/abs/10.2903/j.efsa.2010.1760 (accessed on 21 December 2020).
30. European Food Safety Authority (EFSA). Scientific Opinion on the substantiation of a health claim related to increasing maternal folate status by supplemental folate intake and reduced risk of neural tube defects pursuant to Article 14 of Regulation (EC) No 1924/2006. *EFSA J.* **2013**, *11*, 3328. Available online: https://efsa.onlinelibrary.wiley.com/doi/abs/10.2903/j.efsa.2013.3328 (accessed on 21 December 2020).

31. European Commission. Commission Regulation (EU) No 432/2012 of 16 May 2012 establishing a list of permitted health claims made on food, other than those referring to the reduction of disease risk and to children's development and health. *Off. J. Eur. Union* **2012**, *L136*, 1. Available online: http://eur-lex.europa.eu/legal-content/EN/ALL/?uri=celex:32012R0432 (accessed on 22 December 2020).
32. European Commission. Guidance Document for Competent Authorities for the Control of Compliance with EU Legislation on Regulation (EU) No 1169/2011, Council Directive 90/496/EEC and Directive 2002/46/EC with Regard to the Setting of Tolerances for Nutrient Values Declared on a Label. Available online: https://ec.europa.eu/food/safety/labelling_nutrition/labelling_legislation/nutrition-labelling_en (accessed on 13 December 2020).

MDPI AG
Grosspeteranlage 5
4052 Basel
Switzerland
Tel.: +41 61 683 77 34

Nutrients Editorial Office
E-mail: nutrients@mdpi.com
www.mdpi.com/journal/nutrients

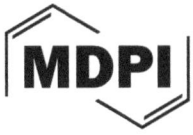

Disclaimer/Publisher's Note: The title and front matter of this reprint are at the discretion of the Collection Editors. The publisher is not responsible for their content or any associated concerns. The statements, opinions and data contained in all individual articles are solely those of the individual Editors and contributors and not of MDPI. MDPI disclaims responsibility for any injury to people or property resulting from any ideas, methods, instructions or products referred to in the content.

www.ingramcontent.com/pod-product-compliance
Lightning Source LLC
LaVergne TN
LVHW072353090526
838202LV00019B/2533